CHILD NEUROPSYCHOLOGY

Volume 2

Clinical Practice

This is a volume in

PERSPECTIVES IN
**NEUROLINGUISTICS, NEUROPSYCHOLOGY, AND
PSYCHOLINGUISTICS: A Series of Monographs and Treatises**

A complete list of titles in this series is available from the publisher on request.

CHILD NEUROPSYCHOLOGY
Volume 2
Clinical Practice

Edited by

JOHN E. OBRZUT

Department of Educational Psychology
College of Education
University of Arizona
Tucson, Arizona

GEORGE W. HYND

Departments of Educational Psychology and Psychology
University of Georgia
Athens, Georgia
and Department of Neurology
Medical College of Georgia
Augusta, Georgia

1986

ACADEMIC PRESS, INC.
Harcourt Brace Jovanovich, Publishers
Orlando   San Diego   New York   Austin
Boston   London   Sydney   Tokyo   Toronto

ACADEMIC PRESS, INC.
Orlando, Florida 32887

United Kingdom Edition published by
ACADEMIC PRESS INC. (LONDON) LTD.
24–28 Oval Road, London NW1 7DX

Library of Congress Cataloging in Publication Data

Child neuropsychology.

(Perspectives in neurolinguistics, neuropsychology,
and psycholinguistics series)
Includes indexes.
Contents: v. 1. Theory and research — v. 2.
Clinical practice.
1. Pediatric neurology. 2. Neuropsychology.
I. Obrzut, John E. II. Hynd, George W. III. Series:
Perspectives in neurolinguistics, neuropsychology, and
psycholinguistics. [DNLM: 1. Child Development Disorders.
2. Nervous System Diseases—in infancy & childhood.
3. Neuropsychology—in infancy & childhood. WS 340 C5357]
RJ486.C458 1986 618.92'89 86-3433
ISBN 0–12–524042–2 (hardcover) (v. 2: alk. paper)
ISBN 0–12–524044–9 (paperback) (v. 2: alk. paper)

PRINTED IN THE UNITED STATES OF AMERICA

86 87 88 89   9 8 7 6 5 4 3 2 1

To all the special colleagues and students who have both stimulated and encouraged this particular project from its inception. Also, special thanks to Krystopher, who provides the motivation to continue these professional endeavors.

J.E.O.

To W. Louis Bashaw, who provided the time, support, and friendship; and to Alphonse Buccino, who continues to facilitate our efforts to prepare psychologists to work with neurologically impaired children.

G.W.H.

Contents

Part II Neuropsychological Evaluation: Perspectives

Part III   Intervention and Treatment

Chapter 10   **Educational Intervention
in Children with
Developmental Learning
Disorders**
Cynthia R. Hynd

Chapter 11   **Behavioral Neuropsychology with
Children**
*Arthur MacNeill Horton, Jr., and
Antonio E. Puente*

Contributors

Numbers in parentheses indicate the pages on which the authors' contributions begin.

Richard A. Berg* (113), Psychiatry/Psychology Division, St. Jude Children's Research Hospital, Memphis, Tennessee 38101

John F. Bolter (59), Clinical Psychology Service, Silas B. Hays Army Community Hospital, Fort Ord, California 93941

Thomas A. Boyd (15), Department of Psychology, Bradley Hospital, East Providence, Rhode Island 02915, and Department of Psychiatry and Human Behavior, Brown University, Providence, Rhode Island 02912

Raymond S. Dean (83), Neuropsychology Laboratory, Ball State University, Muncie, Indiana 47306, and Indiana University School of Medicine, Muncie, Indiana 47306

Stephen R. Hooper (15), Department of Psychology, Bradley Hospital, East Providence, Rhode Island 02915, and Department of Psychiatry and Human Behavior, Brown University, Providence, Rhode Island 02912

Arthur MacNeill Horton, Jr. (299), Veterans Administration Medical Center, Baltimore, Maryland 21212, and The Johns Hopkins University, Baltimore, Maryland 21218

Cynthia R. Hynd (265), Division of Developmental Studies, Georgia State University, Atlanta, Georgia 30303

George W. Hynd (3), Departments of Educational Psychology and Psychology, University of Georgia, Athens, Georgia 30602, and Department of Neurology, Medical College of Georgia, Augusta, Georgia 30912

---

* Present address: Department of Behavioral Medicine, West Virginia University Medical Center, Charleston, West Virginia 25330.

Robert M. Knights (229), Department of Psychology, Carleton University, Ottawa, Ontario, Canada KlS 5B6

John E. Obrzut (3), Department of Educational Psychology, College of Education, University of Arizona, Tucson, Arizona 85721

Antonio E. Puente (299), Department of Psychology, University of North Carolina at Wilmington, Wilmington, North Carolina 28403

Clare Stoddart (229), Department of Psychology, Carleton University, Ottawa, Ontario, Canada KlS 5B6

Phyllis Anne Teeter (187), Department of Educational Psychology, University of Wisconsin at Milwaukee, Milwaukee, Wisconsin 53201

David E. Tupper (139), Cognitive Rehabilitation Department, LIFEstyle Institute, Edison, New Jersey 08820

W. Grant Willis (245), School of Education, University of Colorado at Denver, Denver, Colorado 80202

Preface

D. O. Hebb (1949) once suggested that the psychologist and neurophysiologist chart the same bay. While both psychologist and neurophysiologist may use the same fixed reference points, they may pursue different but potentially complementary endeavors. The research in the area of child neuropsychology, as discussed in Volume 1, reflects well the potential interface between the efforts of psychologists and those interested in the neurophysiological basis of behavior. Clearly, significant progress has been made in correlating neurodevelopmental behavior to its neurophysiological basis. In this regard, the future for those who attempt to chart the waters between neurobiology and cognitive developmental neuropsychology has never looked more promising.

For the applied psychologist, the challenge of providing clinical neuropsychological services to children is likely to increase in proportion to the advances made in understanding the neurophysiological basis of disorders. However, it is becoming increasingly more difficult to keep abreast of both the research in the area of developmental neuropsychology and the efforts of psychologists in the applied or clinical domain.

The clinical child or pediatric neuropsychologist must have available a source of clear and current information on issues germane to the provision of neurological services to children. In this volume, the editors place strong emphasis on understanding the research in developmental neuropsychology such that the provision of clinical services may rest on a firm conceptual foundation. Thus, for the clinician, the broader and deeper the understanding of the neurophysiological and neuropsychological bases of behavior, the greater the probability that the services provided will reflect current and appropriate conceptualizations of brain–behavior relations in children. In this light, the volume attempts to bridge the gap between neurodevelopmental theory and clinical practice with a pediatric population.

Compiled with this broad objective in mind, this volume is relevant to clinical child or pediatric neuropsychologists, child or school psychologists, physicians interested in pediatric neuropsychological disorders, and other professionals who provide services to children with neurologically based disorders. The book may also serve as a reference for audiologists, speech and language therapists, or educators.

The chapters have been organized into three major parts. In the first, the focus is on some of the more common neuropsychological disorders encountered in children. After a brief introductory chapter by Hynd and Obrzut, Hooper and Boyd present an overview of the neurodevelopmental disorders. Bolter, in the next chapter, discusses epilepsy in children. Dean then provides a critical overview of the neuropsychological basis of psychiatric disorders in children, and Berg addresses closed-head injury in children. The second part offers an overview of different approaches and issues relevant to neuropsychological evaluation of children. Tupper addresses the importance of soft signs and neuropsychological screening, while Teeter discusses the more traditional approaches to neuropsychological assessment with children. Stoddart and Knights offer a more contemporary perspective to assessment, while Willis discusses a topic often ignored in the pediatric literature, actuarial and clinical assessment practices. The final part addresses what eventually must concern all who work with patients suffering from neuropsychological disturbance, i.e., intervention and treatment. Only two chapters are included in this part, since so little research has documented or evaluated the effectiveness of different intervention strategies with children who experience neurologically based behavioral disorders. C. R. Hynd presents an overview of how one might conceptualize and integrate differential diagnosis of neurodevelopmental learning disabilities with appropriate curriculum-based intervention strategies. In the final chapter, Horton and Puente discuss the broader applications of behavioral neuropsychology.

In no fashion can the chapters in this volume be considered as completely representative of the current status of clinical child neuropsychology. This has not been our intent. As suggested previously, we have attempted to provide a bridge between theory and research on the one hand and applied practice on the other. The chapters included are those representative of the multifaceted nature of potential applied concerns. We hope that our efforts and those of our exceptionally well qualified contributors offer a current and balanced perspective on clinical neuropsychology with children.

George W. Hynd

John E. Obrzut

REFERENCE

Hebb, D. O. (1949). *The organization of behavior*. New York: Wiley.

CHILD NEUROPSYCHOLOGY

Volume 2

Clinical Practice

Part I

Neuropsychological Disorders in Children

Chapter 1

Clinical Child Neuropsychology: Issues and Perspectives

GEORGE W. HYND

Departments of Educational Psychology and Psychology
University of Georgia
Athens, Georgia 30602
and
Department of Neurology
Medical College of Georgia
Augusta, Georgia 30912

JOHN E. OBRZUT

Department of Educational Psychology
College of Education
University of Arizona
Tucson, Arizona 85721

INTRODUCTION

Since the mid-1970s, significant efforts have been directed at understanding brain–behavior relations in children. A number of factors have been responsible for the increase in these efforts to articulate the exact nature and relations between developing neuropsychological organization in children and deficits in performance reflective of either deviant development or some trauma. Certainly, the efforts of researchers in the neurosciences have resulted in a better understanding of the neurophysiology associated with deficits in neurocognitive development (e.g., Duffy, Denckla, Bartels, & Sandini, 1980; Duffy, Denckla, Bartels, Sandini, &

3

CHILD NEUROPSYCHOLOGY, VOL. 2
Copyright © 1986 by Academic Press, Inc.
All rights of reproduction in any form reserved.

Kiessling, 1980; Galaburda & Eidelberg, 1982; Galaburda & Kemper, 1979). Also, the effect of federal legislation (e.g., Public Law 94-142; The Education for All Handicapped Children Act) helped focus national efforts in education on understanding and educating children with handicapping conditions.

Another significant factor in the growth of interest in clinical child neuropsychology is the recognition that the survival rates for children suffering neurological trauma has increased to the point that the incidence rates for children so afflicted will increase considerably through the 1980s and 1990s. Two examples may serve to illustrate this point and thus draw attention to the possible implications.

Children of very low birthweight (<1500 grams) now have a reasonable chance for survival, due to the proliferation of neonatal intensive care facilities. For those children whose birthweight is between 500 to 999 grams, approximately 25% will survive. For those infants whose weight at birth is between 1000 to 1500 grams, nearly 80% will leave the hospital alive (Horwood, Boyle, Torrance, & Sinclair, 1982). While mortality rates are decreasing significantly in this population, morbidity continues to be a significant concern. Nickel, Bennett, and Lamson (1982) found that at age 10 years, 64% of the children who received neonatal intensive care were in a special education program at school.

With regard to children who survive acute lymphocytic leukemia, concern exists that the effects of treatment may induce long-lasting neuropsychological deficits. There is some evidence that for those children who receive intrathecal methotrexate and/or intracranial radiation during treatment, deficits seem to exist posttreatment in intellectual abilities (Massari, 1982), memory, visual–motor integration, and in verbal fluency (Goff, 1982). In some children, these deficits prove to be serious enough that they are diagnosed as learning disabled (Elbert, Culbertson, Gerrity, Guthrie, & Bayles, 1985). While these findings may be challenged (e.g., Berg, Tuseth, & Daniel, 1985), it does seem an important consideration if one considers the prediction that by the year 2000, 4 out of every 100 children will be a long-term survivor of childhood cancer.

Most authorities would currently agree that the prevalence of various handicapping conditions is between 10 and 16% of the population (Gaddes, 1980; Hynd & Cohen, 1983; Myklebust & Boshes, 1969). With the two preceding examples, it seems reasonable to project that the incidence rate for various neurodevelopmental behavioral and learning disorders will probably increase significantly in the next several decades. In this context there may indeed be more children diagnosed as learning disabled, behaviorally disordered, or as suffering attentional deficiencies than at present.

Thus, the current interest in clinical child neuropsychology may well represent the beginning of an entirely specialized field of professional endeavor. As the number of children increases who survive previously fatal diseases, traumatic incidents, and neonatal crisis, so too must the services provided to these patients. The sophistication of the clinical services provided children is only as sound as our knowledge regarding neuropsychological processes and organization is reflective of the developing child.

Since 1974, when Reitan and Davison published the first volume in clinical neuropsychology, the vast majority of the literature has focused on neuropsychological disorders in adults. While this trend continues today, there is an increasing realization that neuropsychological disorders in children represent a uniquely different perspective requiring specialized knowledge in developmental, cognitive, and educational psychology. A number of volumes have appeared that attest to this notion (Gaddes, 1980; Hynd & Obrzut, 1981; Rourke, Bakker, Fisk, & Strang, 1983; Spreen, Tupper, Risser, Tuokko, & Edgell, 1984).

The chapters of this volume attempt to fill a void not addressed previously in any great detail. These topics, while most relevant to the practice of clinical child neuropsychology, are of considerable theoretical importance. As advances are made in our theoretical understanding of issues relevant to the topics presented by the contributors, it must be understood that practice in clinical child neuropsychology should in turn be modified. The interplay between the advances in theory presented in Volume I and the clinical issues presented here should not be underestimated.

To highlight some of the important conceptual issues pertaining to the following chapters, a brief overview is presented. Rather than present an overview of each of the chapters to follow, it is the intent here to highlight important theoretical or clinical considerations pertaining to each of the following sections. In this manner, the chapters in this volume can be examined in a critical context as to important perspectives and issues.

NEUROPSYCHOLOGICAL DISORDERS IN CHILDREN

It was Hyrtl (1846) who once suggested that "the internal anatomical structure of the brain is now, and probably always will remain, a book sealed with seven seals, and written, moreover, in hieroglyphics." Although certainly reflective of the state of knowledge in his time, it does seem as though significant advances have been made in understanding not only the internal anatomical structure of the brain, but also the neuropathology associated with disordered development in children. With respect to neuropsychological disorders in children, several important issues deserve consideration.

Neuropathological Basis of Behavioral and Learning Disorders

It has long been recognized that many factors could affect fetal growth and development (Gregg, 1941; Zappert, 1927), and the relation between various cerebral and cortical dysplasias and mental retardation has been well documented (Malamud, 1964). Until recently, however, what has not been established is the exact nature of the neurophysiological anomalies associated with learning or behavioral disorders.

The contribution of Galaburda and Kemper (1979) and Rosen, Sherman, and Galaburda (see Volume 1) in this regard is important. Galaburda and his colleagues have provided convincing evidence that subtle anomalies in the organization and architecture of the cortex may form the foundation of learning and behavioral disabilities. While Hinshelwood (1900) and others (e.g., Bastian, 1898; Morgan, 1896) had suggested that the region of the angular gyrus might be critical in reading disorders, no direct neuropathological evidence in children existed in support of this notion. The work of Galaburda is important because there now seems to be evidence that randomly distributed dysplasias in the left cerebral hemisphere (including the region of the angular gyrus) may be responsible for the subtle cognitive deficits observed in learning disabilities.

These findings are important for two reasons. First, the anomalies seem localized to the left cerebral hemisphere and are distributed in a highly focal but apparently random fashion. Second, more-recent evidence suggests that these anomalies may also be present in subcortical structures such as the thalamus (Galaburda & Eidelberg, 1982).

The fact that these deficits are localized in the left cerebral hemisphere is consistent with the observation that children with learning disabilities often have lower verbal-scale IQs than performance-scale IQs. Unfortunately, no direct evidence exists that ties these two observations together in a developmental context. The seemingly random yet focal nature of the distribution of these anomalies, suggests that depending on the functional system that may be disrupted, each child's neuropsychological profile may be highly unique. Also, the focal nature of these anomalies provides strong evidence as to the futility and irrelevance of attempting to localize cortical dysfunction in developmental disorders. Realistically, all that can be accomplished in assessment with these children is some statement as to the nature of the impaired neuropsychological process.

Also, in the context of the material presented in Hooper and Boyd's chapter, as well as in Dean's chapter, it may well be that, depending on the distribution of the focal anomalies, either behavioral or learning (or both) difficulties might be manifested. In fact, there is correlative evidence that suggests a significant relationship between psychiatric disorders and neurological impairment in children (Hertzig & Birch, 1968; Tramontana, Sherrets, & Golden, 1980).

Clearly, all behavioral or learning deficiencies need not be due to anomalies in neuronal migration or development. Evidence also exists suggesting that the deficits associated with hypoxic–ischemic events may produce similar patterns of behavior. For instance, Lou, Hendriksen, and Bruhn (1984) found focal cerebral hypoperfusion in the frontal cortex as well as the caudate nuclei region in children with attention deficit disorders (ADD). They suggested that this finding was consistent with a hypoxic–ischemic event.

Thus, whether due to anomalies in normal neurological development or due to some early event, evidence exists that developmental learning and behavioral disorders have a neurophysiological basis. While this may seem a strongly stated conclusion, the evidence continues to mount in support of this perspective.

Cortical versus Subcortical Processes

As already mentioned, evidence has been provided by Galaburda and Eidelberg (1982) that subcortical anomalies may also be present in patients with neurodevelopmental disorders (in their case, dyslexia). Dyken and McCleary (see Volume 1) note that in the pediatric neurodegenerative diseases there is no clear evidence as to whether symptoms manifest as primarily cortical or subcortical in nature (as some believe they do in the adult dementias). From a clinical perspective, it is indeed risky practice in light of this observation to be attributing various deficits in children to cortical dysfunction, as the interplay neurodevelopmentally between cortical and subcortical functioning may be obscured. Not only does this conclusion have obvious clinical implications, but also it suggests that research is urgently needed in carefully articulating and correlating the clinical manifestations of the various neurodegenerative disease processes in children at various age levels.

Despite the considerable difficulties associated with research of this nature, it is possible to chart in a developmental context the course and response to treatment of neurodegenerative disease in children. The efforts of Swift, Dyken, and DuRant (1984) are important in this regard, as they provide a well-conceptualized model for future efforts.

Effects of Brain Injury in Children

It is widely recognized that the effects of head trauma in children may be considerably different in children than in adults. Clearly, the plasticity of the young child's skull is important. Because the sutures in very young children have often not fused together, the skull can expand due to trauma and the resulting increased intracranial pressure (Schurr, 1979). For this reason, skull fractures are usually rare in the very young.

It is a popular notion that when young children sustain head trauma that the mechanisms of neural plasticity allow for the recovery of function to occur. In support of this notion, it has been argued by many that damage to the left cerebral hemisphere at an early age allows the remaining cerebral hemisphere to assume linguistic function (Alajouanine & Lhermitte, 1965). At approximately age 5 years or even later, the apparent plasticity of the brain diminishes as cerebral dominance for linguistic competence is established in the left cerebral hemisphere (Lenneberg, 1967). The evidence suggests that by 10 years of age, damage sustained to the left cerebral hemisphere produces long-lasting semantic–linguistic deficits (Fromkin, Krashen, Rigler, & Rigler, 1974). More is stated regarding this topic in Volume 1.

So the theory states. While many mechanisms are involved in the recovery of function after trauma (including diaschisis, reorganization, neural sprouting, etc.), to anyone in clinical practice, the factors associated with recovery or reorganization of function seem inconsistent. When reorganization does occur, often moderate to severe neuropsychological deficits remain even when the trauma is acquired very early (Cohen, Hynd, & Hartlage, 1984).

The essential issue relates to what are those factors that are associated with recovery of function? To date, no national registry exists to aid in the documentation of conclusive cases where either recovery or reorganization has occurred. Needless to say, many difficulties exist in documenting these cases, including estimating premorbid levels of functioning, obtaining reliable neuropsychological data, and verifying the nature of the recovery or reorganization. However, efforts must be made in this regard. But it is only through a more-careful documentation of case history data that a clearer focus on this important issue will emerge.

NEUROPSYCHOLOGICAL EVALUATION

It has been argued that the essential difference between clinical psychology and clinical neuropsychology is that the clinical psychologists' role is to effect behavioral change while the role of the clinical neuropsychologist is to assess change in behavior due to neurological events. Thus, for the clinical neuropsychologist, the vast majority of time is spent in assessing behavioral change (Craig, 1979).

For this reason, the literature in neuropsychology seems to have such a heavy emphasis on clinical assessment. While many deplore the proliferation of neuropsychological test batteries (Satz & Fletcher, 1981), the reality, whether for good or not, is that most clinical neuropsychologists are trained through workshop settings and most frequently administer standardized neuropsychological test batteries (Craig, 1979; McCaffrey, Malloy, & Brief, in press).

For those who work with children, however, the situation may be somewhat different. Because of the short attention span of children, the nature of the deficits they may manifest, and developmental-norming issues, clinical child neuropsychologists may very well be less bound to test batteries than their clinical counterparts who work primarily with adults. It is for this reason that the chapters in the second section of this volume represent such diversity in perspectives regarding assessment. No matter what the approach though, some issues need to be kept in mind.

Lack of a Nosology for Neuropsychological Disorders in Children

While DSM III (American Psychiatric Association, 1980) provides a very basic conceptual framework for many childhood disorders, no accepted nosology for the neuropsychological disorders frequently seen in children currently exists. Typical of this problem is the lack of any accepted empirically based definition of dyslexia (Hynd & Cohen, 1983). Most definitions are exclusionary in nature and are thus criticized for being circular (Satz & Fletcher, 1981). While many medical syndromes are diagnosed by exclusion (e.g., multiple sclerosis), the confusion in neuropsychology is compounded by the use of many psychometrically questionable clinical assessment practices (e.g., Boder & Jerrico, 1982). Thus, it becomes almost impossible for clinicians or researchers to agree on diagnostically distinct neuropsychological syndromes.

Some would advocate a more empirically based approach to deriving meaningful diagnostic classifications (e.g., Rourke & Adams, 1984; Satz & Fletcher, 1981; Satz & Morris, 1981). However, these approaches are confounded by the number of correlated and noncorrelated measures administered to derive the classification rules. Other problems exist as well, and they relate to considerations pertinent to base rates in classification (Willis, see this volume, Chapter 9)—the observation made previously that from a clinical neuroanatomical perspective, each child probably represents a unique profile of abilities and disabilities (thus rendering diagnostic classifications relatively useless), and statistical problems associated with classification theory.

Whether or not a recognized nosology is ever developed, it is critical in practice to adequately and empirically define the parameters used to base clinical judgments. Only in this fashion will it be possible to reach some consensus regarding the precise nature of learning disabilities, dyslexia, and other pediatric neurodevelopmental syndromes.

Effect of g in Neuropsychological Assessment

There exists increasing concern that those tasks employed on standard neuropsychological assessment batteries for children reflect not distinct neuropsychological processes, but g, general cognitive ability. For example, Seidenberg, Giordani, Berent, and Boll (1983) found a significant effect of IQ on the level of performance for 6 of the 14 tests on the Halstead-Reitan Neuropsychological Test Battery for Children. Tramontana, Klee, and Boyd (1984) found a similar significant effect on WISC-R IQ and performance on the Halstead-Reitan and Luria-Nebraska Neuropsychological Battery-Children's Revision. Others have found significant relations between SES and performance on neuropsychological tasks.

While (according to Luria's [1980] theory) one might expect the correlation of IQ with a number of other functional systems, the degree of these findings suggests that many of the tasks employed on neuropsychological batteries are simply redundant and duplicate data obtained from IQ tests. This is indeed a concern if one must work with children who may have seriously compromised attentional abilities due to some neurological syndrome.

Other related issues exist with regard to neuropsychological assessment with children. For instance, there still has not been a national effort aimed at providing adequate and representative cross-sectional norms for any neuropsychological assessment battery. Also, those tasks employed on the batteries often ignore the age-appropriateness of the tasks in clinical evaluation. In this respect, Passler, Isaac, and Hynd (1986) found that performance among normal children on tasks designed to assess behaviors associated with frontal lobe function varied greatly between the ages of 6 and 12 years. These tasks were adopted from the Luria examination as being pertinent to the assessment of frontal lobe functioning. If adequate cross-sectional norms do not exist for children, then it becomes nearly impossible to provide any accurate appraisal of the possible impairment of developing abilities.

Thus, it may seem a reasonable conclusion that with children one may design a neuropsychological assessment battery that not only answers the referral question but also provides for little redundancy in assessment of functional skills. It may also be relevant to suggest that psychophysiological techniques may be relevant and underused in assessment with children (reaction time, evoked potentials, brain electrical activity mapping, etc.). Not only might these techniques provide more basic data regarding the integrity of the nervous system but also they may be interesting and motivating to the child who otherwise may have difficulty in sustaining attention on the more traditional paper and pencil tasks. Clearly, in judging the utility of neuropsychological assessment tasks or batteries, one should be aware of the significant redundancy and correlation with IQ across many tasks employed. Also, the adequacy of norms remains a persistent issue.

INTERVENTION AND TREATMENT

It is in the area of intervention and treatment where the services of the clinical neuropsychologist are not often utilized (Craig, 1979). Most time appears to be spent in assessment and evaluation, and little time is devoted to intervention. There are probably several important factors that contribute to the lack of involvement in treatment.

Perhaps first and foremost, clinical neuropsychologists receive little or no training in intervention. Recommended standards for internships in clinical neuropsychology (Division 40 of APA) emphasize assessment, diagnosis, and consultation. One out of the seven recommended didactic experiences refers to "training in methods of intervention specific to neuropsychology" (Bieliausleas & Boll, 1984). Of interest, those methods specific to neuropsychology are not noted.

With children, it should seem apparent not only that intervention must deal with the attempt to integrate the child into their educational environment but also that the behavioral–affective dimension requires different clinical skills than one might engage in working with an adult. It would seem desirable, for example for a clinical child neuropsychologist to have training in (1) play therapy, (2) educational programming and curriculum, (3) and behavior modification, as well as child development. Unfortunately, this perspective is notably absent from the training standards in clinical neuropsychology.

Another difficulty that may contribute to the lack of training and/or research literature on intervention is that most internship experiences are in hospital settings pertinent primarily to adult populations (McCaffrey et al., in press). While there may be carry-over from the rehabilitation literature as it relates to services to children, there appear at this time to be few successful documented programs of intervention designed for brain-damaged children. Furthermore, the literature on the success of intervention programs designed for children with the neurodevelopmental disorders (e.g., dyslexia) is remarkably impoverished. The concluding section in this volume provides a conceptual framework for designing remedial programs that are at the least conceptually sound. The notion of differential diagnosis is of paramount importance in this conceptualization. It will remain, however, for future investigators to validate the notions advanced in the final section of this volume.

CONCLUSION

It has been the intent here to broadly address some of the issues and perspectives that may be brought to bear in reading the content provided in the following chapters. It is argued that clinical child neuropsychology must be separated from any conceptualization of clinical neuropsychology that does not require considerable education and training in theory of child development and the other aforementioned areas.

Separate training standards must be developed that draw on those relevant experiences in the neurosciences, developmental, clinical, school and cognitive psychology, as well as education (Hynd, 1981). Clinical child neuropsychology shares many of the same techniques found in adult neuropsychology. However, the nature of children must force a recognition that an entirely different set of perspectives must be brought to bear if children are to receive the services they richly deserve.

REFERENCES

Alajouanine, T., & Lhermitte, F. (1965). Acquired aphasia in children. *Brain, 88,* 853–862.
American Psychiatric Association. (1980). *Diagnostic and statistical manual of mental disorders* (3rd ed.). Washington, DC.
Bastian, H. C. (1898). *A treatise on aphasia and other speech defects.* London: H. K. Lewis.
Berg, R. S., Tuseth, S., & Daniel, M. S. (1985, February). *Long-term effects of Leukemia and its treatment: A seven year report.* Paper presented at the annual meeting of the International Neuropsychological Society, San Diego, CA.
Bieliausleas, L., & Boll, T. (1984). Report on the Subcommittee on Psychology Internships. *Division of Clinical Neuropsychology (APA): Newsletter, 40.*
Boder, E., & Jerrico, S. (1982). *The Boder Test of Reading–Spelling Patterns.* New York: Grune & Stratton.
Cohen, M., Hynd, G. W., & Hartlage, L. C. (1984). A shift in language lateralization. *Clinical Neuropsychology, 5,* 129–135.

Craig, D. L. (1979). Neuropsychological assessment in public psychiatric hospitals: The current state of practice. *Clinical Neuropsychology, 1,* 1–7.

Duffy, F. H., Denckla, M. B., Bartels, P. H., & Sandini, G. (1980a). Dyslexia: Regional differences in brain electrical activity by topographic mapping. *Annals of Neurology, 7,* 412–430.

Duffy, F. H., Denckla, M. D., Bartels, P. H., Sandini, G., & Kiessling, L. S. (1980b). Dyslexia: Automated diagnosis by computerized classification of brain electrical activity. *Annals of Neurology, 7,* 421–428.

Elbert, J. C., Culbertson, J. L., Gerrity, K. M., Guthrie, L. J., & Bayles, R. (1985, February). *Neuropsychological and electrophysiologic follow-up of children surviving acute lymphocytic Leukemia.* Paper presented at the annual meeting of the International Neuropsychological Society, San Diego, CA.

Fromkin, V., Krashen, C. S., Rigler, D., & Rigler, M. (1974). The development of language in Genie: A case of language acquisition beyond the "critical period." *Brain and Language, 1,* 81.

Gaddes, W. H. (1980). *Learning disabilities and brain function: A neuropsychological approach.* New York: Springer-Verlag.

Galaburda, A. M., & Eidelberg, D. (1982). Symmetry and asymmetry in the human posterior thalamus: II. Thalamic lesions in a case of developmental dyslexia. *Archives of Neurology, 39,* 333–336.

Galaburda, A. M., & Kemper, T. L. (1979). Cytoarchitectonic abnormalities in developmental dyslexia: A case study. *Annals of Neurology, 6,* 94–100.

Goff, J. R. (1982). *Memory deficits and distractability in survivors of childhood leukemia.* Paper presented at the annual meeting of the American Psychological Association.

Gregg, N. McA. (1941). Congenital cataract following German measles in the mother. *Transactions of the Ophthalmological Society of Australia, 3,* 35.

Hertzig, M. E., & Birch, H. G. (1968). Neurological organization in psychiatrically disturbed adolescents. *Archives of General Psychiatry, 19,* 528–537.

Hinshelwood, J. (1900). Congenital word-blindness. *Lancet, 1,* 1506–1508.

Horwood, S. P., Boyle, M. H., Torrance, G. W., & Sinclair, J. C. (1982). Mortality and morbidity of 500- to 1,499-gram birth weight infants live-born to residents of a defined geographic region before and after neonatal intensive care. *Pediatrics, 69,* 613–620.

Hynd, G. W. (1981). Training the school psychologist in neuropsychology: Perspectives, issues and models. In G. W. Hynd & J. E. Obrzut (Eds.), *Neuropsychological assessment and the school-age child: Issues and procedures* (pp. 379–404). New York: Grune & Stratton.

Hynd, G. W., & Cohen, M. (1983). *Dyslexia: Neuropsychological theory, research and clinical differentiation.* New York: Grune & Stratton.

Hynd, G. W., & Obrzut, J. E. (Eds.). (1981). *Neuropsychological assessment and the school-age child: Issue and procedures.* New York: Grune & Stratton.

Hyrtl, J. (1946). *Lehrbuch.* Cited by Malamud, N. (1970). Ludwig Turck. In W. Haymaker & F. Schiller (Eds.), The *Founders of neurology* (pp. 85–88). Springfield, Illinois: Charles C. Thomas.

Lenneberg, E. H. (1967). *Biological foundations of language.* New York: Wiley.

Lou, H. C., Henriksen, L., & Bruhn, P. (1984). Focal cerebral hypoperfusion in children with dysphasia and/or attention deficit disorder. *Archives of Neurology, 41,* 825–829.

Luria, A. R. (1980). *Higher cortical functions in man.* New York: Basic Books.

Malamud, N. (1964). Neuropathology. In H. A. Stevens & R. Heber (Eds.), *Mental retardation* (pp. 429–452). Chicago: University of Chicago Press.

Massari, D. (1982). *Late neuropsychological effects in children with ALL.* Paper presented at the annual meeting of the American Psychological Association.

McCaffrey, R. J., Malloy, P. F., & Brief, D. J. (in press). Internship opportunities in clinical neuropsychology emphasizing recent INS Training guidelines. *Professional Psychology: Research and Practice.*

Morgan, W. P. (1896). A case of congenital word-blindness. *British Medical Journal, 2,* 1378.

Myklebust, H. R., & Boshes, B. (1969). *Final report, minimal brain damage in children.* Washington, DC: United States Department of Health, Education and Welfare.

Nickel, R. E., Bennett, F. C., & Lamson, F. N. (1982). School performance of children with birth weights of 1,000 g or less. *American Journal of Diseases of Children, 136,* 105–110.

Passler, M., Isaac, W., & Hynd, G. W. (1986). Development of frontal lobe behaviors in children. *Developmental Neuropsychology, 1* (4).

Reitan, R. M., & Davison, L. A. (Eds.). (1974). *Clinical neuropsychology: Current status and applications.* Washington, DC: V. H. Winston & Sons.

Rourke, B. P., & Adams, K. M. (1984). Quantitative approaches to the neuropsychological assessment of children. In R. L. Tarter & G. Goldstein (Eds.), *Advances in clinical neuropsychology* (pp. 79–108). New York: Plenum.

Rourke, B. P., Bakker, D. J., Fisk, J. L., & Strang, J. D. (1983). *Child neuropsychology.* New York: Guilford.

Satz, P., & Fletcher, J. M. (1981). Emergent trends in neuropsychology: An overview. *Journal of Consulting and Clinical Psychology, 49,* 851–865.

Satz, P., & Morris, R. (1981). Learning disabilities subtypes: A review. In F. J. Pirozzolo & M. C. Wittrock (Eds.), *Neuropsychological and cognitive processes in reading.* New York: Academic Press.

Schurr, P. H. (1979). Head injuries. In F. C. Rose (Ed.), *Pediatric neurology.* Oxford: Blackwell.

Seidenberg, M., Giordani, B., Berent, S., & Boll, T. J. (1983). IQ level and performance on the Halstead–Reitan Neuropsychological Test Battery For Older Children. *Journal of Consulting and Clinical Psychology, 51,* 406–413.

Spreen, O., Tupper, D., Risser, A., Tuokko, H., & Edgell, D. (1984). *Human developmental neuropsychology.* New York: Oxford University Press.

Swift, A. V., Dyken, P. R., & DuRant, R. H. (1984). Psychological follow-up in childhood dementia: A longitudinal study of subacute sclerosing panencephalitis. *Journal of Pediatric Psychology, 9,* 469–483.

Tramontana, M. G., Klee, S. N., & Boyd, T. A. (1984). WISC-R interrelationships with the Halstead–Reitan and Childrens' Luria Neuropsychological Batteries. *Clinical Neuropsychology, 6,* 1–8.

Tramontana, M. G., Sherrets, S. D., & Golden, C. J. (1980). Brain dysfunction in youngsters with psychiatric disorders: Application of Selz–Reitan Rules for neuropsychological diagnosis. *Clinical Neuropsychology, 2,* 118–123.

Zappert, J. (1927). Uber rontgenogene fetale mikrocephalie. *Archiv für Kinderheilkunde, 80,* 34.

Chapter 2

Neurodevelopmental Learning Disorders

STEPHEN R. HOOPER
THOMAS A. BOYD

Department of Psychology
Bradley Hospital
East Providence, Rhode Island 02915
and
Department of Psychiatry and Human Behavior
Brown University
Providence, Rhode Island 02912

INTRODUCTION

This discipline of child neuropsychology encompasses brain–behavior relationships as they apply to the developing child. Relatively in its infancy, the field is in much need of theoretical direction from a neurodevelopmental perspective, not to mention the need for improved data-based guidelines for the clinical practice in this specialty area. Although the downward extension of adult neuropsychological theories has broken ground in this regard, the adult models have provided little in the way of basic understanding of the neuropsychological functioning of the developing child. The central nervous system (CNS) of the child is undergoing rapid change, and quantitative as well as qualitative differences should be expected.

This notion becomes particularly important when one begins to engage in the study of the exceptional child. Boll (1974) noted that there are many more factors to consider when performing a neuropsychological evalua-

15

CHILD NEUROPSYCHOLOGY, VOL. 2

tion on a child as compared to an adult. Such factors as chronological age, general developmental status, chronicity of the injury or problem, and age of onset of the difficulties must all be considered conjointly when evaluating a child for brain-based dysfunction. Further, the concept of critical or sensitive periods of development also potentiates difficulties with respect to prognosis and treatment issues (Lenneberg, 1967). Given these factors, it becomes even more problematic in determining the presence of actual deficit versus a developmental delay versus a neuropsychiatric disturbance. Nonetheless, the benefits that can be gained from a neuropsychological perspective with exceptional children seem potentially large. Assessment of a child's relative strengths and weaknesses across basic neuropsychological areas can provide a sound basis for the development and implementation of effective intervention strategies directed toward the child's problems in scholastic, social, and overall adaptive functioning.

The connection between neuropsychology and exceptional children is not a new concept. During the 1940s, Strauss and his colleagues (Strauss & Lehtinen, 1947; Strauss & Werner, 1943) employed a unitary concept of brain damage in their work with exceptional children. They described a behavioral syndrome, the "brain-injured child," which consisted of such behaviors as poor learning, attentional problems, and perceptual difficulties. This syndrome provided the foundation for the later development of terms such as minimal brain dysfunction, attention deficit disorder, and learning disability. However, it is only recently that the importance of brain–behavior relationships has become recognized, especially in regard to exceptional children (Gaddes, 1983). With the advent of Public Law 94–142, the Education for All Handicapped Children's Act (Federal Register, 1976), the importance of the exceptional child was brought to the forefront, with specific areas of exceptionality delineated.

Benton (1970) noted that most of the neuropsychological research with exceptional children focused primarily on the learning-disabled child, a position noted by Rourke, Bakker, Fisk, and Strang (1983) as well. Neuropsychological research in other areas, such as mental retardation, has not progressed as rapidly due to technological and psychometric limitations in evaluating such children. The cognitive, motoric, and other basic functional limitations of children in other areas of exceptionality also have posed evaluative problems. These neurodevelopmental disorders represent a major challenge to the child neuropsychologist providing services to children with various developmental abnormalities. Successfully meeting these challenges also will provide useful contributions to increasing our knowledge of brain–behavior relationships in exceptional children.

Given the numerous concerns that are unique to child neuropsychology, as well as the wide array of factors that can contribute to exceptionality, this chapter focuses on only part of the child-neuropsychology–exceptional-child relationship in discussing several of the more-common neurodevelopmental disorders. Generally, neurodevelopmental disorders describe a heterogeneous group of children who (1) learn at a significantly slower rate, either across many areas or within a specific domain, (2) progress more slowly, and (3) experience more difficulty in learning than their normal peers. It should be noted at the outset that no clear distinction can be made between congenital and acquired disorders of brain functioning in childhood. This is one of the fundamental differences between adult and child neuropsychology, in that a disorder acquired in childhood may result in subsequent disturbances in development and learning. It is this broad view of neurodevelopmental disorders that this chapter addresses.

The ensuing discussion is concerned with the developmental aspects of learning disorders. Included is an overview of particular aspects of the neurodevelopmental sequence, particularly as it relates to learning problems and general cognitive development. Interpretive issues that arise in applying a neurodevelopmental model to assessment are also discussed. Following these sections, several of the more-traditional clinical groupings of neurodevelopmental learning disorders are offered. This section includes a synopsis of the neuropsychology of mental retardation, learning disability, and language disorders. The chapter concludes with a summary of the relationship between neurodevelopmental theory and exceptional children.

NEURODEVELOPMENTAL THEORY

Historically, two opposing theoretical traditions prevailed to describe the functional organization of the brain. *Localization theory* proposed a highly differentiated structure and function to the cerebral cortex, assuming that complex mental activity could be narrowly localized to discrete areas of the brain. In contrast, *equipotential theory* viewed the execution of all complex mental functions as dependent on the equal participation of all areas of the brain. This precluded the need to recognize functional differences among various cortical areas, and brain damage was thought to be directly proportional to the amount of tissue destruction. Needless to say, both of these conceptualizations were fraught with problems and inconsistencies. For example, localization theory could not account for the clinical observations that localized damage to a small area of the cortex did not necessarily result in the loss of a single isolated function, but on the contrary, may contribute to disturbances across many mental processes. On the other hand, equipotential theory could not account for specific deficits associated with localized lesions that were not accompanied by generalized impairment in intellect, abstraction, perception, or other global abilities (Golden, 1981a). As can be surmised, neither localization nor equipotential theory could provide an adequate explanation for various clinical observations of children who have sustained brain damage or those with neurodevelopmental disorders (Wilkening & Golden, 1982).

A third, more integrative theory of brain organization and function has been proposed and extensively developed by the Soviet neuropsychologist Luria (1965, 1970, 1973, 1980). Luria's theory permits the reconciliation of the localizationist and equipotentialist positions. It also is able to account for the various clinical phenomena left unexplained by either of the antecedent theories alone.

Luria's Theory

Generalizing from the knowledge that even basic biological functions, such as respiration, could not be narrowly localized to one particular group of cells within the brain, Luria began his theorizing by examining the role of functional systems in the brain and applying this concept to higher mental activities. A functional system involves the integrated participation of a number of cortical areas and is defined by "the presence of a constant (invariant) task, performed by variable mechanisms, bring the process to a constant (invariant) result" (Luria, 1973, p. 28).

Although a narrowly localized group of cortical cells may actively participate in a number of heterogeneous mental processes, it is not possible to narrowly localize a complex mental function, such as reading, within a discrete cortical region. Higher mental processes are viewed as dynamically organized and involving the integrated activity of functional systems comprising various neuroanatomical substrates. A complex function, such as reading, could be disrupted as a result of damage to many different parts of the cortex. Therefore, localized brain damage will not necessarily result in the loss of a single complex function, but it could create deficits across a wide variety of processes that are partially dependent on the functional integrity of the damaged or malformed area. Awareness of the functional organization of higher mental processes permits the use of sophisticated techniques of syndrome analysis in localizing lesions of the brain.

Functional Units

Luria distinguished three functional units of the brain. These functional units are hierarchically organized and functionally integrated, making them essential to the execution of any type of mental activity. The *first unit* is concerned with arousal and is located primarily in the upper and lower parts of the brainstem. Through reciprocal connections with the cortex, this unit is responsible for regulating cortical tone. The *second unit* is located on the convexity of the posterior regions of the two hemispheres, which includes the occipital (visual), temporal (auditory), and parietal (somatosensory) areas. It is responsible for receiving, analyzing, and storing information. The *third unit,* consisting of the frontal lobes, is responsible for the programming, regulation, and verification of activity (Luria, 1980).

Cortical Zones

Each of the three basic functional units of the brain is itself hierarchical in its organization, and consists of three cortical zones (Luria, 1973). The *primary area* either receives impulses from, or sends impulses to, the periphery. *Secondary areas* are responsible for processing incoming information. *Tertiary areas,* or overlapping zones, receive input from two or more of the secondary areas. The tertiary regions are ". . . in a position to carry out extremely complex forms of mental activity" (Luria, 1965, p. 696).

Neurodevelopmental Stages

Implicit to Luria's system of the hierarchical organization of the brain's functional units and their respective cortical zones is a theory of sequential neurological development. The sequence of development is dependent on the physiological and functional changes that occur with normal maturation of various cortical areas. Progression through each stage is paralleled by qualitative organizational changes in the child's adaptive intellectual abilities—a notion that is highly compatible with Piaget's approach to cognitive development. This neurodevelopmental sequence encompasses five major stages, including (1) development of the arousal unit, (2) development of the primary motor and sensory cortical areas, (3) development of the secondary motor and sensory cortical areas, (4) development of the tertiary cortical regions of the second functional unit, and (5) development of the tertiary cortical regions of the third functional unit.

Stage 1 development involves the arousal unit. The reticular activating system (RAS) forms the basis for Luria's first functional unit. The RAS is generally operative at birth and should be fully functional by about 12 months following conception. The RAS is considered essential for arousal from sleep, and is necessary for wakefulness, focusing of attention, perceptual associations, and directed introspection (Chusid, 1982). It is most vulnerable to injury during the prenatal period when it is being formed. Damage to the RAS or its aberrant functioning has been implicated in hyperkinesis (Satterfield & Dawson, 1971; Zentall, 1975) and attention deficits related to learning disabilities (Douglas, 1983; Dykman, Ackerman, Clements, & Peters, 1971; Rutter, 1983a; Schain, 1972, 1983). Rutter (1983a) has drawn a distinction between early (prior to 12 months post-conception) and late onset injury to the RAS, suggesting that true hyperkinesis results from injuries occurring during the earlier period. Despite the known importance of the RAS to processes of attention, the exact pathophysiology of attentional disturbances remains hypothetical (Mesulam, 1981) and poorly understood (Newlin & Tramontana, 1980; Rosenthal & Allen, 1978).

Stage 2 development involves the three primary sensory areas (somesthetic, visual, auditory) and the primary motor area of the cerebral cortex. Stage 2 follows a similar ontogenetic timetable as Stage 1. Spinal reflexes can be detected during the second fetal month, while responses to tactile stimulation can be elicited as early as the third fetal month. All reflexes, except functional respiration and vocalization, are present by the fourth fetal month (Reinis & Goldman, 1980). The dichotomy of motor and sensory functions reflects, in part, the differential rates of cortical maturation. Specifically, motor layers of the cortex mature earlier than the development and differentiation of the sensory cortex (Rhawn, 1982).

By birth, the primary areas are fully operational and account for the repertoire of characteristic reflexes that are indicative of intact functioning of the CNS in the newborn. These reflexive behaviors are genetically predetermined and not the result of environmentally based learning. This is consistent with Piagetian theory, in that early sensorimotor activities and their subsequent elaboration provide the ultimate basis of intelligence and thought (Piaget, 1952).

Injuries to the primary areas during this period of development will have differential effects depending on the child's age and the extent of the damage. Early unilateral injuries to primary areas that occur before or shortly after birth can be compensated through the adoption of the disrupted function by the opposite hemisphere. However, unilateral injuries occurring after this period, or bilateral injuries occurring at any time, may preclude the possibility of such compensatory plasticity. It is in this latter instance that early brain injury may result in the failure of a basic functional unit to develop adequately, and the child may consequently demonstrate a generalized deficit in abilities regardless of the primary location of the injury (Golden, 1981a).

Stage 3 development is characterized by the functional maturation of the secondary cortical areas associated with, and adjacent to, each of the primary areas. These developmental events are initiated concurrently with those of the first two stages, but continue through about the fifth year of life. During this period, as the more primitive reflex-based sensorimotor behaviors of stage 2 begin to recede, the secondary areas gain a gradual ascendancy and are clearly dominant by about age 2. It is at this time that the child begins to develop consistent verbal skills (Golden, 1981a). Development of the secondary areas also marks the beginning of the progressive lateralization of function, with language and motor skills typically being associated with the left hemisphere (Luria, 1973).

With respect to the development of these secondary cortical regions, Luria (1965) described these areas as "intrinsic" structures. The major reason for this description centers around the conceptualization that these regions are only indirectly connected with the periphery as compared to the primary areas, which are directly related to the periphery. The secondary areas receive fibers from subcortical substrates as well as from their respective primary cortical areas, and thus, are in a position to synthesize and act on information. These areas provide the basis for the diverse functional systems necessary for complex perceptual and motor processes (Luria, 1980). Stage 3 marks the transition from simple sensory–motor processes to the more mature modes of perceptual–motor activity. From a Piagetian perspective, this stage parallels the transition to representational thought that is characteristic of the preoperational period (Piaget, 1951).

Many theories have evolved that emphasize sensory–motor and perceptual–motor approaches to the remediation of learning disorders (Ayres, 1973; Delacato, 1966; Doman, 1967; Getman, 1965; Kephart, 1967; Valet, 1973). Although these theories lack a neuropsychological basis (Gaddes, 1980), their common denominator is the assumption that later conceptual abilities are dependent on the child's successful negotiation of more fundamental sensory–motor and perceptual–motor tasks (Lerner, 1976).

From a neuropsychological perspective, during the child's first 5 years the secondary cortical areas are the primary site of learning, and this typically occurs *within* single modalities rather than among them (Golden, 1981b). The brain undergoes qualitative changes during stage 3 due to the increasing specialization of the hemispheres (DeRenzi & Piercy, 1969; Dikemen, Matthews, & Harley, 1975; Golden, 1981b). In general, the more a unilateral injury to the left hemisphere precedes the age of 2 years, the greater the potential for transfer of verbal abilities to the right hemisphere. By age 2 years, the results of childhood brain damage increasingly begin to resemble the effects of brain damage acquired during adulthood. However, even with early injuries, cerebral reorganization of function only occurs with significant injuries to the secondary areas, thus creating the apparent paradox that smaller injuries may produce greater deficits than larger injuries (Golden, 1981b). Such small injuries prenatally or during the birth process may be a primary factor contributing to specific neurodevelopmental learning disorders involving a single modality (Golden & Anderson, 1979).

Stage 4 development involves the maturation of the tertiary areas of the second functional unit, which are located in the parietal regions. This zone is intermediate to the modality-specific secondary areas and permits crossmodal integration and production of supramodal (symbolic) schemes. The tertiary regions form the basis for complex mental activity (Luria, 1973).

The similarity between Luria's Stage 4 period of development and Piaget's period of concrete operations is remarkable. The representational cognitive actions characteristic of the Stage 3 preoperational child gradually combine to form increasingly complex integrated systems of action which Piaget (1950) called *operations*. The child between ages 5 and 12 demonstrates an increasing cognitive decentration from the perceptual aspects of experience, such that multiple dimensions of an event can be represented in thought (Grala, 1976).

The integrative, multimodal functions associated with the tertiary parietal area form the foundation for the acquisition of most formal academic skills such as reading, spelling, and arithmetic. Injuries or anomalies in this area can lead to severe impediments to learning. Deficits in bimodal integration, specific to the precise location of dysfunction within the tertiary region, may be the cause of specific learning disabilities or higher-order language difficulties (Golden & Anderson, 1979). Larger injuries to this area may lead to more profound and global deficits such as mental retardation (Golden, 1981a, 1981b).

Stage 5 development (the final stage) is characterized by development of the tertiary regions of the third functional unit. These prefrontal regions are phylogenetically and ontogenetically the latest of the cerebral structures to develop. However, there is some controversy as to when this stage of development occurs. Luria (1973) believed that this region of the brain did not become functional until the age range of 4 to 7 years, with development continuing through early adulthood. Although this latter point has not been disputed, Golden (1981a, 1981b) estimated that the prefrontal area did not become functionally significant until adolescence.

Recent evidence has emerged, however, suggesting that the development of behaviors associated with frontal lobe functioning is a multistage process, with the greatest period of development occurring between the ages of 6 and 8 years, and the mastery of most tasks evident by age 12 (Passler, Isaac, & Hynd, 1985).

The prefrontal areas possess a rich network of afferent and efferent fibers, which place them in intimate communication with nearly all other cortical zones. Accordingly, Luria assigned this region the role of a "superstructure above all other parts of the cortex" (Luria, 1973, p. 89). The tertiary regions of the prefrontal lobes perform a more universal integrative and regulatory function than do the tertiary areas of the second functional unit (Luria, 1973). These aspects of tertiary frontal functions have obvious parallels to the activities described by Piaget during his discussion of the period of formal operations. Formal operations are dependent on the development of a superordinate cognitive structure which requires the combination and integration of four logical operations. These include *identity, negation, reciprocity,* and *correlativity* (Inhelder & Piaget, 1958). The complex coordination between these operations permits the use of propositional thinking, and allows the child both to simultaneously consider all possible relationships between elements of a situation and to evaluate his or her decisions.

Injuries to the prefrontal regions have been associated with deficits in attention, abstraction, mental and behavioral flexibility, planning sequences of behavior, self-evaluation of performance, and visuoconstructive abilities (Stuss & Benson, 1984). Golden (1981a) asserted, however, that the results of early prefrontal injuries may not be apparent until the child encounters failure meeting the age-appropriate social, behavioral, and cognitive demands of adolescence. With the findings of Passler et al. (1985), this assertion may even be extrapolated downward to include the latency-age child.

Neurodevelopmental Issues

During the ontogenetic development of higher mental processes the child gradually becomes increasingly automatized in the execution of complex behaviors. Along with this, the cortical constituents of complex functional systems also are gradually changing (Wilkening & Golden, 1982). This sequence of change in cortical organization of complex mental process is regular and predictable (Luria, 1980), and it has strong implications for better understanding neurodevelopmental learning disorders. The fact that there are differential effects of childhood brain injury at various ages has been well documented (Boll, 1974; Boll & Barth, 1981; Chelune & Edwards, 1981; Dikemen et al., 1975; Reed & Reitan, 1969;

Reed, Reitan, & Klöve, 1965; Reitan, 1974). Consequently, the awareness of developmental norms is crucial in the evaluation of neurodevelopmental disorders (Rourke, 1978a, 1978b, 1981). Further, the nature, extent, and persistence of a learning disorder depend on a variety of factors including the developmental stage at which the injury occurred, the significance of the disturbed functional system(s) to the learning process, and the availability of alternate functional systems to compensate for resultant deficits (Golden, 1981a). In addition, knowledge of prenatal CNS development may prove useful in elucidating a neurodevelopmental disorder (Dobbing, Hopewell, & Lynch, 1971).

For example, during the embryonic development of the human brain, two significant periods of growth result in a rapid increase in brain weight. There is a minor growth spurt occurring about 10 to 18 weeks from gestation, and a major growth spurt extending from about the fourth to fifth prenatal month to about the end of the fourth year of life (Dobbing & Sands, 1973). The earlier period of brain growth is most vulnerable to severe developmental disorders related to genetic and chromosomal defects, viral infections, and the effects of irradiation and other teratogens.

During the second growth period, the developing brain appears most vulnerable to permanent dysfunction related to malnutrition (Dobbing et al., 1971). During the perinatal period, most of the neurological sequelae are associated with hypoxic–ischemic and hemorrhagic lesions that occur in the newborn infant (Volpe, 1983). Cerebrovascular asymmetries are such that the left hemisphere is likely to be affected sooner and more severely than the right hemisphere, possibly contributing to developmental learning difficulties (Carmon, Harishanu, Louringer, & Lavy, 1972; LeMay & Culebras, 1972). In addition, most of the major neurological disorders of the neonatal period can result in convulsive phenomena, possibly resulting in disturbances in neuronal migration and creating a wide variety of neurodevelopmental aberrations (Volpe, 1983).

For the child neuropsychologist, understanding neurodevelopmental theory becomes crucial to understanding neurodevelopmental learning disorders. This foundation permits one to evaluate a child's neuropsychological performance against developmental expectancies and thereby establish a profile of the child's areas of strength and deficiency. However, it should be noted that the neurodevelopmental model presented does not readily permit greater prognostic accuracy beyond the use of actuarial methods. For example, a child with an early injury or malformation of the tertiary parietal region may demonstrate age-appropriate abilities when evaluated at age 4, using Stage 3 criteria; however, by age 8, this same child may show considerable learning impairment when evaluated against Stage 4 expectations. Transitional phases between Luria's stages of development require further study, particularly as they may relate to diagnosis, prognosis, and early intervention of neurodevelopmental disorders.

From a clinical perspective, an additional issue posed by this model concerns the interpretive significance attached to abnormal neuropsychological performance in the developing child. In interpreting a child's neuropsychological results, the four levels of inference espoused by Reitan (1974) probably compose the most strategic methods of interpretation. These include the child's level of performance, pattern of performance, right–left differences, and the presence of pathognomonic signs. However, the identification of brain dysfunction becomes more complex with children. One must distinguish whether the impaired performance reflects a neuropsychological deficit versus a psychiatric disturbance versus a developmental delay (Tramontana, 1983b).

The distinction between psychiatric disturbance and neuropsychological deficit is often difficult to untangle. Many children with neurodevelopmental learning disorders experience secondary, if not co-existing primary, emotional difficulties. These emotional problems, in turn, can assert their effects in a neuropsychological evaluation by producing an impaired level of performance. In children with neurodevelopmental or chronic learning problems, this is even more problematic. Not only will their present functioning appear impaired, but typically these children also will not master the prerequisite skills and abilities necessary for more advanced learning. It is important for the child neuropsychologist to include measures of lateralizing and localizing value in an evaluation, as significant findings on these measures will strengthen the inference of neuropsychological deficits with this population of children.

The distinction between developmental delay and neuropsychological deficit also presents interpretive difficulty for the child neuropsychologist. Instances of delay will frequently result from irregularities in cortical maturation which postpone the child's readiness for school achievement. Although evidence has shown correspondence between neuroanatomical indices of delayed brain maturation and abnormal neuropsychological performance (Tramontana & Sherrets, 1985), other research has not supported a delay concept of learning problems (Satz & Fletcher, 1981). Moreover, it appears that the prognosis for disabled learners is poor, in that these children do not catch up to age level on either academic or neuropsychological tasks (Schonhaut & Satz, 1983).

Summary

This section has attempted to provide an overview of neurodevelopmental theory and its various components, with some parallels being drawn between neurodevelopmental theory and Piagetian thinking. In addition, some of the main interpretive issues with respect to neurodevelopmental concerns and the practice of child neuropsychology were enumerated. The following sections discuss three of the more common neurodevelopmental learning disorders with which the child neuropsychologist will become involved. These disorders include mental retardation, learning disabilities, and speech and language problems.

MENTAL RETARDATION

Definitional Issues

Mental retardation is a collective term that is used to describe a heterogeneous population. It is a social or behavioral classification, typically defined in psychometric terms, thus not a medical diagnosis (Benton, 1970). The American Association on Mental Deficiency has defined mental retardation in terms of low intelligence (at least two standard deviations below the mean on an individually administered test of intelligence), deficits in adaptive behavior, and with the retardation occurring before the 18th birthday (Grossman, 1977). The current version of the Diagnostic and Statistical Manual (DSM-III) has adopted this definition as well (American Psychiatric Association, 1980).

The definition and psychometric criteria for mental retardation tend to be more arbitrary than empirical in nature. Historically, there has been a tendency to view mental retardation in a dichotomous fashion as opposed to a homogeneous entity (Baumeister & MacLean, 1979). Within this conceptualization, all mentally retarded individuals fall between a range of 0 (or typically less than 20) to 70 on standardized intelligence scores. One group has been characterized as nonorganic, or cultural–familial retardation, with intelligence quotients usually ranging from 50 to 70. This subgroup has been described as biologically intact with their abnormalities being the result of a normally distributed polygenetic controlled set of attributes and/or the product of impoverished surroundings and a lack of cultural opportunities. This subgroup is estimated to compose about 80% of the mentally retarded population (Heber, 1970).

A second subgroup, representing the remaining 20% of the population of retarded individuals, has been described as comprising its own unique normal distribution at the tail end of the traditional normal curve (Zigler, 1967). This variant in the normal distribution has become known as the "bump of pathology" because these individuals evidence clear manifestations of brain damage beyond the expected polygenetic expression of intelligence at this level (Baumeister & MacLean, 1979).

Although of historical value, this dichotomous perspective on mental retardation has been contested. Tredgold and Soddy (1963) stated that mental retardation is nearly always accompanied by defective development of the brain. Prior to this, Masland (1958) put forth the thought that brain injury is present in all mentally retarded individuals, with mild injury being more prevalent than severe injury. More recently, Baumeister and MacLean (1979) proposed that any sort of dichotomous description of mental retardation is incorrect, and that mental retardation should be conceptualized as falling along a continuum of neurological impairment. They stated that there is very little information contributing to a dichotomous view of mental retardation. In support of this contention, Luria (1963) noted that no distinction should be made between retarded individuals having known organic impairment and that larger group whose retardation is of unknown etiology. This thinking reflects more contemporary views regarding mental retardation and suggests that brain pathology and CNS dysfunction should always be considered variables in this population.

Neuroanatomical Factors

Given the current view that brain dysfunction is a concomitant of mental retardation, it stands to reason to expect neurostructural defects to be associated with this population. In fact, postmortem studies have documented neuropathology in retarded individuals not diagnosed as having brain dysfunction. As early as 1960, Crome (1960) performed necropsies on a large sample of institutionalized retarded individuals. Various kinds of structural damage, ranging from mild to severe, were found in nearly all of the patients. Other postmortem studies, using patients exhibiting a continuum of maladaptive functioning, added strength to this finding (Freytag & Lindenberg, 1967; Jellinger, 1972; Malamud, 1964). Jellinger (1972), in examining over 1000 institutionalized cases, found that more than 90% evidenced some degree of brain damage, with a tendency for the less severe cases of retardation to exhibit milder brain anomalies.

In the largest postmortem study to date, Malamud (1964) demonstrated that over 97% of the patients ($N = 1410$) showed neurostructural pathology at autopsy. Given this finding, Malamud concluded that brain pathology is present at all levels of mental retardation. Similar findings were documented by Freytag and Lindenberg (1967), although they did show that 17% of their sample ($N = 359$) exhibited no detectable neuroanatomical abnormalities. In addition, cortical biopsies taken from retarded children have shown significant anomalies in axonal, dendritic, and synaptic processes (Gonatas, Evangelista, & Walsh, 1967; Huttenlocher, 1975), particularly in the number, length, and spatial arrangements of these structures. Other anomalies have implicated the pyramidal motor neurons (Huttenlocher, 1974; Purpura, 1974), suggesting the disruption of motor functions, and the hippocampal regions of the brain, possibly leading to memory and intellectual impairment (Sylvester, 1983).

These data are supportive of the notion that brain dysfunction is pervasive throughout the range of mental retardation, and that it is due to developmental deviation. However, there are few data directly connecting these documented neuroanatomical deficits to behavioral and cognitive difficulties in the mentally retarded child. These findings also must be tempered by the cases reporting hemispherectomies in children with no apparent adverse effects on cognitive functioning (Kennedy & Ramirez, 1964). In addition, aberrations in the neuroanatomical structures of the child's brain may produce behaviors qualitatively distinct from those resulting from malfunctioning neuronal processes. Comparison of cases of retardation arising from neurodevelopmental factors to cases of acquired damage also should proceed with caution.

Neurophysiological Factors

The tendency for neurostructural impairment to be somewhat related to the severity of mental retardation also may be seen when neurophysiological factors in the retarded are explored. Specifically, with increasing severity of mental retardation in children and adolescents there is an increase in electroencephalographic (EEG) abnormalities (Beckett, 1956; LaVeck & de la Cruz, 1963; Matthews & Manning, 1964; Pevzner, 1961). However, there is some evidence to suggest that children with Down's Syndrome (Trisomy 21), a relatively genetically homogeneous group of mentally retarded individuals, are an exception to this rule. Generally, there are significantly less EEG aberrations found in Down's Syndrome than in other forms of mental deficiency (Ellingson, Eisen, & Ottersberg, 1973; Ellingson, Menolascino, & Eisen, 1970; Frühmann & Roth, 1963; Levinson, Friedman, & Stamps, 1955). When EEG anomalies are found, they tend to be observed more frequently during the childhood years (Ellingson et al., 1970, 1973; Frühmann & Roth, 1963) or later in life when neuronal degeneration is present (Crapper, Dalton, Skopitz, Scott, & Hachinski, 1975).

EEG abnormalities are difficult to detect during the first 2 years of life in nonepileptic mentally retarded infants; however, when abnormalities are present, they are suggestive of poor prognosis with respect to growth and development (Friedman & Pampiglione, 1970, 1971). Particular abnormal EEG patterns identified early in life have been shown to be somewhat sensitive indicators of progressive neurological processes, such as neurometabolic storage disease (Pampiglione & Harden, 1974), Tay-Sachs disease (Pampiglione, Privett, & Harden, 1974), and Batten's disease (Zeaman & Dyken, 1969). However, EEG patterns have not been conclusively linked to the functional end of the structural–functional continuum (e.g., intelligence) in this population of children.

One promising feature of the EEG in this regard is the event-related potential (ERP). Generally, the ERP is a background pattern that can be extracted from the EEG in relation to behaviors in which the individual may be engaged. They can be used to investigate differential activation of brain regions relative to a particular stimulus or task. In relation to mentally retarded children, various types of ERPs have been differentially sensitive to stages of sensory processing (Sohmer & Student, 1978), subgroups of mental retardation such as Hurler's Syndrome (Borda, 1977), agenesis of the corpus callosum (Galbraith, 1976), and levels of intelligence (Gasser, von Lucadow-Miller, Verleger, & Bächer, 1983; Karrer & Ivins, 1976). Generally, mentally retarded children show a different topographical representation of brain activity for behavioral tasks when compared to their normal counterparts. In fact, broad-band spectral parameters have accounted for approximately 95% of the topographical variation between normal and mildly retarded children (Gasser, Möcks, & Bächer, 1983). With the technological advances of neurophysiological measures, such as John's neurometric battery (John, 1977; Prichep, John, Ahn, & Kaye, 1983), and Duffy's Brain Electrical Activity Mapping (BEAM) procedure (Duffy, 1981), relationships between neurophysiological activity and neuropsychological functioning in this population will become further articulated.

Neuropsychological Factors

As noted earlier, the neuropsychological aspects of mental retardation have not received the attention that other neurodevelopmental disorders have been afforded (Benton, 1970). This is unfortunate, in that a thorough neuropsychological evaluation could provide a specific analysis of the motoric, perceptual, mnestic, and cognitive functioning of the mentally retarded child. Not only would this information be useful in educational/vocational rehabilitation planning, but it also would prove useful in bridging the gap between the neuroanatomical–neurophysiological aspects of the retarded and their behavioral correlates (Gordon, 1977). Benton (1970) further speculated that there may even be subtypes of mental retardation that show specific deficit patterns, possibly in conjunction with specific etiologies.

To date, much of the research with the mentally retarded has been concerned with the cognitive aspects of their functioning, such as memory (Kamizono, 1983; Ross & Ward, 1978) and information-processing strategies (Ashman, 1982; Camara-Resendiz & Fox, 1983; Das, Kirby, & Jarman, 1975, 1979; Stanovich, 1978). Although extraordinarily useful in the attempt to better understand the mentally retarded child, developing brain–behavior correlates is not necessarily a goal of cognitive psychology. Consequently, the state of knowledge with respect to brain-behavior relationships in the mentally retarded child is definitely in its infancy. Reasons for this lag in a neuropsychological knowledge base for the retarded child include (1) the difficulties in administering neuropsychological tests to this population, (2) the few specific neuroanatomical and neurophysiological correlates of behavior in this population, and (3) uncertainties with respect to neuropsychological normative data (Benton, 1970; Tramontana, 1983a). More generally, consideration must be given to the lack of lateralizing and focal findings that are believed by many researchers to typify the adaptive behavior deficits of the mentally retarded child. With general adaptive behavior deficits, the utility of a thorough neuropsychological evaluation and the subsequent clinical time involved would need to be weighed against the clinical benefits of such a task.

In spite of the numerous methodological and clinical issues related to neuropsychological investigation of children with mental retardation, it remains feasible to investigate the neuropsychological functioning of this population (Benton, 1970; Matthews, 1974; Tramontana, 1983a), particularly the higher-functioning individuals. Further, many of the aforementioned concerns pertaining to the neuropsychological investigation of the mentally retarded child have begun to be addressed.

Some normative data are available for retarded children, ages 9 to 14 years, on the Halstead–Reitan Neuropsychological Battery (Matthews, 1974). Dividing 81 children into moderately retarded (IQ = 40–54), mildly retarded (IQ = 55–69), and borderline to low average (IQ = 70–84) groups, Matthews found nearly all of the neuropsychological variables to be significantly related to full scale IQ as defined by the Wechsler Intelligence Scale for Children (WISC). Only time on the tactual performance test, dynamometer grip strength, auditory and visual imperception errors, and finger tapping were not significantly related to full-scale IQ. Matthews noted that it would be important to collect normative data on younger mentally retarded children, as well as to begin to investigate neuropsychological functioning relative to the etiology of mental retardation.

With respect to specificity of neuropsychological functions for the retarded child, research has been accumulating to suggest that implicit strengths, weaknesses, and patterns of performance can be uncovered. Specifically, certain patterns of performance have been associated with particular types of mental retardation. Money (1973) noted that individuals with Turner's Syndrome, a chromosomal abnormality associated with mental retardation, frequently demonstrated differential difficulty on visuoconstructive tasks such as the Bender–Gestalt, Benton Visual Retention Test, and the WISC-R Block Design and Object Assembly subtests. Performance on these measures tended to be inferior when compared to these children's verbal abilities. Money speculated that Turner's Syndrome individuals were more susceptible to right parietal dysfunction than other mentally retarded children.

Mentally retarded children have been shown to have a right-ear advantage for speech on dichotic listening tasks, but the advantage is reduced in comparison to their normal-functioning counterparts (Pipe, 1983; Pipe & Beale, 1983). A replication of this finding also is found in the tachistoscopic literature, with mentally retarded children having a typical right visual field advantage for language stimuli (Shihazaki, 1983). However, in Down's Syndrome children, the opposite appears to be true. Using sequential and simultaneous processing tasks, Hartley (1982, 1983) demonstrated that Down's Syndrome children, ages 9 to 13, performed more poorly on sequential tasks than a matched set of non-Down's-Syndrome retarded children and normals matched for mental age. Although both mentally retarded groups were significantly lower than the normal children, the mentally retarded children exhibited similar functioning on simultaneous tasks. This may be suggestive of right hemisphere dominance for language in the Down's Syndrome population (Hartley, 1983).

Attentional deficiencies also are prominent in the mentally retarded population. Ager (1983), in reviewing 12 studies, concluded that failure to attend to appropriate features of a task is an important component of learning difficulties in this population. Further, as with their learning disabled counterparts (Hynd, Cohen, & Obrzut, 1983; Hynd, Obrzut, Weed, & Hynd, 1979), mentally retarded children have been found to be able to significantly shift their attention from a right-ear advantage to a left-ear advantage on a directed dichotic listening task, whereas normal children seem to be unable to do this (Žekulin-Hartley, 1982). Similarly, other evidence has been found for incomplete lateralization of brain function.

Kuroda and Kobayaski (1984) demonstrated that mentally retarded children will exhibit an indistinguishable hand preference pattern more frequently and for a longer duration than normal children. Bradshaw-McAnulty, Hicks, and Kinsbourne (1984) also have presented evidence of increased familial sinistrality, which corresponded with greater severity of mental retardation. Neuropsychological deficits have been found in mentally retarded children's language skills (Ashman, 1982; Hartley, 1982; Pipe & Beale, 1983; Walton, Ellis, & Court, 1962), somesthetic functioning (Reed, 1967), and psychomotor functioning (Niihara & Kusano, 1984) when compared normatively as well as ipsatively. These findings suggest the utility of a complete neuropsychological evaluation in prescriptive planning for a mentally retarded youngster's educational/ vocational program.

As might be expected, the mentally retarded child has shown deficient performance on nearly all basic neuropsychological functions when compared to their normal peers; however, it appears that qualitative and quantitative differences in ability levels exist not only between genetically different types of mental retardation, but within the general population of mentally retarded children as well. One can also observe relative performance variability in the individual child. The neuropsychology of the mentally retarded child is an old concern, but a relatively unresearched area. Moreover, it seems that the neuropsychological study of the mentally retarded child would make a theoretical as well as a clinical contribution to the increased understanding of brain–behavior relationships in children in general.

SPECIFIC LEARNING DISABILITIES

While the neuropsychological study of mental retardation in children has only begun, the neuropsychological study of learning disabilities has been fervently explored. Indeed, the past 20 to 25 years have witnessed tremendous growth with respect to the neuropsychology of the learning disabled child (Gaddes, 1980; Hynd & Obrzut, 1981; Rourke, 1985; Rutter, 1983b). This growth has resulted largely from the complex nature of specific learning disabilities, and it has encompassed the fields of psychology, education, neurology, pediatrics, and ophthalmology to mention a few. Further, the growth has been fueled by the estimate that this population of children, particularly those who would be classified as dyslexic, exceeds the combined population of children who have seizure disorders, cerebral palsy, or severe mental retardation (Duane, 1979). Clinically, this translates into an expected incidence rate of approximately 20 to 30 children in every 1000 (Hynd, Obrzut, Hayes, & Becker, in press), making this an extremely important area for the child neuropsychologist.

Definitional Issues

Kirk (1963) is originally credited with the coining of the term "learning disability." However, the conceptualization of childhood learning disorders has spanned nearly 100 years, dating back to Morgan's (1896) case of congenital word blindness. It was not until 1975 that the 94th U.S. Congress put forth the first widely accepted definition of learning disabilities. This definition stated that the learning disabled child experiences

> a disorder in one or more of the basic psychological processes involved in understanding or in using language, spoken or written, which may manifest itself in an imperfect ability to listen, think, speak, read, write, spell, or do mathematical calculations. The term includes such conditions as perceptual handicaps, brain injury, minimal brain dysfunction, dyslexia, and developmental aphasia. (Federal Register, 1976, p. 56977)

This definition was adopted by most state education departments, and being a legal mandate, carried with it numerous due-process procedures and regulations. Although not fully detailed, this definition did allude to the involvement of some form of neurological dysfunction in the learning disabled child. McCarthy (1975) attempted to operationalize this definition by noting that (1) these children do not learn despite average intellectual potential (usually IQs above 85) and adequate opportunities; (2) a discrepancy must exist between their demonstrated academic aptitude and their academic achievement; and (3) this discrepancy must be significant enough to warrant specialized treatment. Although this definition was important in setting the tone for the nature of learning disabilities, it remained sufficiently general in its description that the definition was considered inadequate. Part of this vagueness was attributable to the interest and concern of multiple disciplines in defining this concept.

In an effort to generate more clear and acceptable guidelines for this neurodevelopmental disorder, the National Joint Committee for Learning Disabilities (NJCLD) was formed. This Committee consisted of representatives from organizations concerned with speech and language, learning disability, communication disorders, and reading (Hammill, Leigh, McNutt, & Larsen, 1981). This committee generated the following definition:

> Learning disability is a generic term that refers to a heterogeneous group of disorders manifested by significant difficulties in the acquisition and use of listening, speaking, reading, writing, reasoning, or mathematical abilities. These disorders are instrinsic to the individual and presumed to be due to central nervous system dysfunction. Even though a learning disability may occur concomitantly with other handicapping conditions (e.g., sensory impairment, mental retardation, social and emotional disturbance) or environmental influences (e.g., cultural differences, insufficient/inappropriate instruction, psychogenic factors), it is not the direct result of those conditions or influences (Hammill et al., 1981, p. 336).

This definition widens the scope of the learning-disability concept. Specifically, the definition acknowledges the heterogeneous nature of learning disabilities and opens the door for subtype analysis for this group of disorders. Further, placing the term within a neurological framework implicates the need for neuropsychological investigation of this population, not to mention a greater need for practitioners working with learning-disabled children to have at least a basic working knowledge of CNS functioning. Finally, the definition allows for a learning disability to exist concurrently with psychiatric disturbance, a concept that the former definition did not fully address. This definition is not without its problems, but it does represent a refinement over the previous attempts.

Subtypes of Specific Learning Disability

Probably the biggest contributions of the new definition of learning disability are the acceptance of both the heterogeneous nature of the disorder and the presumed etiology to be of a neurological nature. Support for this latter point has been generated from electrophysiological studies (Duffy, 1981; Duffy, Burchfield, & Lombroso, 1979; Duffy, Denckla, Bartels, & Sandini, 1980; Duffy, Denckla, Bartels, Sandini, & Kiessling, 1980), neuroanatomical postmortem studies (Drake, 1968; Galaburda & Kemper, 1979; Galaburda, Sherman, & Geschwind, in press), as well as studies of the hemispheric functioning of children (Bakker, 1983; Obrzut, Hynd, Obrzut, & Pirozzolo, 1981; Pirozzolo & Rayner, 1979).

Much of the earlier work with children experiencing learning problems sought to identify the single deficient process that was contributing to the learning difficulties. As might be expected, this resulted in multiple, typically conflictual, single-factor theories of learning disabilities. Some of these models included deficits in cerebral dominance (Orton, 1928, 1937; Satz, Rardin, & Ross, 1971; Yeni-Komshian, Isenberg, & Goldstein, 1975; Zurif & Carson, 1970), perceptual processes (Lyle, 1969; Lyle & Goyen, 1968, 1975), temporal-order recall (Bakker, 1972), bisensory memory (Senf, 1969; Senf & Freundl, 1971), perceptual–motor matching (Kephart, 1967), and crossmodal integration (Birch & Belmont, 1964, 1965). It was this proliferation of single-factor theories that provided the impetus for conceptualizing learning disabilities in a multidimensional fashion (Hynd & Cohen, 1983).

To date, numerous subtype models have been presented in an effort to better refine the field. Many of these models have been concerned with subtypes of reading disability, or dyslexia, due to the frequency of reading problems in school-age children. However, spelling subtypes (Naidoo, 1972; Nelson & Warrington, 1974; Sweeney & Rourke, 1978) and arithmetic subtypes also have been described (Rourke & Finlayson, 1978; Rourke & Strang, 1978). Many different subtypes of learning disability are believed to exist, and to exemplify this, some investigators have identified as many as six different reading patterns (Lyon & Watson, 1981). Further, if one agrees with the conceptualization of the functional system as described by Luria (1980), then the potential number of subtypes of learning disability is limited only by the sophistication and variability of the neuropsychological procedures employed (Hynd et al., in press). Table 1 provides an overview of the studies, employing statistical and clinical methods of grouping, that have revealed various subtypes of learning disability.

Reading Subtypes

Within the reading domain, there is support for at least two different subgroups of developmental dyslexia (Bakker, 1983; Pirozzolo, 1977, 1979). The first subtype that seems to be consistently described demonstrates auditory–linguistic deficits, but relatively adequate visual–spatial skills. This group of deficient readers experiences primary deficits in letter–sound integration and poor use of phonetic word-decoding strategies. Linguistic deficits also may be found in this particular subtype pattern. This tends to be the largest group of dyslexics (Boder, 1970; Mattis, Erenberg, & French, 1978; Mattis, French, & Rapin, 1975).

A second subtype that has been described manifests the opposite pattern of the auditory–linguistic group. In this subtype, auditory processing and linguistic abilities are relatively intact, but visual–spatial difficulties are pronounced. These children experience primary deficiencies in perceiving whole words as gestalts, and may even overphoneticize in their word decoding. This subtype tends to be more rare than the auditory–linguistic subtype (Boder, 1970; Mattis et al., 1975), perhaps because of the emphasis on auditory and linguistic strategies in traditional classroom instruction.

Some investigators have insisted on a third diagnostic subtype, incorporating characteristics of the auditory–linguistic and visual–spatial subtypes (Bateman, 1968; Boder, 1970, 1973; Doehring & Hoshko, 1977; Ingram, Mason, & Blackburn, 1970; Omenn & Weber, 1978; Satz & Morris, 1981), while others have attempted to include motor and sensory deficits in their subtype models (Fisk & Rourke, 1979; Lyon & Watson, 1981; Mattis et al., 1975).

TABLE 1

Statistical and clinical studies investigating subtypes of learning disabilities

Date	Investigator(s)	Description of Subtype(s)
1963	Kinsbourne & Warrington	Verbally deficient readers
		Spatially deficient readers
1964	Quiros	Auditory dyslexia
		Visual dyslexia
1966	Bannatyne	Neurological dyslexia
		Genetic dyslexia
1967	Johnson & Myklebust	Audiophonic dyslexia
		Visuospatial dyslexia
1968	Bateman	Auditory memory subgroup
		Visual memory subgroup
		Combined subgroup
1970	Boder	Dysphonetic dyslexia
		Dyseidetic dyslexia
		Alexic
1970	Ingram, Mason, & Blackburn	Audiophonetic subtype
		Visual–spatial subtype
		Combined subtype
1971	Rourke, Young, & Flewelling	Performance IQ > Verbal IQ
		Performance IQ < Verbal IQ
		Performance IQ ≈ Verbal IQ
1972	Naidoo	Reading/spelling deficits
		Spelling deficits only
1974	Nelson & Warrington	Reading/spelling deficits
		Spelling deficits only
1975	Mattis, French, & Rapin	Language disordered
		Articulatory and graphomotor dyscoordination
		Visual perception deficits
1977	Doehring & Hoshko	Linguistic deficits
		Phonological deficits
		Intersensory integration deficits
		Visual perceptual deficits
1977	Smith, Coleman, Dokecki, & Davis	High IQ group
		Low IQ group
1978	Sweeney & Rourke	Reading/spelling deficits
		Spelling deficits
1978	Rourke & Finlayson	Reading, spelling, and arithmetic deficits
		Reading and spelling deficient group
		Arithmetic deficient group
1978	Omenn & Weber	Auditory deficits
		Visual deficits
		Mixed subtype

TABLE 1 (*Continued*)

Date	Investigator(s)	Description of Subtype(s)
1978	Mattis, Erenberg, & French	Phonemic sequencing deficits Language deficits Articulatory–graphomotor deficits Visual–perceptual deficits Subtypes with two of the preceding deficits
1979	Petrauskas & Rourke	Left temporal lobe deficits Posterior left hemisphere deficits
1979	Fisk & Rourke	Auditory–verbal processing, visual sequencing, and finger localization deficits Auditory–verbal processing and motor deficits Word blending, memory, and fingertip number writing deficits
1979	Pirozzolo	Auditory–linguistic subtype Visual–spatial subtype
1980	Coltheart, Patterson, & Marshall	Deep dyslexia
1981	Satz & Morris	Global language subtype Specific language subtype Visual perceptual subtype Mixed subtype
1981	Lyon & Watson	Language comprehension, auditory and visual memory, sound blending, and visual spatial deficits Language comprehension, auditory memory, and visual–motor integration deficits Aphasic subtype Expressive and receptive language deficits Visuoperceptive deficits Normal pattern with low reading achievement
1982	Deloche & Andreewsky	Surface dyslexia
1983	Sevush	Surface dyslexia Deep dyslexia Phonological dyslexia
1983	Watson, Goldgar, & Ryschon	Language-disordered subtype Visual processing subtype Minimal deficits subtype
1984	Meacham & Fisher	Reading disabled Language disabled

Arithmetic Subtypes

Subtypes of arithmetic disability have not been explored as extensively as reading problems. However, as early as 1971, Cohn stated that difficulties in mathematics could be attributable to a more pervasive language disorder. Rourke and Finlayson (1978), and Rourke and Strang (1978), have since provided evidence for subtypes of arithmetic disability. Using a wide range of instruments selected to tap the neuropsychological areas of tactile perception, visual perception, auditory perception, motor function, conceptual thinking, and academic achievement, Rourke and his colleagues described two statistically derived subtypes of arithmetic disability.

The first subtype provided support for Cohn's (1971) speculation that language deficits were primarily responsible for difficulties in mathematics. This group manifested relatively adequate understanding of basic arithmetic processes in the presence of deficits in reading and/or spelling skills. These children exhibited neuropsychological deficits on verbally based tasks, but adequate visual–perceptual processing abilities. Mathematical errors were characterized by inadequate comprehension of word problems and instructions, difficulties memorizing facts and step-by-step procedures, and inexperience with subject material, largely because of grade retentions and special education intervention focusing on other areas, such as reading. However, these children did seem to have an adequate understanding of basic arithmetic processes (Rourke & Strang, 1983).

The second subtype of arithmetic disabilities identified by Rourke (1978b) evidenced adequate reading and spelling skills, but deficient arithmetic. These children had adequately developed auditory–perceptual skills, but deficient visual–perceptual, psychomotor, and tactile–perceptual abilities. In contrast to the first subtype, this arithmetic subtype had difficulties with the mechanical aspects of calculation, such as misreading procedural signs, misaligning columns of numbers, neglecting numbers in the arithmetic process, and poorly forming their numerals. In addition, these children were poorly organized in performing arithmetical calculations, they did not check their work, and they did not always understand the arithmetic principle that they were using (Rourke & Strang, 1983).

Spelling Disorders

Research in this academic area has consistently yielded two subtypes of disabled spellers (Naidoo, 1972; Nelson & Warrington, 1974; Sweeney & Rourke, 1978). One of the subtypes exhibits reading and spelling deficiencies, suggesting the possibility of a more pervasive language disorder.

Children in the second subtype have managed to overcome their initial reading problems, but they still remain poor spellers. This subtype of deficient spellers has been described as not utilizing lexical, or letter-by-letter, processing in learning to spell, thus implicating phonological processing problems (Frith, 1983). Rourke (1981) elucidated that poor spellers are more effectively discriminated from good spellers across many neuropsychological tasks, particularly at older age levels. Further, those spellers who evidenced the use of phonetic principles, even in their spelling errors, seem to have a better academic prognosis (Sweeney & Rourke, 1978).

Although some dyslexia models would argue for a strong interrelationship between reading and spelling problems (Boder, 1970, 1973; Finucci, Isaacs, Whitehouse, & Childs, 1983), it may be that symptoms associated with disorders of spelling do not implicate, or even correlate with, problems in reading (Hynd & Hynd, 1984; Roeltgen, 1984). Further validation of spelling subtypes, particularly as they relate to prognosis and treatment strategies, is required.

Issues in Subtype Analysis

The definition adopted by the NJCLD (Hammill et al., 1981) acknowledges the neurological basis and heterogeneous nature of learning disabilities. Further, the subtype models generated to date also reflect a refinement of the field to some degree. At present, however, there exist many problems with the subtype literature.

The studies describing subtype models have used either clinical (a priori) or statistical (a posteriori) procedures. Using clinical methodology, subtypes are formed on the basis of a particular performance pattern and then compared on neuropsychological measures. The problem with this procedure is in defining the initial sample from which the subgroups were selected. These selection criteria tend to vary from study to study, making subtype comparisons limited at best. This contributes to the possibility of poor reliability and validity of the subtypes, although it should be noted that Mattis and colleagues (Mattis et al., 1978) were successful in replicating their clinical model for developmental dyslexia.

With multivariate procedures, such as Q-factor analysis and clustering techniques, study-to-study comparisons can be flawed by methodological decisions, such as what to include in the variables to be grouped or clustered. The old adage regarding factor analytic strategies, "you get out what you put in," rings true in this regard. The inclusion of tests with low reliability and validity only serves to cloud the subtype picture with unnecessary error variance. Using clustering procedures, Meacham and Fisher (1984) also questioned the reliability of subtypes, and thus their persistence over time. If such classification procedures are employed in generating subtypes, careful selection of reliable and valid measures known to be sensitive to the functional integrity of the brain is absolutely essential (Fisk & Rourke, 1979). Satz and Morris (1981) and Morris, Blashfield, and Satz (1981) have presented several approaches for assessing and validating group classification schemes. Until these methodological concerns are better addressed, model-to-model comparisons will be tenuous at best.

In spite of the problems, the subtype literature points to new directions for the child neuropsychologist working with learning disabled children, particularly with respect to improved treatment for such children. Given the neurodevelopmental basis of learning disabilities, and its relationship to subtyping, it should be possible to provide for a specific child's learning needs through a modification of the attribute × treatment paradigm (Kaufman & Kaufman, 1983). By using a general subtyping model for classification of a child's strengths and weaknesses, and further delineating specific needs based on a qualitative assessment of the child's performance, an appropriate treatment strategy should be viable. These subtype × attribute × treatment interactions could then be subjected to empirical validation, thus providing further verification for the utility of diagnosing subtypes of learning-disabled children (Boder, 1970, 1973; Petrauskas & Rourke, 1979; Rourke, 1985).

SPEECH AND LANGUAGE DISORDERS

From the preceding discussion on learning disabilities, it can be seen that language disorders are not mutually exclusive diagnostically from specific learning disabilities, or even mental retardation. However, language disorders do seem more intimately related to learning disabilities than many of the other types of neurodevelopmental learning disorders. Although the area of language dysfunction has been generally viewed under the auspices of speech and language pathology, language disorders can have far-reaching effects on the growth of a child. Not only can these disorders interfere with cognitive and scholastic performance, but also they can significantly disrupt the adaptive social–emotional growth of the child (de Hirsch, 1976). The concerns presented by developmental language disorders are quite relevant to the child neuropsychologist.

Definitional Issues

Language disorders of a developmental nature have been assigned a variety of labels, including word deafness, developmental aphasia, congenital auditory imperception, and idiopathic language retardation. More traditionally, this group of disorders has been referred to as developmental, or childhood, dysphasia. With respect to this discussion, the term *dysphasia* is used instead of aphasia, in an effort to illustrate the *partial acquisition* of language that many of these children demonstrate. Although somewhat of a paradoxical term, childhood dysphasia refers to a group of children who acquire language at a slower rate, at a later age, and with less success than their peers with normal language functioning (Kail, Hole, Leonard, & Nippold, 1984). In many of these children basic language skills do develop, but their language is characterized by unconventional grammar, atypical order of skill acquisition, and unusual production–comprehension relationships (Wilkening & Golden, 1982).

One definition of this population of children extends back to 1960 from the Proceedings of the Institute on Childhood Aphasia (West, 1962). This definition reads as follows:

> Impairment of language function (expressive and receptive) resulting from maldevelopment or injury to the central nervous system, prenatally, perinatally, or postnatally (not later . . . than the normal time for the development of speech . . .). The language deficiency may or may not be associated with other cerebral or neurological pathology or dysfunction. Excluded are language problems associated primarily with (1) mental deficiency, (2) hearing impairment, (3) central nervous system damage affecting the peripheral speech mechanism, (4) emotional disturbance, and (5) delayed maturation in language development resulting from social and emotional factors or physical factors not primarily due to central nervous system involvement. (p. 1)

This definition has been the subject of much controversy as well as a shifting emphasis, such as using formulae or multiple criteria (Bloom & Lahey, 1978; Leonard, 1979; Monsees, 1972; R. E. Stark & Tallal, 1981; West, 1962). Nonetheless, the term childhood dysphasia has been used to differentiate acquired aphasia (the loss of already established language skills) from a developmental disorder. Of course, as with other acquired disturbances impacting on learning, instances of acquired dysphasia in childhood may impede further normal language development. The term *childhood dysphasia* also concurs with adult aphasia, in that this primary language disorder is the result of CNS dysfunction (Bloom & Lahey, 1978). Currently, this term is used more as a clinical category, as the study of childhood language disorders is becoming more interested in the structure and use of language as opposed to global clinical descriptions such as aphasia.

Several types of childhood dysphasia have been presented in the literature. These include *receptive dysphasia,* which involves difficulties in understanding speech, and *expressive (motor) dysphasia,* which is defined by impairment in speech production in the absence of damage to the speech mechanism. Telford and Sawrey (1972) also have defined another set of symptoms called *conceptual dysphasia,* which involves the inability to formulate concepts. Luria (1973) has described another type, *semantic dysphasia,* which is characterized by difficulty in associating individual words and ideas into a meaningful whole. *Conduction dysphasia,* which is the inability to repeat oral language on command, and *global (mixed) dysphasia,* in which all forms of language are disrupted, have been discussed in the adult literature, but have not been applied to children.

Supporting evidence for childhood dysphasia and developmental language disorders in general has come from postmortem neuroanatomical studies (Drake, 1968; Landau, Goldstein, & Kleffner, 1960; Roberts, 1962), which have shown bilateral anomalies, primarily in the region of the planum temporale. Further support also has come from neurophysiological research implicating the left cerebral hemisphere (Roberts, 1962). However, children suffering from childhood dysphasia often do not evidence a history of cerebral insult, nor do they necessarily show positive signs on the classic pediatric neurological examination. This does not imply that there is not CNS dysfunction or anomaly, as these effects can be subtle, less circumscribed, and more diffuse in their disruption of language in children than in adults (de Hirsch, 1976).

Neurolinguistic Processes and Childhood Dysphasia

Neurolinguistics is a broad-based discipline encompassing the neurological, biological, and linguistic aspects of speech and language. As such, its importance to understanding childhood language disorders, or more specifically, childhood dysphasia, is evident. Historically, childhood dysphasia has been related to the child's difficulty in processing auditory stimuli (Eisenson & Ingram, 1972). Many different aspects of this functional system have been implicated, including the integrative capacity of the brain in the management of acoustic information (Hardy, 1965), deficient auditory verbal memory and temporal sequencing (J. Stark & Poppen, 1967), difficulty in discriminating letter sounds in context (McReynolds, 1966, 1967; Rees, 1973a), and problems with categorizing linguistic relations (Menyuk, 1971).

Current thinking with respect to childhood dysphasia implicates the child's inability to manage linguistic sequences (Eisenson, 1968, 1969; Tallal & Newcombe, 1978). The dysphasic child typically exhibits adequate isolated phoneme discrimination, but the child is unable, or at least inefficient, in making similar discriminations when the sounds are incorporated into a dynamic and complex linguistic structure. Eisenson (1968,

1969) noted that these functional deficits coincide with the secondary divisions of the auditory cortex and the postcentral kinesthetic regions as defined by Luria (1973).

Although Johnston and Schery (1976) and Morehead and Ingram (1973) presented evidence to suggest that the linguistic forms employed by childhood dysphasics and normal children are qualitatively similar, there are several important differences. First, these children make less frequent use of particular grammatical structures (e.g., subject–verb agreement, pronoun clarity). Second, as with learning-disabled and mentally retarded children, the language-disordered children are less creative and more inefficient in their overall use of language. Finally, language-disordered children have demonstrated linguistic deficits in syntax (Johnston & Schery, 1976; Leonard, 1972; Menyuk, 1964; Morehead & Ingram, 1973), semantics (Freedman & Carpenter, 1976; Leonard, Bolders, & Miller, 1976), pragmatics (Snyder, 1975), and the interactional aspects of content, form, and use in functional language (Bloom & Lahey, 1978).

Speech Disorders

Developmental speech disorders in children tend to fall into three broad areas. These areas include speech-sound disorders (articulation), voice problems, and speech dysfluencies.

Speech-sound disorders refer to the mispronunciation of oral speech sounds. At a more complex level, this group of disorders has been included within the area of phonology, which is concerned with the structure and function of sound systems within language (Hyman, 1975). Procedures for conceptualizing, classifying, and assessing phonological disorders have been cogently outlined by Shriberg and Kwiatkowski (1982). Although the child neuropsychologist should be familiar with phonological disorders, the speech and language pathologist should be consulted on matters regarding phonological patterns and analysis.

Correct speech articulation is dependent on complex processes that control and coordinate the speech neuromusculature (Espir & Rose, 1976). In addition, the child must have a working knowledge, even if it is at an automatic level, of the phonological aspects of speech (Locke, 1983). Specific types of articulation errors include sound substitutions, sound omissions, sound distortions, and addition of inappropriate and unnecessary sounds (Pirozzolo & Campanella, 1981). Although one of these errors will tend to dominate, a child may manifest more than one type of misarticulation. It should be noted that children who evidence articulation errors do not necessarily have neurological impairment. In fact, misarticulation of particular speech sounds (e.g., /sh/, /z/, /v/) at certain ages is developmentally normal (Templin, 1957; Winitz, 1969). Sex differences also are evident with females achieving correct articulation sooner than males (Menkes, 1980). Typically by age 8, nearly all phonemes should be mastered at least in isolated sounds.

There are many reasons why some children experience speech-sound difficulties. One reason, mentioned here earlier, is that it is developmentally normal for certain speech sounds to be misarticulated. These misarticulations may be secondary to immaturity in the development of the oral–motor musculature. A second reason is that some children fail to learn, and become competent with, phonological rules. These types of misarticulation arise from deficiencies in pitch and general auditory discrimination and, as a group, have been labelled phonological disorders (Crary, 1980; Edwards & Shriberg, 1983). A third reason children exhibit articulation errors is that there is neurological impairment contributing to poor coordination of the speech mechanism, such as dysarthria or developmental dyspraxia. The neurological causes of dysarthria and oral–motor dyspraxia are grouped according to which part of the neuromuscular system is affected. Some of these include the musculature, upper and lower motor neurons, the extrapyramidal system, the cerebellum and its various connections, and of course, the motor speech area of the cerebral cortex (Espir & Rose, 1976). The prevalence of speech-sound disorders is closely related to age. They are most common in young children, reaching an incidence of about 15% in kindergarten children. Of children younger than age 8, 90% outgrow their speech defects, but those who still have defective speech by adolescence can expect to improve only with speech therapy (Travis, 1971).

The second category of speech problems is voice disorders. Voice disorders are usually described in terms of their pitch, loudness, or quality of vocal production. They can be the result of either organic or functional involvement, including hearing loss, social–emotional difficulties, hormonal problems, tension, or laryngeal anomalies (Boone, 1971; G. P. Moore, 1971). Although the child neuropsychologist should be familiar with the various types of voice disorders, this category of speech problems in and of itself has minimal implications for a child's learning.

The third category of speech problems is speech dysfluency. Speech dysfluency refers to any behavior, such as repetitions or prolongation of sounds, syllables, or words, that disrupts the rhythm and flow of speech. Abnormally long pauses, or blocks, also are included as contributing to speech dysfluency. When these behaviors become severe, this abnormal speech pattern is referred to as stuttering. Stuttering is defined by the International Classification of Diseases as disorders in the rhythm of speech, in which the individual knows precisely what he wished to say, but at that time is unable to say it because of an involuntary, repetitive prolongation or cessation of a sound (World Health Organization, 1977, p. 202).

This topic has been extensively reviewed by Andrews et al. (1983), and the interested reader is referred there for a more complete discussion of this disorder.

As with the development of articulation skills, some speech dysfluency is expected to occur as part of the normal development and mastery of speech processes (Bloodstein, 1981; Sheehan & Martyn, 1970; Van Riper, 1972). However, it is when these dysfluent behaviors continue, usually beyond the age of 5 (Menkes, 1980), that the child in question should be followed by a speech and language pathologist.

With respect to speech dysfluencies, and in particular stuttering, research has been reported describing alteration of EEG activity (Sayles, 1971), bilateral hemispheric representation for speech in patients with organic brain lesions (Andrews, Quinn, & Sorby, 1972; Luessenhop, Boggs, Laborwit, & Walle, 1973), dilation of the pupils (Gardner, 1937), eye-movement abnormalities (Kopp, 1963), decreases in blood-sugar levels (W. E. Moore, 1959), anomalies in the dynamics of articulation (Zimmerman, 1980a, 1980b), variations in regional cerebral blood flow (Wood, Stump, McKeehan, Shelton, & Proctor, 1980), and differences in laryngeal behavior between the various types of stuttering (Conture, McCall, & Brewer, 1977). In addition, stuttered speech reportedly can be significantly distinguished from normal speech even when written transcriptions of speech samples are used (Wingate, 1977), although this requires further validation. Bloodstein (1981) estimated that the prevalence of stuttering in preadolescent children is about 1%, with it dropping to about .8% during adolescence. As with most neurodevelopmental learning disorders, more males stutter than females, at a ratio of about 3 to 1, and this proportion increases with age.

Summary

This section presented three of the more common neurodevelopmental learning disorders that the child neuropsychologist may encounter. Although the categories of neurodevelopmental learning disorders reviewed here have been described as clinical entities, the child neuropsychologist must recognize the heterogeneous nature of each. Attempting to conceptualize neurodevelopmental learning disorders along a continuum of neurological impairment may prove useful in differentiating the numerous features that children experiencing learning difficulties can present.

CONCLUSIONS

This chapter has covered the neurodevelopmental foundations of learning difficulties and discussed three of the more-common neurodevelopmental disorders confronted by the clinical child neuropsychologist. It should be noted that the neurodevelopmental aspects of learning difficulties also can be applied to other developmental disorders such as attention-deficit disorder, autism, seizure disorders, neuromuscular disorders, and sensory disorders (e.g., deaf, hearing impaired, visually impaired, blind). It is imperative that the child neuropsychologist have a firm working knowledge of neurodevelopmental theory in evaluating and planning for a child's specific educational and adaptive behavior needs. At present, the clinical child neuropsychologist can make a valuable contribution to a child's functioning by further identifying and refining patterns of spared and impaired abilities, particularly as they may help to determine specific rehabilitative efforts. This contribution may even be enhanced with the further delineation of more homogeneous subtypes of learning problems across all areas of exceptionality.

From a theoretical perspective, the field of child neuropsychology requires better integration of developmental theory (e.g., Piaget) and neuropsychological functioning, not to mention greater substantiation of the correspondencies between neuroanatomical, neurophysiological, and neuropsychological findings. A better understanding of these relationships, in conjunction with stronger theoretical underpinnings of a developmental nature, will contribute to helping the clinical child neuropsychologist differentially diagnose and treat the child with neuropsychological deficits and the children experiencing developmental delay or neuropsychiatric disturbance.

REFERENCES

Ager, A. K. (1983). An analysis of learning and attentional processes in mentally handicapped individuals. *International Journal of Rehabilitative Research, 6,* 369–370.

American Psychiatric Association. (1980). *Diagnostic and statistical manual of mental disorders* (3rd ed.). Washington, DC: Author.

Andrews, G., Craig, A., Feyer, A. M., Hoddinott, S., Howie, P., & Neilson, M. (1983). Stuttering: A review of research findings and theories circa 1982. *Journal of Speech and Hearing Disorders, 48,* 226–246.

Andrews, G., Quinn, P. T., & Sorby, W. A. (1972). Stuttering: An investigation into cerebral dominance for speech. *Journal of Neurology, Neurosurgery, and Psychiatry, 35,* 414–418.

Ashman, A. F. (1982). Strategic behavior and linguistic functions of institutionalized moderately retarded persons. *International Journal of Rehabilitation Research, 5,* 203–214.

Ayres, A. J. (1973). *Sensory integration and learning disorders.* Los Angeles: Western Psychological Services.

Bakker, D. J. (1972). *Temporal order in disturbed reading.* Rotterdam: University Press.

Bakker, D. J. (1983). Hemispheric specialization and specific reading retardation. In M. Rutter (Ed.), *Developmental neuropsychiatry.* New York: Guilford Press.

Bannatyne, A. (1966). The color phonics system. In J. Money & G. Schiffman (Eds.), *The disabled reader.* Baltimore: Johns Hopkins University Press.

Bateman, B. (1968). *Interpretation of the 1961 Illinois Test of Psycholinguistic Abilities.* Seattle: Special Child Publications.

Baumeister, A. A., & MacLean, W. E. (1979). Brain damage and mental retardation. In N. R. Ellis (Ed.), *Handbook of mental deficiency, psychological theory and research.* Hillsdale, NJ: Lawrence Erlbaum Associates.

Beckett, P. G. (1956). The electroencephalogram and various aspects of mental deficiency. *American Journal of Diseases of Childhood, 92,* 374–381.

Benton, A. L. (1970). Neuropsychological aspects of mental retardation. *Journal of Special Education, 4,* 3–11.

Birch, H. G., & Belmont, S. (1964). Auditory–visual integration in normal and retarded readers. *American Journal of Orthopsychiatry, 34,* 852–861.

Birch, H. G., & Belmont, L. (1965). Auditory–visual integration, intelligence, and reading ability in school children. *Perceptual and Motor Skills, 20,* 295–305.

Bloodstein, O. (1981). *A handbook on stuttering.* Chicago: National Easter Seal Society.

Bloom, L., & Lahey, M. (1978). *Language development and language disorders.* New York: Wiley.

Boder, E. (1970). Developmental dyslexia: A new diagnostic approach based on the identification of three subtypes. *Journal of School Health, 40,* 289–290.

Boder, E. (1973). Developmental dyslexia: A diagnostic approach based on three atypical reading–spelling patterns. *Developmental Medicine and Child Neurology, 15,* 663–687.

Boll, T. J. (1974). Behavioral correlates of cerebral damage in children aged 9 through 14. In R. M. Reitan & L. A. Davison (Eds.), *Clinical neuropsychology: Current status and applications.* Washington, DC: Hemisphere.

Boll, T. J., & Barth, J. T. (1981). Neuropsychology of brain damage in children. In S. B. Filskov & T. J. Boll (Eds.), *Handbook of clinical neuropsychology.* New York: Wiley.

Boone, D. R. (1971). *The voice and voice therapy.* Englewood Cliffs, NJ: Prentice-Hall.

Borda, R. P. (1977). Visual evoked potentials to flash in the clinical evaluation of the optic pathways. In J. E. Desmedt (Ed.), *Visual evoked potentials in man: New developments.* London: Oxford University Press.

Bradshaw-McAnulty, G., Hicks, R. E., & Kinsbourne, M. (1984). Pathological left handedness and familial sinistrality in relation to degree of mental retardation. *Brain and Cognition, 3,* 349–356.

Camara-Resendiz, P. S., & Fox, R. (1983). Impulsive versus inefficient problem solving in retarded and nonretarded Mexican children. *Journal of Psychology, 114,* 187–191.

Carmon, A., Harishanu, Y., Louringer, E., & Lavy, S. (1972). Asymmetries in hemispheric blood flow and cerebral dominance. *Behavioral Biology, 7,* 853–859.

Chelune, G. T., & Edwards, P. (1981). Early brain lesions: Ontogenetic–environmental considerations. *Journal of Consulting and Clinical Psychology, 49,* 777–790.

Chusid, J. G. (1982). *Correlative neuroanatomy and functional neurology.* Los Angeles: Lange Medical Publications.

Cohn, R. (1971). Arithmetic and learning disabilities. In H. R. Mykleburst (Ed.), *Progress in learning disabilities* (Vol. 2). New York: Grune & Stratton.

Coltheart, M., Patterson, K., & Marshall, J. C. (Eds.). (1980). *Deep dyslexia*. London: Routledge & Kegan Paul.

Conture, E., McCall, G., & Brewer, D. (1977). Laryngeal behavior during stuttering. *Journal of Speech and Hearing Research, 20,* 661–668.

Crapper, D. R., Dalton, A. G., Skopitz, M., Scott, J. W., & Hachinski, V. C. (1975). Alzheimer degeneration in Down's Syndrome. Electrophysiologic alterations and histopathologic findings. *Archives of Neurology, 32,* 618–623.

Crary, M. (1980). *Phonological intervention. Concepts and procedures*. San Diego: College Hill Press.

Crome, L. (1960). The brain and mental retardation. *British Medical Journal, 1,* 897–904.

Das, J. P., Kirby, J. R., & Jarman, R. F. (1975). Simultaneous and successive synthesis: An alternative model for cognitive abilities. *Psychological Bulletin, 82,* 87–103.

Das, J. P., Kirby, J. R., & Jarman, R. F. (1979). *Simultaneous and successive cognitive processes*. New York: Academic Press.

de Hirsch, K. (1976). Language disabilities. In A. M. Freedman, H. I. Kaplan, & B. J. Saddock (Eds.), *Comprehensive textbook of psychiatry*. Baltimore: Williams & Wilkins.

Delacato, C. (1966). *Neurological organization and reading*. Springfield, IL: Charles C. Thomas.

Deloche, G., & Andreewsky, E. (1982). Surface dyslexia: A case report and some theoretical implications to reading models. *Brain and Language, 15,* 12–31.

DeRenzi, E., & Piercy, M. (1969). The Fourteenth International Symposium of Neuropsychology. *Neuropsychologia, 7,* 383–386.

Dikeman, S., Matthews, C. G., & Harley, J. P. (1975). The effects of early versus late onset of major motor epilepsy upon cognitive–intellectual performance. *Epilepsia, 16,* 73.

Dobbing, J., Hopewell, J., & Lynch, A. (1971). Vulnerability of developing brain: VIII. Permanent deficits of neurons in cerebral and cerebellar cortex following early mild undernutrition. *Experimental Neurology, 32,* 439–447.

Dobbing, J., & Sands, J. (1973). Quantitative growth and development of human brain. *Archives of Diseases in Childhood, 48,* 757–767.

Doehring, D. G., & Hoshko, I. M. (1977). Classification of reading problems by the Q-technique of factor analysis. *Cortex, 13,* 281–294.

Doman, R. (1967). Children with severe brain injuries: Neurological organization in terms of mobility. In E. Frierson & W. Barbe (Eds.), *Educating children with learning disabilities*. New York: Appleton-Century-Crofts.

Douglas, V. (1983). Attentional and cognitive problems. In M. Rutter (Ed.), *Developmental neuropsychiatry*. New York: Guilford Press.

Drake, W. (1968). Clinical and pathological findings in a child with a developmental learning disability. *Journal of Learning Disabilities, 1,* 468–475.

Duane, D. D. (1979). Toward a definition of dyslexia: A summary of views. *Bulletin of the Orton Society, 29,* 56–64.

Duffy, F. H. (1981). Brain electrical activity mapping (BEAM): Computerized access to complex brain function. *International Journal of Neuroscience, 13,* 55–65.

Duffy, F. H., Burchfield, J. L., & Lombroso, C. T. (1979). Brain electrical activity mapping (BEAM): A method for extending the clinical utility of EEG and evoked potential data. *Annals of Neurology, 5,* 309–321.

Duffy, F. H., Denckla, M. B., Bartels, P. H., & Sandini, G. (1980). Dyslexia: Regional differences in brain electrical activity by topographical mapping. *Annals of Neurology, 7,* 412–420.

Duffy, F. H., Denckla, M. B., Bartels, P. H., Sandini, G., & Kiessling, L. S. (1980). Dyslexia: Automated diagnosis by computerized classification of brain electrical activity. *Annals of Neurology, 7,* 421–428.

Dykman, R., Ackerman, P., Clements, S., & Peters, J. (1971). Specific learning disabilities: An attentional deficit. In H. R. Myklebust (Ed.), *Progress in learning disabilities* (Vol. 2). New York: Grune & Stratton.

Edwards, M. L., & Shriberg, B. (1983). *Phonology: Applications in communicative disorders.* San Diego: College Hill Press.

Eisenson, J. (1968). Developmental aphasia: A speculative view with therapeutic implications. *Journal of Speech and Hearing Research, 33,* 3.

Eisenson, J. (1969). Developmental aphasia (dyslogia)—a postulation of a unitary concept of the disorder. *Cortex, 4,* 184–200.

Eisenson, J., & Ingram, D. (1972). Childhood aphasia: An updated concept based on recent research. *Acta Symbolica, 3,* 108.

Ellingson, R. J., Eisen, J. D., & Ottersberg, G. (1973). Clinical electroencephalograph observations on institutionalized Mongoloids confirmed by karyotype. *Electroencephalography and Clinical Neurophysiology, 34,* 193–196.

Ellingson, R. J., Menolascino, F. J., & Eisen, J. D. (1970). Clinical EEG relationships in Mongoloids confirmed by karotype. *American Journal of Mental Deficiency, 74,* 645–650.

Espir, M. L. E., & Rose, F. C. (1976). *The basic neurology of speech.* Oxford: Blackwell.

Federal Register. (1976). *Education of handicapped children and incentive grants program.* U.S. Department of Health, Education, and Welfare. Vol. 41, p. 56977.

Finucci, J. M., Isaacs, S. D., Whitehouse, C. C., & Childs, B. (1983). Classification of spelling errors and their relationship to reading ability, sex, grade placement, and intelligence. *Brain and Language, 20,* 340–355.

Fisk, J. L., & Rourke, B. P. (1979). Identification of subtypes of learning disabled children at three age levels: A neuropsychological, multivariate approach. *Journal of Clinical Neuropsychology, 1,* 289–310.

Freedman, P., & Carpenter, R. (1976). Semantic relations used by normal and language impaired children at stage I. *Journal of Speech and Hearing Research, 19,* 784–795.

Freytag, E., & Lindenberg, R. (1967). Neuropathologic findings in patients of a hospital for the mentally deficient. A study of 359 cases. *Johns Hopkins Medical Journal, 121,* 379–392.

Friedman, E., & Pampiglione, G. (1970). Hypsarrhythmic EEG patterns in the first year of life: A 6–12 year clinical outcome. *Electroencephalography and Clinical Neurophysiology, 29,* 326.

Friedman, E., & Pampiglione, G. (1971). Prognostic implications of electroencephalographic findings of hypsarrhythmia in first year of life. *British Medical Journal, iv,* 323–325.

Frith, U. (1983). The similarities and differences between reading and spelling problems. In M. Rutter (Ed.), *Developmental neuropsychiatry.* New York: Guilford Press.

Frühmann, E., & Roth, G. (1963). Monoglismus and EEG versuch einer korrelation vom klinischen austanbsbild und EEG-befund. *Proceedings of the Second International Congress on Mental Retardation* (Part I, pp. 381–386).

Gaddes, W. (1983). Applied educational neuropsychology: Theories and problems. *Journal of Learning Disabilities, 16,* 511–514.

Gaddes, W. (1980). *Learning disabilities and brain function: A neuropsychological approach.* New York: Springer-Verlag.

Galaburda, A. M., & Kemper, T. L. (1979). Cytoarchitectonic abnormalities in developmental dyslexia: A case study. *Annals of Neurology, 6,* 94–100.

Galaburda, A. M., Sherman, G. F., & Geschwind, N. (in press). Developmental dyslexia: A third consecutive case with cortical abnormalities. *Science.*

Galbraith, G. C. (1976). Computer analysis of the electroencephalogram and sensory evoked responses. In J. W. Prescott, M. S. Read, & D. B. Coursin (Eds.), *Brain function and malnutrition.* New York: Wiley.

Gardner, W. H. (1937). Study of the pupillary reflex with special reference to stuttering. *Psychological Monographs, 49,* 1–31.

Gasser, T., Möcks, J., & Bächer, P. (1983). Topographic factor analysis of the EEG with applications to development and to mental retardation. *Electroencephalography and Clinical Neurophysiology, 55,* 445–463.

Gasser, T., von Lucadow-Miller, I., Verleger, R., & Bächer, P. (1983). Correlating EEG and IQ. A new look at an old problem using computerized EEG parameters. *Electroencephalography and Clinical Neurophysiology, 55,* 493–504.

Getman, G. (1965). The visuomotor complex in the acquisition of learning skills. In J. Hellmuth (Ed.), *Learning disorders* (Vol. 1). Seattle: Special Child Publications.

Golden, C. J. (1981a). *Diagnosis and rehabilitation in clinical neuropsychology.* Springfield, IL: Charles C. Thomas.

Golden, C. J. (1981b). The Luria–Nebraska Children's Battery: Theory and formulation. In G. W. Hynd & J. E. Obrzut (Eds.), *Neuropsychological assessment and the school-age child: Issues and procedures.* New York: Grune & Stratton.

Golden, C. J., & Anderson, S. (1979). *Learning disabilities and brain dysfunction.* Springfield, IL: Charles C. Thomas.

Gonatas, N. K., Evangelista, I., & Walsh, G. O. (1967). Axonal and synaptic changes in a case of psychomotor retardation: An electron microscopic study. *Journal of Neuropathology and Experimental Neurology, 26,* 179–199.

Gordon, J. E. (1977). Neuropsychology and mental retardation. In I. Bialer & M. Sternlicht (Eds.), *The psychology of mental retardation: Issues and approaches.* New York: Psychological Dimensions.

Grala, C. (1976). *Implications of the psychoanalytic and Piagetian theories of thinking for diagnostic psychological testing.* Unpublished master's thesis, Hahnemann University, Philadelphia.

Grossman, H. J. (Ed.). (1977). *Manual on terminology and classification in mental retardation.* Washington, DC: American Association on Mental Deficiency.

Hammill, D. D., Leigh, J. E., McNutt, G., & Larsen, S. C. (1981). A new definition of learning disabilities. *Learning Disability Quarterly, 4,* 336–342.

Hardy, W. G. (1965). On language disorders in young children: A reorganization of thinking. *Journal of Speech and Hearing Disorders, 30,* 3.

Hartley, X. (1982). Receptive language processing of Down's syndrome children. *Journal of Mental Deficiency Research, 26,* 263–269.

Hartley, X. (1983). Receptive language processing and hemispheric dominance of Down's syndrome children. *International Journal of Rehabilitative Research, 6,* 357–358.

Heber, R. (1970). *Epidemiology of mental retardation.* Springfield, IL: Charles C. Thomas.

Huttenlocher, P. R. (1974). Dendritic development in neocortex of children with mental defect and infantile spasms. *Neurology 24,* 203–210.

Huttenlocher, P. R. (1975). Synaptic and dendritic development and mental defect. In N. A.

Buchwald & M. A. Brazier (Eds.), *Brain mechanisms in mental retardation*. New York: Academic Press.

Hyman, L. (1975). *Phonology: Theory and analysis*. New York: Holt, Rinehart, & Winston.

Hynd, G. W., & Cohen, M. (1983). *Dyslexia: Neuropsychological theory, research, and clinical differentiation*. New York: Grune & Stratton.

Hynd, G. W., Cohen, M., & Obrzut, J. E. (1983). Dichotic CV testing in the diagnosis of learning disabilities in children. *Ear and Hearing, 4*, 283–287.

Hynd, G. W., & Hynd, C. R. (1984). Dyslexia: Neuroanatomical/neurolinguistic perspectives. *Reading Research Quarterly, 19*, 482–498.

Hynd, G. W., & Obrzut, J. E. (Eds.). (1981). *Neuropsychological assessment and the school-age child: Issues and procedures*. New York: Grune & Stratton.

Hynd, G. W., Obrzut, J. E., Hayes, F., & Becker, M. G. (in press). Neuropsychology of childhood learning disabilities. In D. Wedding, A. M. Horton, & J. S. Webster (Eds.), *Handbook of clinical and behavioral neuropsychology*. New York: Springer.

Hynd, G. W., Obrzut, J. E., Weed, W., & Hynd, C. R. (1979). Development of cerebral dominance: Dichotic listening asymmetry in normal and learning disabled children. *Journal of Experimental Child Psychology, 28*, 415–454.

Ingram, T. S., Mason, A. W., & Blackburn, I. (1970). A retrospective study of 82 children with reading disability. *Developmental Medicine and Child Neurology, 12*, 271–281.

Inhelder, B., & Piaget, J. (1958). *The growth of logical thinking from childhood to adolescence*. New York: Basic Books.

Jellinger, J. (1972). Neuropathological features of unclassified mental retardation. In J. B. Cavanaugh (Ed.), *The brain in unclassified mental retardation*. Baltimore: Williams & Wilkins.

John, E. R. (1977). *Functional neuroscience: Vol. 2. Neurometrics*. Hillsdale, NJ: Lawrence Erlbaum Associates.

Johnson, D., & Myklebust, H. (1967). *Learning disabilities: Educational principles and practices*. New York: Grune & Stratton.

Johnston, J., & Schery, T. (1976). The use of grammatical morphemes by children with communication disorders. In D. Morehead & A. Morehead (Eds.), *Normal and deficient child language*. Baltimore: University Park Press.

Kail, R., Hole, C. A., Leonard, L. B., & Nippold, M. A. (1984). Lexical storage and retrieval in language-impaired children. *Applied Psycholinguistics, 5*, 37–49.

Kamizono, S. (1983). Organization of memory in the mentally retarded. Developmental characteristics. *Japanese Journal of Special Education, 21*, 1–11.

Karrer, R., & Ivins, J. (1976). Steady potentials accompanying perceptions and responses in mentally retarded and normal children. In R. Karrer (Ed.), *Developmental psychophysiology of mental retardation*. Springfield, IL: Charles C. Thomas.

Kaufman, N. L., & Kaufman, A. S. (1983). Remedial intervention in education. In G. W. Hynd (Ed.), *The school psychologist: An introduction*. Syracuse: Syracuse University Press.

Kennedy, C., & Ramirez, L. S. (1964). Brain damage as a cause of behavioral disturbance in children. In H. G. Birch (Ed.), *Brain damage in children: The biological and social aspects*. Baltimore: Williams & Wilkins.

Kephart, N. (1967). Perceptual–motor aspects of learning disabilities. In E. Frierson & W. Barbe (Eds.), *Educating children with learning disabilities*. New York: Appleton-Century-Crofts.

Kinsbourne, M., & Warrington, E. K. (1963). Developmental factors in reading and writing backwardness. *British Journal of Psychology, 54,* 145–146.

Kirk, S. A. (1963). Behavioral diagnosis and remediation of learning disabilities. In *Conference on exploration into the problems of the perceptually handicapped child.* Evanston, IL: Fund for the Perceptually Handicapped Child.

Kopp, H. G. (1963). Eye movements in reading as related to speech dysfunction in male stutterers. *Speech Monographs, 30,* 248.

Kuroda, N., & Kobayaski, H. (1984). Development of handedness in moderate mentally retarded children. *Japanese Journal of Special Education, 21,* 36–43.

Landau, W., Goldstein, R., & Kleffner, F. (1960). Congenital aphasia: A clinicopathologic study. *Neurology, 10,* 915–921.

LaVeck, G. D., & de la Cruz, F. (1963). Electroencephalographic and etiologic findings in mental retardation. *Pediatrics, 31,* 478–485.

LeMay, M., & Culebras, A. (1972). Human brain morphologic differences in the hemispheres demonstrable by carotid arteriography. *New England Journal of Medicine, 287,* 168–170.

Lenneberg, E. H. (1967). *The effect of age on the outcome of central nervous system disease in children.* New York: Wiley.

Leonard, L. (1972). What is deviant language? *Journal of Speech and Hearing Research, 37,* 427–446.

Leonard, L. (1979). Language impairment in children. *Merrill Palmer Quarterly, 25,* 205–232.

Leonard, L., Bolders, J., & Miller, J. (1976). An examination of the semantic relations reflected in the language usage of normal and language disordered children. *Journal of Speech and Hearing Research, 19,* 371–392.

Lerner, J. W. (1976). *Children with learning disabilities.* Boston: Houghton Mifflin.

Levinson, A., Friedman, A., & Stamps, F. (1955). Variability of mongolism. *Pediatrics, 16,* 43–51.

Locke, J. L. (1983). Clinical phonology: The explanation and treatment of speech sound disorders. *Journal of Speech and Hearing Disorders, 48,* 339–341.

Luessenhop, A. J., Boggs, J. S., Laborwit, L. J., & Walle, E. L. (1973). Cerebral dominance in stutterers determined by Wada testing. *Neurology, 23,* 1190–1192.

Luria, A. R. (1963). *The mentally retarded child.* New York: Pergamon Press.

Luria, A. R. (1965). Neuropsychological analysis of focal brain lesions. In B. B. Wolman (Ed.), *Handbook of clinical psychology.* New York: McGraw-Hill.

Luria, A. R. (1970). The functional organization of the brain. *Scientific American, 222,* 66–78.

Luria, A. R. (1973). *The working brain.* New York: Basic Books.

Luria, A. R. (1980). *Higher cortical functions in man.* New York: Basic Books.

Lyle, J. G. (1969). Reading retardation and reversal tendency: A factorial study. *Child Development, 40,* 833–843.

Lyle, J. G., & Goyen, J. (1968). Visual recognition development lag and strephosymbolia in reading retardation. *Journal of Abnormal Psychology, 73,* 25–29.

Lyle, J. G., & Goyen, J. (1975). Effects of speed and exposure and difficulty of discrimination on visual recognition of retarded readers. *Journal of Abnormal Psychology, 8,* 673–676.

Lyon, R., & Watson, B. (1981). Empirically derived subgroups of learning disabled readers: Diagnostic characteristics. *Journal of Learning Disabilities, 14,* 256–261.

Malamud, N. (1964). Neuropathology. In H. A. Stevens & R. Heber (Eds.), *Mental retardation: A review of research.* Chicago: University of Chicago Press.

Masland, R. L. (1958). The prevention of mental subnormality. In R. L. Masland, S. B. Sarason, & T. Gladwin (Eds.), *Mental subnormality*. New York: Basic Books.

Matthews, C. G. (1974). Applications of neuropsychological test methods in mentally retarded subjects. In R. M. Reitan & L. A. Davison (Eds.), *Clinical neuropsychology: Current status and applications*. Washington, DC: Hemisphere.

Matthews, C. G., & Manning, G. C. (1964). Psychological test performances in three electroencephalographic classifications of mentally retarded subjects. *American Journal of Mental Deficiency, 68,* 485–492.

Mattis, S., Erenberg, G., & French, J. H. (February, 1978). *Dyslexia syndromes: A cross validation study*. Paper presented at the sixth annual meeting of the International Neuropsychological Society, Minneapolis.

Mattis, S., French, J. H., & Rapin, I. (1975). Dyslexia in children and young adults: Three independent neuropsychological syndromes. *Developmental Medicine and Child Neurology, 17,* 150–163.

McCarthy, J. M. (1975). Children with learning disabilities. In J. J. Gallager (Ed.), *The application of child development research to exceptional children*. Reston, VA: Council for Exceptional Children.

McReynolds, L. V. (1966). Operant conditioning for investigating speech sound discrimination in aphasic children. *Journal of Speech and Hearing Research, 9,* 519–528.

McReynolds, L. V. (1967). Verbal sequence discrimination training for language impaired children. *Journal of Speech and Hearing Disorders, 32,* 249.

Meacham, M. L., & Fisher, G. L. (1984). The identification and stability of subtypes of disabled readers. *International Journal of Clinical Neuropsychology, 4,* 269–274.

Menkes, J. H. (1980). *Textbook of child neurology*. Philadelphia: Lea & Febiger.

Menyuk, P. (1964). Comparison of grammar of children with functionally deviant and normal speech. *Journal of Speech and Hearing Research, 7,* 109–121.

Menyuk, P. (1971). *The acquisition and development of language*. Englewood Cliffs, NJ: Prentice-Hall.

Mesulam, M. (1981). A cortical network for directed attention and unilateral neglect. *Annals of Neurology, 10,* 309–325.

Money, J. (1973). Turner's syndrome and parietal lobe functions. *Cortex, 9,* 387–393.

Monsees, E. K. (1972). *Structural language for children with special language learning problems*. Washington, DC: Children's Hospital of District of Columbia.

Moore, G. P. (1971). *Organic voice disorders*. Englewood Cliffs, NJ: Prentice-Hall.

Moore, W. E. (1959). A study of blood chemistry of stutterers under two hypnotic conditions. *Speech Monographs, 26,* 64–68.

Morehead, D., & Ingram, D. (1973). The development of base syntax in normal and linguistically deviant children. *Journal of Speech and Hearing Research, 16,* 330–352.

Morgan, W. P. (1896). A case of congenital word blindness. *British Medical Journal, ii,* 1978.

Morris, R., Blashfield, R., & Satz, P. (1981). Neuropsychology and cluster analysis: Potential and problems. *Journal of Clinical Neuropsychology, 3,* 79–99.

Naidoo, S. (1972). *Specific dyslexia*. New York: Wiley.

Nelson, H. E., & Warrington, E. K. (1974). Developmental spelling retardation and its relation to other cognitive abilities. *British Journal of Psychology, 65,* 265–274.

Newlin, D., & Tramontana, M. (1980). Neuropsychological findings in a hyperactive adolescent with subcortical brain pathology. *Clinical Neuropsychology, 2,* 178–183.

Niihara, T., & Kusano, K. (1984). Temporal accuracy of rhythmic movement in mentally retarded children. *Japanese Journal of Educational Psychology, 32,* 18–24.

Obrzut, J. E., Hynd, G. W., Obrzut, A., & Pirozzolo, F. (1981). Effects of selective attention on cerebral asymmetries in normal and learning disabled children. *Developmental Psychology, 17,* 118–125.

Omenn, G. S., & Weber, B. A. (1978). Dyslexia: Search for phenotypic and genetic heterogeneity. *American Journal of Medical Genetics,* 1, 333–342.

Orton, S. T. (1928). Specific reading disability—strephosymbolia. *Journal of the American Medical Association, 90,* 1095–1099.

Orton, S. T. (1937). *Reading, writing, and speech problems in children.* New York: Norton.

Pampiglione, G., & Harden, A. (1974). An infantile form of neuronal "storage" disease with characteristic evolution of neurophysiological features. *Brain, 97,* 355–360.

Pampiglione, G., Privett, G., & Harden, A. (1974). Tay–Sachs Disease: Neurophysiological studies in 20 children. *Developmental Medicine and Child Neurology, 16,* 201–208.

Passler, M. A., Isaac, W., & Hynd, G. W. (1985). Neuropsychological development of behavior attributed to frontal lobe functioning in children. *Developmental Neuropsychology, 1,* 349–370.

Petrauskas, R., & Rourke, B. (1979). Identification of subgroups of retarded readers: A neuropsychological multivariate approach. *Journal of Clinical Neuropsychology, 1,* 17–37.

Pevzner, M. S. (1961). *Oligophrenia: Mental deficiency in children.* New York: Consultants Bureau.

Piaget, J. (1950). *The psychology of intelligence.* New York: Harcourt Brace.

Piaget, J. (1951). *Play, dreams, and imitation in childhood.* New York: Norton.

Piaget, J. (1952). *The origins of intelligence in children.* New York: International Universities Press.

Pipe, M. E. (1983). Dichotic listening performance following auditory discrimination training in Down's syndrome and developmentally retarded children. *Cortex, 19,* 481–491.

Pipe, M. E., & Beale, I. L. (1983). Hemispheric specialization for speech in retarded children. *Neuropsychologia, 21,* 91–98.

Pirozzolo, F. J. (1977). *Visual–spatial and oculomotor deficits in developmental dyslexia: Evidence for two neurobehavioral syndromes of reading disability.* Unpublished doctoral dissertation, University of Rochester, Rochester, New York.

Pirozzolo, F. J. (1979). *The neuropsychology of developmental reading disorders.* New York: Praeger.

Pirozzolo, F. J., & Campanella, D. J. (1981). The neuropsychology of developmental speech disorders, language disorders, and learning disorders. In G. W. Hynd & J. E. Obrzut (Eds.), *Neuropsychological assessment and the school-age child: Issues and procedures.* New York: Grune & Stratton.

Pirozzolo, F. J., & Rayner, K. (1979). Cerebral organization and reading disability. *Neuropsychologia, 17,* 485–491.

Prichep, L., John, E. R., Ahn, H., & Kaye, H. (1983). Neurometrics: Quantitative evaluation of brain dysfunction in children. In M. Rutter (Ed.), *Developmental neuropsychiatry.* New York: Guilford Press.

Purpura, D. P. (1974). Dendritic spine "dysgenesis" and mental retardation. *Science, 186,* 1126–1128.

Quiros, J. B. (1964). Dysphasia and dyslexia in school children. *Folia Phoniatrica, 16,* 201.

Reed, J. C. (1967). Lateralized finger agnosia and reading achievement at ages 6 and 10. *Child Development, 38,* 213–220.

Reed, J. C., & Reitan, R. M. (1969). Verbal and performance differences among brain injured children with lateralized motor deficits. *Perceptual and Motor Skills, 29,* 747.

Reed, H. B., Reitan, R. M., & Klöve, H. (1965). Influence of cerebral lesions on psychological test performance of older children. *Journal of Consulting Psychology, 29,* 247.

Rees, N. (1973a). Auditory processing factors in language disorders: A view from Procrustes bed. *Journal of Speech and Hearing Disorders, 38,* 304–315.

Reinis, S., & Goldman, J. M. (1980). *The development of the brain: Biological and functional perspectives.* Springfield, IL: Charles C. Thomas.

Reitan, R. M. (1974). Psychological effects of cerebral lesions in children of early school age. In R. M. Reitan & L. A. Davison (Eds.), *Clinical neuropsychology: Current status and applications.* Washington: DC: Hemisphere.

Rhawn, J. (1982). The neuropsychology of development: Hemispheric laterality, limbic language, and the origin of thought. *Journal of Clinical Psychology, 38,* 4–33.

Roberts, L. (1962). Childhood aphasia and handedness. In R. West (Ed.), *Childhood aphasia.* San Francisco: California Society for Crippled Children and Adults.

Roeltgen, D. (1984). Agraphia. In K. M. Heilman & E. Valenstein (Eds.), *Clinical neuropsychology.* New York: Oxford University Press.

Rosenthal, R., & Allen, T. (1978). An examination of attention, arousal, and learning dysfunctions of hyperkinetic children. *Psychological Bulletin, 85,* 689–715.

Ross, L. E., & Ward, T. B. (1978). The processing of information from short-term visual store: Developmental and intellectual level differences. In N. R. Ellis (Ed.), *International review of research in mental retardation* (Vol. 9). New York: Academic Press.

Rourke, B. P. (1978a). Neuropsychological research in reading retardation. A review. In A. L. Benton & D. Pearl (Eds.), *Dyslexia: An appraisal of current knowledge.* New York: Oxford University Press.

Rourke, B. P. (1978b). Reading, spelling, and arithmetic disabilities: A neuropsychological perspective. In H. R. Myklebust (Ed.), *Progress in learning disabilities* (Vol. IV). New York: Grune & Stratton.

Rourke, B. P. (1981). Neuropsychological assessment of children with learning disabilities. In S. B. Filskov & T. J. Boll (Eds.), *Handbook of clinical neuropsychology.* New York: Wiley.

Rourke, B. P. (1983). Reading and spelling disabilities: A developmental neuropsychological perspective. In U. Kirk (Ed.), *Neuropsychology of language, reading, and spelling.* New York: Academic Press.

Rourke, B. P. (1985). *Neuropsychology of learning disabilities: Essentials of subtype analysis.* New York: Guilford Press.

Rourke, B. P., Bakker, D. J., Fisk, J. L., & Strang, J. D. (1983). *Child neuropsychology.* New York: Guilford Press.

Rourke, B. P., & Finlayson, M. A. J. (1978). Neuropsychological significance of variations in patterns of academic performance: Verbal and visual–spatial abilities. *Journal of Abnormal Child Psychology, 6,* 121–133.

Rourke, B. P., & Strang, J. D. (1978). Neuropsychological significance of variations in patterns of academic performance: Motor, psychomotor, and tactile–perceptual abilities. *Journal of Pediatric Psychology, 3,* 62–66.

Rourke, B. P., & Strang, J. D. (1983). Subtypes of reading and arithmetic disabilities: A neuropsychological analysis. In M. Rutter (Ed.), *Developmental neuropsychiatry.* New York: Guilford Press.

Rourke, B. P., Young, G. C., & Flewelling, R. W. (1971). The relationship between WISC verbal-performance discrepancies and selected verbal, auditory–perceptual, visual–perceptual, and problem-solving abilities in children with learning disabilities. *Journal of Clinical Psychology, 27,* 475–479.

Rutter, M. (1983a). Behavioral studies: Questions and findings on the concept of a distinctive syndrome. In M. Rutter (Ed.), *Developmental neuropsychiatry*. New York: Guilford Press.

Rutter, M. (Ed.) (1983b). *Developmental neuropsychiatry*. New York: Guilford Press.

Satterfield, J., & Dawson, M. (1971). Electrodermal concepts of hyperactivity in children. *Psychophysiology, 8,* 191–197.

Satz, P., & Fletcher, J. (1981). Emergent trends in neuropsychology: An overview. *Journal of Consulting and Clinical Psychology, 49,* 851–865.

Satz, P., & Morris, R. (1981). Learning disabilities subtypes: A review. In F. J. Pirozzolo & M. C. Wittrock (Eds.), *Neuropsychological and cognitive processes in reading*. New York: Academic Press.

Satz, P., Rardin, D., & Ross, J. (1971). An evaluation of a theory of specific developmental dyslexia. *Child Development, 42,* 2009–2021.

Sayles, D. G. (1971). Cortical excitability, perseveration, and stuttering. *Journal of Speech and Hearing Research, 14,* 463–475.

Schain, R. J. (1972). *Neurology of childhood learning disorders*. Baltimore: Williams & Wilkins.

Schain, R. J. (1983). Learning disorders. In T. W. Farmer (Ed.), *Pediatric neurology*. Philadelphia: Harper & Row.

Schonhaut, S., & Satz, P. (1983). Prognosis of children with learning disabilities: A review of follow-up studies. In M. Rutter (Ed.), *Developmental neuropsychiatry*. New York: Guilford Press.

Senf, G. M. (1969). Development of immediate memory for bisensory stimuli in normal children, and children with learning disabilities. *Developmental Psychology, 6,* 28.

Senf, G. M., & Freundl, P. C. (1971). Memory and attention factors in specific learning disabilities. *Journal of Learning Disabilities, 4,* 94–106.

Sevush, S. (1983, February). *The neurolinguistics of reading: Anatomic and neurologic correlates*. Paper presented at the annual meeting of the International Neuropsychological Society, Mexico City.

Sheehan, J. G., & Martyn, M. M. (1970). Stuttering and its disappearance. *Journal of Speech and Hearing Research, 13,* 279–289.

Shihazaki, M. (1983). Development of hemispheric function in hiragana, kanji, and figure processing for normal and mentally retarded children. *Japanese Journal of Special Education, 21,* 1–9.

Shriberg, L. D., & Kwiatkowski, J. (1982). A diagnostic classification system. *Journal of Speech and Hearing Disorders, 47,* 226–241.

Smith, M. D., Coleman, J. M., Dokecki, P. R., and Davis, E. E. (1977). Recategorized WISC-R scores of learning disabled children. *Journal of Learning Disabilities, 10,* 444–449.

Snyder, L. S. (1975). *Pragmatics in language disabled children: Their prelinguistic and early verbal performatives and presuppositions*. Unpublished doctoral dissertation, University of Colorado, Boulder.

Sohmer, H., & Student, M. (1978). Auditory nerve and brainstem evoked responses in normal, autistic, minimal brain dysfunction and psycho-motor retarded children. *Electroencephalography and Clinical Neurophysiology, 44,* 380–388.

Stanovich, K. E. (1978). Information processing in mentally retarded individuals. In N. R. Ellis (Ed.), *International review of research in mental retardation* (Vol. 9). New York: Academic Press.

Stark, J., & Poppen, R. (1967). Effects of alterations of prosodic features on the sequencing performance of aphasic children. *Journal of Speech and Hearing Research, 10,* 189.

Stark, R. E., & Tallal, P. (1981). Selection of children with specific language deficits. *Journal of Speech and Hearing Disorders, 46,* 114–122.

Strauss, A. A., & Lehtinen, M. A. (1947). *Psychopathology and education of the brain-injured child.* New York: Grune & Stratton.

Strauss, A. A., & Werner, H. (1943). Comparative psychopathology of the brain-injured child and the traumatic brain-injured adult. *American Journal of Psychiatry, 99,* 835–888.

Stuss, D. T., & Benson, D. F. (1984). Neuropsychological studies of the frontal lobes. *Psychological Bulletin, 95,* 3–28.

Sweeney, J. E., & Rourke, B. P. (1978). Neuropsychological significance of phonetically inaccurate spelling errors in younger and older retarded spellers. *Brain and Language, 6,* 212–225.

Sylvester, P. E. (1983). The hippocampus in Down's syndrome. *Journal of Mental Deficiency Research, 27,* 227–236.

Tallal, P., & Newcombe, F. (1978). Impairment of auditory perception and language comprehension in dysphasia. *Brain and Language, 5,* 13–24.

Telford, C. W., & Sawrey, J. M. (1972). *The exceptional individual.* Englewood Cliffs, NJ: Prentice-Hall.

Templin, M. (1957). *Certain language skills in children.* Minneapolis: University of Minnesota Press.

Tramontana, M. G. (1983a). Application of neuropsychological methods in the evaluation of coexisting mental retardation and mental illness. In F. J. Menolascino & B. M. McCann (Eds.), *Mental health and mental retardation: Bridging the gap.* Baltimore: University Park Press.

Tramontana, M. G. (1983b). Neuropsychological evaluation of children and adolescents with psycopathological disorders. In C. J. Golden & P. J. Vicente (Eds.), *Foundations of clinical neuropsychology.* New York: Plenum Press.

Tramontana, M. G., & Sherrets, S. D. (1985). Brain impairment in child psychiatric disorders: Correspondencies between neuropsychological and CT scan results. *Journal of the American Academy of Child Psychiatry, 24,* 590–596.

Travis, L. E. (1971). *Handbook of speech pathology and audiology.* New York: Appleton-Century-Crofts.

Tredgold, R. F., & Soddy, K. (1963). *Textbook of mental deficiency.* Baltimore: Williams & Wilkins.

Valet, R. E. (1973). *Learning disabilities. Diagnostic prescriptive instrument.* Belmont, CA: Lear Siegler-Fearon.

Van Riper, C. (1972). *The nature of stuttering.* Englewood Cliffs, NJ: Prentice-Hall.

Volpe, J. J. (1983). Perinatal disorders. In T. W. Farmer (Ed.), *Pediatric neurology.* Philadelphia: Harper & Row.

Walton, J. N., Ellis, E., & Court, S. D. (1962). Clumsy children: Developmental apraxia and agnosia. *Brain, 85,* 603–612.

Watson, B. U., Goldgar, D. E., & Ryschon, K. C. (1983). Subtypes of reading disability. *Journal of Clinical Neuropsychology, 5,* 377–399.

West, R. (Ed.). (1962). *Childhood aphasia: Proceedings at the Institute on Childhood Aphasia Conference, 1960.* San Francisco: California Society for Crippled Children and Adults.

Wilkening, G. N., & Golden, C. J. (1982). Pediatric neuropsychology: Status, theory, and research. In P. Karoly, J. Steffen, & D. Grady (Eds.), *Child health psychology. Concepts and issues*. New York: Pergamon Press.

Wingate, M. E. (1977). Criteria for stuttering. *Journal of Speech and Hearing Research, 20*, 596–607.

Winitz, H. (1969). *Articulatory acquisition and behavior*. New York: Appleton-Century-Crofts.

Wood, F., Stump, D., McKeehan, A., Shelton, S., & Proctor, J. (1980). Patterns of regional cerebral blood flow during attempted reading aloud by stutterers both on and off haloperidol medication: Evidence for inadequate left frontal activation during stuttering. *Brain and Language, 9*, 141–144.

World Health Organization. (1977). *Manual of the international statistical classification of diseases, injuries, and causes of death* (Vol. 1). Geneva: Author.

Yeni-Komshian, G. H., Isenberg, P., & Goldstein, H. (1975). Cerebral dominance and reading disability: Left visual-field deficit in poor readers. *Neuropsychologia, 13*, 83–94.

Zeaman, W., & Dyken, P. (1969). Neuronal ceroidlipofuscinosis (Batten's Disease): Relationship to amaurotic family idiocy. *Pediatrics, 44*, 470–583.

Žekulin-Hartley, X. Y. (1982). Selective attention to dichotic input of retarded children. *Cortex, 18*, 311–316.

Zentall, S. (1975). Optimal stimulation as theoretical basis of hyperactivity. *American Journal of Orthopsychiatry, 45*, 549–561.

Zigler, E. (1967). Familial mental retardation: A continuing dilemma. *Science, 155*, 292–299.

Zimmerman, G. (1980a). Articulatory behaviors associated with stuttering: A cinefluorographic analysis. *Journal of Speech and Hearing Research, 23*, 108–121.

Zimmerman, G. (1980b). Articulatory dynamics of fluent utterances of stutterers and nonstutters. *Journal of Speech and Hearing Research, 23*, 95–107.

Zurif, E. G., & Carson, G. (1970). Dyslexia in relation to cerebral dominance and temporal analysis. *Neuropsychologia, 8*, 351–361.

Chapter 3

Epilepsy in Children: Neuropsychological Effects

JOHN F. BOLTER

Clinical Psychology Service
Silas B. Hays Army Community Hospital
Fort Ord, California 93941

Epilepsy is considered by many to represent the most prevalent chronic neurological disorder of childhood. It is a rather unique neurological disorder in that the clinical presentation, progression, and underlying etiology appears to vary from case to case. More importantly, however, is the fact that the organ of pathology in epilepsy is the brain itself and accordingly, epilepsy has long been implicated as a cause of impaired behavioral, emotional, and cognitive functioning in seizure-prone children. The present chapter is an overview of epilepsy as it pertains to understanding its role in determining the psychological status of an epileptic child. Consistent with that intention, the chapter is structured to provide information on the nature of epilepsy, its adaptive implications, and its component elements identified as potential contributors of neuropsychological impairment in epileptic children.

THE NATURE OF EPILEPSY

Definition

Although epilepsy has been recognized as a clinical syndrome for centuries, it was not until the late nineteenth century than an adequate definition was introduced by Jackson (1925, 1931). Jackson described epilepsy

59

as an occasional excessive and disorderly discharge of neurons in various parts of the brain. Glaser (1979) added to the definition by noting that such paroxysmal events develop suddenly, usually cease spontaneously and demonstrate a strong tendency to recur. In physiological terms, it appears that these excessive and disorderly discharges arise in neurons when their threshold for firing is decreased beyond the capacity of their membrane-threshold-stabilizing mechanism to prevent firing.

While the physiological event underlying seizures at a cellular level appears uniform, the disease process of epilepsy is not. Epilepsy can arise as the result of a variety of pathological brain states. The excessive discharges may be restricted to a localized brain region, or spreading throughout the brain can occur. When the discharges from these hyperexcitable neurons propagate along neural pathways, or sufficient local recruitment of neighboring neurons occurs, a multitude of clinical manifestations may appear in the form of a seizure, including sudden alterations in motor, sensory, affective, cognitive, or autonomic functions. The symptoms accompanying a particular epileptic attack are therefore thought to be a direct function of the presumed brain region(s) interrupted by the excessive neural discharges. For example, loss of consciousness reflects involvement of the upper brainstem, and nuclei of the diffuse thalamic projection system while whole somatic muscular contractions are associated with involvement of frontal motor areas.

Prevalence and Incidence

Epilepsy is considered a major health problem, which affects millions of people of all races, geographic localities, and both sexes alike (Forster & Booker, 1984; Lishman, 1978). While factually accurate epidemiological data cannot be obtained, estimates from various sources indicate that the prevalence of recurrent seizures among the general population is approximately 1–2% (Epilepsy Foundation of America, 1975). Available evidence (Kurtzke & Kurland, 1984) indicates that the annual incidence of new cases is approximately 50 per 100,000 with an average duration of active seizures lasting approximately 13 years. In the United States alone, with its estimated population of nearly 230 million, one can expect to find more than 100,000 new cases of epilepsy per year. It is important to note, however, that the overall prevalence of epilepsy is greatest among children.

Approximately 70% of the persons suffering from recurrent seizures will manifest their first attack during childhood or adolescence (Dreisbach, Ballard, Russo, & Schain, 1982; Lennox & Lennox, 1960). In one survey (Pond, Bidwell, & Stein, 1960), it was reported that 25% of 245 outpatient epileptics suffered their first attack prior to the age of 5 years, 25% during early childhood (5–14 years), and 10% during adolescence (15–19 years). Generally, there appears to be two peak ages for the onset of epilepsy. The first is found during the first 2 years of life and the second occurs at the age of puberty (Bridge, 1949; Glaser, 1979). From these data, it is not difficult to understand why many clinicians consider epilepsy predominantly a disorder of childhood, as well as the most common chronic neurological disorder of childhood (Meighan, Queener, & Weitman, 1976; Rose, Penry, Markush, Radloff, & Putman, 1973; Weinberg, 1972). It is also easy to assume that with the age of onset being relatively early in life and the duration of the disorder being long, the opportunities to impact on a child's development and life adjustment would be great.

Classification

Epilepsy can be classified on the basis of several features, including the presumed site of the abnormal activity within the brain, electroencephalographic (EEG) patterns, clinical manifestations of the seizure attacks, or the etiology of the disorder. To date, no single or comprehensive classification system has proven entirely satisfactory. In an effort to standardize a grouping system of seizures, the International League against Epilepsy (Gastaut, 1970) formulated a scheme based on clinical and EEG manifestations. The International Classification of Epileptic Seizures (ICES) is the most widely accepted classification scheme of seizures in use today.

Consistent with the ICES system, the majority of all seizures can be classified as some form of a partial or generalized seizure (Dodrill, 1981). In partial seizures (also known as focal), the epileptogenic activity usually begins in a circumscribed brain area and, unless secondary generalization occurs, the abnormal EEG activity is restricted to that area of the scalp corresponding to the cortical region involved. The symptomatology of a partial seizure may be limited to *elementary* sensory or motor processes without an accompanying loss of consciousness, or it may include more *complex* disturbances of consciousness, behavior, cognition, or affect.

The epileptogenic focus of generalized seizures, however, involves both cerebral hemispheres and their subcortical connections and structures simultaneously. The abnormal EEG patterns in generalized seizures are bilateral, synchronous, and symmetrical over the two hemispheres. The clinical presentation does not entail symptoms associated with localized brain disturbances, but instead consists of impaired consciousness that is frequently accompanied by abnormal bilateral motor activity. Generalized seizures are occasionally further divided on the basis of the presence or the absence of major motor disturbances (e.g., tonic, clonic, and

TABLE 1

International classification of seizures

I. Partial (Focal) Seizures
    A. Simple-partial seizures with elementary symptomatology
        1. Motor symptoms
        2. Special sensory or somatosensory symptoms
        3. Autonomic symptoms
        4. Compound forms
    B. Complex-partial seizures with complex symptomatology
        1. Impaired consciousness only
        2. Cognitive symptoms
        3. Affective symptoms
        4. Psychomotor symptoms (automatisms)
        5. Psychosensory symptoms
        6. Compound forms
    C. Partial seizures secondarily generalized
II. Generalized Seizures
    A. Absence (petit mal)
    B. Myoclonic
    C. Clonic
    D. Tonic
    E. Tonic–clonic (grand mal)
    F. Infantile spasms
    H. Akinetic
III. Unilateral Seizures (predominantly)
IV. Unclassified Seizures

tonic–clonic versus absence attacks). Without specific regard for age, it appears that tonic-clonic, simple partial, and complex partial seizures are the most common types of seizures found (Browne & Feldman, 1983).

Etiology

A variety of causes for epilepsy have been identified. Traditionally, however, the etiology of epilepsy has been divided into two broad categories: (1) *symptomatic* (also known as secondary or acquired) and (2) *idiopathic* (also known as primary or essential). In symptomatic epilepsy, the onset of seizures is directly attributed to an acquired cerebral or general systemic disease. Such seizures are therefore described as symptoms of another disease process. At least nine major disease entities have been identified as direct causes in the presentation of clinical seizures; these include infections, trauma, fluid and electrolyte imbalances, metabolic disorders, anoxia, drugs and toxins, congenital malformations, neoplasms, and cerebrovascular anomalies (Forster & Booker, 1984; Green & Sidell, 1982).

Symptomatic epileptics appear to reveal age-specific patterns in terms of underlying pathological processes. For instance, prior to or immediately following birth, the principle causes for seizures include toxemia and infections during pregnancy, congenital defects, metabolic deficiencies and difficult birth was either mechanical trauma, premature placenta separation or inadequate respiration. During the school years, however, high fevers, infectious diseases, and cerebral trauma take over as the major etiological factors underlying seizures. By adulthood, the major etiologies of seizures involve neoplasms, cerebrovascular problems, and cerebral trauma.

In approximately two-thirds of epileptic cases, no evidence can be found in the history or on physical examination for an underlying cause (Balaschak & Mastofsky, 1982; Lishman, 1978; Merritt, 1979). In the absence of an identifiable cause, which may be more a function of our technological limitations than a true state, such seizures have been termed *idiopathic*. The vast majority of these seizures are generalized and in particular, absence (petit mal) and tonic–clonic variants (grand mal) are the most frequently observed. Interestingly, absence seizures usually appear between the ages of 5 and 12 years and rarely after the age of 20 (Browne & Feldman, 1983; Merritt, 1979). The incidence of tonic–clonic seizures, however, does not appear to vary with age. While the etiology of idiopathic seizures remains unknown, there does seem to be a genetic component involved. Patients with idiopathic epilepsy more often report a positive family history of seizures than patients suffering from symptomatic seizures (Forster & Booker, 1984; Lishman, 1978). Moreover, there appears to be a higher concordance rate for idiopathic seizures among monozygotic than dyzygotic twin pairs (Lennox, 1947, 1951).

Age Factor

The type of epilepsy seen is to a large extent a function of the patient's brain maturation at the time of injury (Green & Sidell, 1982). For instance, the neonate's brain (0–15 days) is highly excitable and generally incapable of discharging in its entirety as a unit. During this stage of development, the brain has a limited capacity for spreading discharges, and epileptogenic discharges are erratic and unevenly distributed. Seizures manifested during this period accordingly present as brief tonic or clonic convulsions with markedly unstable EEG patterns. During infancy (15 days to 2 years), the brain retains its hyperexcitable state but becomes more capable of discharging through one or both cerebral hemispheres.

Thus, seizures arising during infancy are usually unilateral or generalized. Unilateral seizures are, however, more common during this period, and generalized seizures that do appear most often present as tonic attacks or infantile spasms. Toward 2 to 3 years of age, the brain becomes less excitable, and there seems to be a significant decline in the frequency of seizures overall. From this age of early childhood until adolescence, generalized seizures are the most common form of attacks seen, and unilateral and partial seizures are infrequent. With the onset of puberty, however, generalized seizures become less frequent and partial seizures become more common.

By way of simplification, the immature brain tends to react with a diffuse irritative response, while the adult brain demonstrates more localized reactions. Generalized dysrrhythmias are therefore more commonly found in children, whereas focal dysrrhythmias are more characteristic of adult epileptics. Moreover, epileptic seizures tend to change with advancing age to a form more characteristic of the age the patient has attained (Boshes & Gibbs, 1972). For instance, a child with absence seizures may cease to have such attacks upon reaching adulthood only to have them replaced with partial seizures (e.g., psychomotor).

ADAPTIVE IMPLICATIONS

The potential for psychological problems arising in association with epilepsy is thought to be greatest during childhood (Dreisbach et al., 1982). Childhood is quite obviously a period of considerable emotional–behavioral, intellectual, and cognitive development. The presence of recurrent seizures could possibly interfere with the normal developmental process through a number of means, including negative social reactions, parental anxieties and apprehensions, learning difficulties, and altered brain functions. Historically, there has been considerable interest in the psychological concomitants of childhood epilepsy. And despite the efforts of many investigators, no specific pattern of psychological dysfunction has been identified (Boll, 1978; Dikmen, 1980; Dodrill, 1981). While it appears that epilepsy is compatible with normal psychological functioning, a large body of evidence does indicate that psychological difficulties of varying types and degrees are overrepresented in children suffering from recurrent seizures.

Emotional–Behavioral

The frequency estimates of emotional–behavioral problems in epileptic children have been found to vary across studies. For example, Henderson

(1953) reported that 12% of a sample of school children suffering from epilepsy were emotionally disturbed or badly behaved, whereas Pond and Bidwell (1960) reported that 25% of school-age epileptics reveal significant emotional problems. Rutter, Graham, and Yule (1970) reported that 29% of their epileptic children studied revealed psychiatric problems, in contrast to 12% of a chronically ill comparison group. Bridge (1949), however, reported that only 9% of his sample manifested severe personality disturbances, while another 37% revealed moderate personality problems. Several other studies have also reported relatively high but variable frequencies of emotional–behavioral problems among epileptic children (Bolter, Berg, Ch'ien, & Cummins, 1984; Corbett & Trimble, 1977; Green & Hartlage, 1971; Halstead, 1957; Hoare, 1984a; Keating, 1961; Mellor, Lowit, & Hall, 1974; Mignone, Donnelly, & Sadowski, 1970; Pazzaglia & Frank-Pazzaglia, 1976; Price, 1950; Richman, 1964; Stores, 1978; Tizard, 1962; Whitehouse, 1976).

Variations in the frequency of emotional–behavioral problems reported in the aforementioned studies probably reflect differences with respect to criteria for psychopathology employed, as well as populations studied. Despite the fact that the question of exact frequency has yet to be resolved, it is generally held that epileptic children reveal higher rates of psychopathology (roughly 20–35%) than is the probable distribution of such problems in the general population (Dreisbach et al., 1982; Keating, 1961; Lishman, 1978; Werry, 1979; Stores, 1980). It is also quite evident from these studies that the range of psychological problems revealed by epileptic children include all those found in the general population. For the most part, there does not appear to be anything unique or characteristic of the emotional–behavioral difficulties manifested by epileptic children.

Educational

Epilepsy also appears to be compatible with the whole range of educational accomplishments. Nonetheless, epileptic children attending ordinary schools are at greater risk of developing learning problems than other children. In one study of 85 school children with recurrent seizures, it was reported that 16% of the children were regarded as falling seriously behind and 53% were functioning at a below-average educational level (Holdsworth & Whitmore, 1974). It was also noted in the same study that 42% of the children were described as inattentive by their teachers, and that inattentiveness was associated with poorer school performance. In the Isle of Wight study (Rutter, Tizard, & Whitmore, 1970), it was reported that more than twice as many epileptic children revealed serious reading comprehension problems when compared to similar-aged nonepileptic children. Moreover, reading problems in the children were unrelated to their level of intelligence. Support for the overrepresentation of educational problems among epileptic children comes from a number of other studies (Bagley, 1970; Green & Hartlage, 1971; Long & Moore, 1979; Pazzaglia & Frank-Pazzaglia, 1976; Stores, 1978; Stores & Hart, 1976). In fact, Yule (1980) concluded, from reviewing a number of studies, that epileptic children are usually reading 1 year below expected levels by 10 to 11 years of age.

While educational progress in epileptic children has largely been examined in terms of reading skills (Stores, 1980), there is evidence suggesting that arithmetic skills are particularly at risk in these children (Bagley, 1970; Green & Hartlage, 1971). This conclusion was strongly supported in a study of 31 children with chronic generalized epilepsy (Bolter, 1984). The results of the study indicated that impaired performances on the Wide Range Achievement Test (WRAT) occurred in 3% of the children for word recognition reading, in 13% for spelling, and in 26% for mechanical arithmetic. In each case, an impaired performance was defined as earning a standard score equivalent one or more standard deviations below an expected level, based on the child's full-scale IQ (FSIQ).

Cognitive Abilities

Overall, epilepsy is poorly correlated with intelligence, and epileptic children manifest a range of cognitive abilities from retarded to above average (Folsom, 1953; Halstead, 1957; Keating, 1961; Rodin, 1968; Schmidt & Wilder, 1968). While epileptics as a group tend to fall within the normal range of intelligence, the distribution of their scores is skewed toward the lower end of functioning. That is, there tend to be fewer bright epileptics than there are those with lower intelligence (Bagley, 1970; Collins, 1951; Klove & Matthews, 1966; Matthews & Klove, 1967). For example, Bolter (1984) observed, in a study of epileptic children, that as a group the children fell within the average range of intelligence on the WISC-R (FSIQ: $\bar{X} = 92.74$, $SD = 14.21$). The individual scores were, however, clearly skewed toward the lower end of functioning, with only 13% of 31 cases earning scores above average (FSIQ > 110), while 48% earned scores below average (FSIQ < 90). It is important to note that while epilepsy may in some instances be associated with intellectual limitations, the presence of the disorder in a child is not equated with diminished capacity. Moreover, global measures of intelligence provide little information regarding the specific nature of cognitive deficits or educational needs of an epileptic child.

With respect to other areas of cognitive functioning, most notably those evaluated with standard neuropsychological measures (i.e., motor, sensory, language, visuospatial, memory, and complex integrative functions), no specific pattern of impairment has yet been identified as characteristic of children with epilepsy (Boll, 1978; Boll & Barth, 1981; Schwartz & Dennerll, 1970). Some support for a specific attentional deficit in epileptic children has been reported (Holdsworth & Whitmore, 1974; Stores, 1978; Stores & Hart, 1976), but the general conclusion is that these children as a group reveal mild and nonspecific impairments, none of which are found in every case. This conclusion is not surprising in light of the multifaceted nature of epilepsy, including variations across cases with respect to etiology, clinical type, and underlying brain integrity.

CONTRIBUTING FACTORS

A variety of factors have been implicated as significant in the development of cognitive–behavioral problems in children suffering with recurrent seizures, some of which are unique to epilepsy, while others may be characteristic of any child presenting with psychological problems (Corbett & Trimble, 1983; Dodrill, 1981; Dreisbach et al., 1982; Halstead, 1957; Hoare, 1984a, 1984b, 1984c; Holdsworth & Whitmore, 1974; Klove & Matthews, 1974; Lindsay, Ounsted, & Richards, 1979a, 1979b, 1979c; Stores, 1980). For instance, Grunberg and Pond (1957) aptly demonstrated the major contribution adverse family conditions play in the development of behavioral problems in epileptic children. They reported that a comparison between epileptic children without behavioral problems, epileptic children with behavioral problems, and nonepileptic children with behavioral problems revealed that the crucial determinant of behavioral difficulties related to the presence of family disturbance and was unrelated to epilepsy. For the epileptic child, however, there do appear to be other factors in the development of psychological difficulties related to the psychosocial consequences of epilepsy, as well as neuropsychological impairments accompanying altered brain functions, recurrent epileptogenic discharges and prolonged treatment with anticonvulsant medications. At the present time, it would be of little value to speculate on the relative contribution each of these makes in determining the overall cognitive–behavioral functioning of an epileptic child because research in the area has tended to evaluate each in relative isolation without regard for potential interactive effects. What does follow, however, is a general discussion of each as they pertain to their implicated role in the functioning of an epileptic child.

Psychosocial Effect

The psychosocial consequences of epilepsy during childhood are not expected to directly contribute to cognitive or learning deficits. Their influence appears to be more indirect through such things as impaired educational progress, faulty learning experiences, and/or motivation–behavioral problems. It is not too difficult to imagine how the presence of recurrent seizures may affect the extent to which a child can achieve a satisfactory psychological adjustment (Bridge, 1949; Lishman, 1978; Whitehouse, 1976). For example, parental and peer reactions, as well as the child's own reactions to the disorder, may have significant impact on a child's interpersonal stability and the degree to which he or she responds to normal social influences.

Parental misconceptions concerning the causes and consequences of seizures would also seem to be a source of significant, possibly unnecessary, anxieties that lead to altered and often maladjusted patterns of relating to a seizure-prone child (Tavriger, 1966). Anxious parents of epileptic children seem to foster excessive dependency, and they frequently accept lower standards of achievement from these children (Bagley, 1970; Hartlage & Green, 1972; Stores, 1980; Stores and Piran, 1978). In fact, Long and Moore (1979) reported that parents of an epileptic child tend to be less optimistic about that child's future than about their nonepileptic siblings, which in turn appears to be related to poor self-esteem and poor academic achievement in the epileptic child.

In addition to the negative effects of parental anxieties, several studies have observed that epileptic children often suffer from social isolation and have few friends (Golding, Perry, Margolin, Stotsky, & Foster, 1971; Mulder & Sourmeijer, 1977). The results of a recent survey reported by the Epilepsy Foundation of America (1975) clearly reveals the high incidence of negative social experiences associated with childhood epilepsy. Thirty-six percent of the parents surveyed reported that the greatest problems faced by their epileptic child were stigma, poor social acceptance, and negative public opinion. Moreover, 24% reported that ridicule, cruelty, and physical abuse from peers and teachers had been experienced by their epileptic child. In view of the evidence, there appears to be little doubt that the psychosocial consequences of epilepsy during childhood are sufficiently grave to impinge on a child's psychological welfare.

Altered Brain Functions

The results of several experimental studies have documented that pathological cellular changes arise in the central nervous system (CNS) in response to recurrent seizures (Wasterlain, 1974a, 1974b; Wasterlain & Plum, 1973a, 1973b). During an epileptic seizure, the brain appears to have exaggerated metabolic demands, and local ischemic cellular changes arise secondary to hypoxia, hypoglycemia, arterial hypotension, hyperthermia, and acidosis. Moreover, there appears to be a general inhibition of brain protein synthesis and cell growth in response to recurrent seizures. Some identified morphological changes within epileptic brain foci include depopulation of neurons, decreased neuron size and dendritic spines, and astrocytic gliosis within the seizure foci (Ward, 1969).

While the aforementioned findings clearly indicate that seizures alter brain functioning at a cellular level, it is not absolutely certain whether these cellular changes are responsible for cognitive–behavioral deficits found in epileptic children. Theoretically, however, they do provide a basis for assuming a potential brain-related mechanism underlying deficient functioning in epileptic children, and they thereby support the use of neuropsychological measures to elucidate and quantify aspects of brain–behavior relationships potentially effected by recurrent seizures. As alluded to previously, no specific pattern of neuropsychological deficits has been identified as characteristic of epileptic children that could account for the range of cognitive–behavioral difficulties seen in these children.

Hermann (1982) has, however, attempted to directly link the extent of neuropsychological impairment to manifested behavioral problems in epileptic children. Unfortunately, cross-validation work has failed to support such a simple linear relationship (Bolter, 1984). At present, it is widely accepted that several variables related to seizure history, electroencephalographic (EEG) patterns, and anticonvulsant medications contribute to altered brain functions and associated neuropsychological deficits among epileptic children (Dodrill, 1981; Halstead, 1957; Holdsworth & Whitmore, 1974; Ounsted, 1969; Pritchard, Lombroso, & McIntyre, 1980; Rutter, Graham, & Yule, 1970; Stores, 1978, 1980; Tarter, 1972).

Seizure History

A number of factors associated with the history of recurrent seizures have been identified as possible predictors of neuropsychological deficits in epileptic children. The most commonly cited in the literature include age at seizure onset, duration of the disorder, frequency of attacks, type of clinical seizure and etiology of the disorder. Results from several studies have generally conflicted regarding their relative contributions in neuropsychological deficits revealed among epileptics (Chaudhry & Pond, 1961; Chevrie & Aicardi, 1978; Dodrill, 1981; Halstead, 1957; Hartlage & Green, 1972; Holdsworth & Whitmore, 1974; Ounsted, 1969; Pond & Bidwell, 1960; Pritchard et al., 1980; Rutter, Graham & Yule, 1970). Differences across studies with respect to various methodological issues (e.g., populations studied, criteria for subject inclusion, methods of data collection, measures utilized, and range of variables sampled) have no doubt added to variances in their results. Despite these differences, several useful statements can be made regarding the implicated role of seizure-history variables in neuropsychological impairment among epileptics.

Investigations on the age of onset and duration of disorder generally suggest that the earlier the age at onset of seizures and the longer the duration of the disorder, the greater the impairment one is likely to observe (Dikmen, Matthews, & Harley, 1975; Klove & Matthews, 1966). This conclusion is particularly relevant when considering generalized tonic attacks (DeHaas & Magnus, 1958; Lennox & Lennox, 1960), infantile spasms (Corbett, Harris, & Robinson, 1975), and attacks following perinatal brain damage (Bagley, 1972; Gudmusson, 1966; Halstead, 1957). While it appears that early onset and long duration of recurrent seizures identify children at risk for cognitive–behavioral problems, such information does not answer the question of whether recurrent seizures over a prolonged period lead to functional deterioration or whether severe brain damage from the onset underlies recurrent intractible seizures with functional impairment. Furthermore, as aptly pointed out by Dodrill (1981), the magnitude of impairment accounted for by these variables is small, and it appears more reasonable to assume that there are many factors involved in the determination of a child's ultimate level of functioning.

Although conclusive evidence is lacking, it is generally accepted that a high frequency of seizures is associated with greater neuropsychological impairment (Corbett & Trimble, 1983; Dodrill, 1981; Halstead, 1957, Hartlage & Green, 1972; Holdsworth & Whitmore, 1974; Keating, 1960; Pond & Bidwell, 1960; Tarter, 1972). The inconclusive quality of these findings probably reflects, to a large extent, the inherent difficulty in collecting accurate data on frequency of attacks. Many epileptics have seizures during the night when they are likely to occur unbeknownst to the patient or unobserved by others. Only 40–50% of all epileptics have their attacks limited to daytime hours while some 15–20% only have their attacks during the night (Forster & Booker, 1984).

With respect to the type of clinical seizure manifested, it appears that epileptics who have primarily major-motor attacks demonstrate the greatest neuropsychogical impairment (Halstead, 1957; Klove & Matthews,

1974; Matthews & Klove, 1967; Tarter, 1972). In other words, individuals suffering from partial seizures tend to be less impaired than those with generalized tonic–clonic attacks. It has also been suggested that in contrast to a single seizure type, mixed clinical seizures have a greater detrimental impact on the psychological functioning of an epileptic child (Lennox & Lennox, 1960; Schwartz & Dennerll, 1970; Tarter, 1972). A major problem with this conclusion is that in clinical studies, the effects of seizure severity have not been controlled for. It is widely known among clinicians that patients carrying the same seizure diagnosis differ with respect to the severity of their attacks. For instance, tonic–clonic seizures tend to be much longer in some individuals than in others, and in some, respiratory arrest occurs with regularity, whereas in others it is virtually nonexistent.

The relationship between seizure etiology and neuropsychological functioning has proven to be the best single correlate of impairment among the seizure history variables. Results from several studies (Chevrie & Aicardi, 1978; Halstead, 1957; Klove & Matthews, 1974; Lennox & Lennox, 1960; Tarter, 1972) have demonstrated that epileptics with seizures of known etiology typically reveal greater deficits in functioning than is found in those whose seizures are idiopathic. It is important to recognize, however, that epileptics who have suffered sufficient insult to the brain to establish an etiological basis for their attacks may have also suffered more impairment in brain functions. Moreover, while the degree of impairment increases when brain damage is present, the presence of seizures does not appear to significantly add to the degree of impairment found.

Electroencephalographic Patterns

The relationship between higher cortical brain functions and indices of abnormalities on the EEG has been investigated in a large number of studies (Dikmen, 1980; Dodrill & Wilkus, 1976, 1978; Hudges, 1968; Kaufman, Harris, & Schaffer, 1980; Klonoff & Low, 1974; Lennox & Lennox, 1960; Nuffield, 1961a, 1961b; Ritvo, Arnitz, & Walter, 1970; Stores & Hart, 1976; Tarter, 1972; Tymchuk, Knights, & Hinton, 1970; Wilkus & Dodrill, 1976). Although the psychological measures employed vary from study to study, the results suggest that both ictal and interictal EEG epileptiform discharges are associated with a deterioration in cognitive abilities. In particular, measures of attention, memory, and timed performance have been found to be negatively affected by the presence of subclinical EEG epileptiform discharges. Unfortunately, the majority of studies have limited their investigations to only a few indices of EEG abnormality rather than assessing the effects of a broad spectrum of concomitant EEG variables.

In a series of studies, Dodrill and Wilkus investigated the relationship between several measures of EEG abnormality and multiple measures of neuropsychological functioning in a group of adult epileptics (Dodrill & Wilkus, 1976, 1978; Wilkus & Dodrill, 1976). Among the EEG parameters included in their investigation were topographic distribution and rate of epileptiform discharges, as well as dominant waking posterior rhythm frequency. The results of their investigation indicated that for 11 of 15 neuropsychological tests administered, increasing impairment was associated with increasing topographical involvement of the epileptiform discharges. Similarly, an orderly rate of deterioration on neuropsychological measures was found when patients having no abnormal discharges, a low rate of epileptiform discharges (fewer than one per minute) and a high rate of epileptiform discharges (more than one per minute) were successively contrasted. Also, patients with low posterior rhythm frequency (5.1 to 7.7 Hz), in comparison to those with medium (7.8 to 8.7 Hz) and high (8.8 to 11 Hz), were impaired on a number of variables related to concentrated attention, mental flexibility, and motor functions. The authors concluded from their studies that impaired neuropsychological functioning in epileptics is systematically and lawfully related to the presence of interictal EEG abnormalities.

In a similar study, Bolter (1982) investigated the relationship between a battery of neuropsychological measures and interictal EEG abnormalities in a group of 21 children (average age of 11.7 years) with chronic generalized idiopathic seizures. The EEG parameters examined in the study included topographical distribution of epileptiform discharges, rate of discharges per minute, type of discharges, dominant waking parieto-occipital rhythm frequency, and a composite rating of overall EEG abnormality. Unlike the findings reported by Dodrill and Wilkus with adult epileptics, however, interictal EEG abnormalities were not found to be systematically and lawfully associated with neuropsychological impairment in the epileptic children studied. This contradictory outcome may in part reflect the small sample size of epileptic children studied. The small sample size also precluded analyzing any potential interactions among the various indicies of EEG abnormality. For instance, the type of epileptiform discharge may interact with the topographical site of the abnormality to produce a reduction in cognitive efficiency that would not otherwise be apparent through examining each in isolation of the other.

In spite of the few significant findings observed in the Bolter (1982) study, several trends revealed in the data are worthy of discussion. First, of the five EEG parameters investigated, the average rate of epileptiform discharges, type of discharge, and overall rating of EEG abnormality were more clearly related to neuropsychological functioning in the epileptic children. In particular, a high average rate of epileptiform discharges (more than 1/minute) appeared to be associated with reduced functioning across a broad spectrum of neuropsychological measures. With respect to type of discharge, spikes in the EEG record were more often associated with a poorer performance than spike-waves or an absence of epileptiform discharges. Similarly, the electroencephalographer's summary impression of extent of abnormality in the child's interictal EEG record frequently corresponded with the relative degree of neuropsychological impairment. Slowing in the dominant waking parieto-occipital rhythm was not found to be consistently associated with impaired neuropsychological functioning, and no clear distinction was found with regard to the extent or type of deficits manifested for children having either focal or diffuse discharges. Interestingly, the cognitive–behavioral dimensions studied did not appear to be equally sensitive to the effects of EEG abnormalities. For example, deficits in emotionality, intelligence, academic achievement, incidental memory, visual–spatial, auditory perceptual, motor, and verbal functions only rarely revealed an association with the various EEG parameters, while those related to tactile perception, tactile–motor problem solving, and immediate alertness more often accompanied EEG disturbances. Also, poor performance on a digit-span test was found to be systematically related to extent of abnormality on four of the five EEG parameters investigated. This finding is particularly intriguing in light of the measure's sensitivity to attentional difficulties and the hypothesized attentional deficit underlying problematic behaviors in epileptic children advanced by Stores, Hart, and Piran (1978).

Anticonvulsant Medications

Treatment of recurrent seizures primarily relies on the administration of anticonvulsant medications. Approximately 50% of all epileptics obtain complete seizure relief with these medications, while another 30–40% experience only partial relief (Green & Sidell, 1982). A wide variety of anticonvulsant medications are currently available for the treatment of seizures, and undoubtedly more will be developed. The principal drugs used in the treatment of tonic–clonic generalized seizures include phenytoin (Dilantin), phenobarbital, carbamazepine (Tegretol), and primidone (Mysoline). Absence attacks of all types are generally treated with ethosuximide (Zarontin), valproic acid (Depakene), clonazepam (Clonopin), trimethadione (Tridione), and methsuximide (Celontin). Partial seizures with complex or elementary symptomatology usually respond favorably to the same medications effective in controlling generalized convulsions.

It is important to realize, however, that none of the available antiepileptic drugs are truly seizure specific in their effects but instead appear relatively more effective against one type of seizure over another. The selection of an anticonvulsant medication for treatment purposes only in part depends on its seizure specificity and consideration of (1) the potential untoward side effects, (2) general ease of administration, and (3) individual patient responsiveness must be included in that decision process.

While it has long been suspected that anticonvulsant medications potentiate cognitive–behavioral deficits in epileptics, many of the early studies reported in the literature conflicted regarding the relative impact anticonvulsants had on the mental functioning of epileptics (Chaudhry & Pond, 1961; Holdsworth & Whitmore, 1974; Keating, 1960; Lennox, 1942; Lennox & Lennox, 1960; Loveland, Smith, & Forster, 1957; Rayo & Martin, 1959; Stores, 1975). The toxic side effects of anticonvulsant medications have been clinically recognized for a number of years, and sluggishness, depression, excitability, irritability, and aggression are commonly reported (Myklebust, 1978). The subclinical effects on higher cortical functions are, however, only beginning to be appreciated, through the appearance of more carefully controlled studies in the literature (Corbett & Trimble, 1983; Reynolds, 1983; Trimble & Reynolds, 1976; Trimble & Thompson, 1983).

Reynolds (1983) concluded, from reviewing the available literature, that most of the major anticonvulsant medications (i.e., phenytoin, phenobarbital, valproate, and ethosuximide) interfere in subtle ways with various cognitive functions, including attention, concentration, motor speed, memory, and mental processing. Additionally, there appears to be some evidence (especially with phenobarbital and phenytoin) for a relationship between higher serum levels of drugs and more severe impairment, as well as affective and cognitive improvement following a reduction of polytherapy (Trimble & Thompson, 1983). Studies with children (Corbett & Trimble, 1983) have also supported an association between impaired cognitive functions and anticonvulsant levels within therapeutic dose ranges. Moreover, carbamazepine has repeatedly been identified as the least detrimental among the anticonvulsants with respect to cognitive functions (Reynolds, 1983; Trimble & Thompson, 1983). In fact, at least one study has identified cognitive improvements in epileptic children given carbamazepine in substitution for their usual seizure medication (Schain, Ward, & Guthrie, 1977).

The mechanisms by which anticonvulsant medications may induce cognitive–behavioral deficits remains unknown at present. Hypothesized mechanisms include direct neuron damage (Dam, 1983; Shorvon & Reynolds, 1982) and secondary injurious effects accompanying folate defi-

ciency (Reynolds, 1976; Trimble, Corbett, & Donaldson, 1980), disturbances in monoamine metabolism (Chadwick, Jenner, & Reynolds, 1977;
Chadwick, Reynolds, & Marsden, 1976; Trimble, Chadwick, Reynolds, &
Marsden, 1975), or endocrine disturbances (London, 1980). More systematic research concerning the various drug parameters (e.g., dosage, serum
blood level, history of toxicity, selective side effects, and serum half-life)
will need to be completed prior to developing definitive statements regarding the interrelationships between the different anticonvulsant medications and neuropsychological deficits in epileptic children. While the
available evidence does suggest that increased serum levels of anticonvulsant medications can contribute to impaired neuropsychological functions, the magnitude of the effect appears small and varies from case to
case. More importantly, however, the potentially negative impact prolonged anticonvulsant therapy on the neuropsychological functioning of
an epileptic child has to be balanced with the risk of seizure continuation
in the absence of drug therapy.

SUMMARY

Recurrent seizures during childhood represent a potentially negative
impact on the emotional, behavioral, educational, and neuropsychological functioning in a seizure-prone child. In general, however, there does
not appear to be any specific pattern of deficits associated with childhood
epilepsy, and the disorder is compatible with a wide range of abilities.
Instead, there are a number of factors that have been identified as causally
related to the manifestation of cognitive–behavioral impairments in epileptic children. Among these are included the psychosocial effects of
recurrent seizures (e.g., parental and peer responses), historical features
of the disorder (e.g., age at onset, duration, frequency of attacks, type of
attacks, and etiology), EEG abnormalities (e.g., type, rate, topography,
and dominant posterior frequency slowing), and the prolonged use of
anticonvulsant medications. The neuropsychological implications of epilepsy appear to vary from case to case, and all of the aforementioned
factors need to be considered in evaluating an epileptic child.

REFERENCES

Bagley, C. R. (1970). The educational performance of children with epilepsy. *British Journal
of Educational Psychology, 40,* 82–83.
Bagley, C. R. (1972). Social prejudice and adjustment of people with epilepsy. *Epilepsia, 13,*
33–45.
Balaschak, B. A., & Mastofsky, D. I. (1982). Seizure disorders. In E. J. Mash & L. G.
Terdal (Eds.), *Behavioral assessment of childhood disorders.* New York, Guilford
Press.

Boll, T. J. (1978). Diagnosing brain impairment. In B. Wolman (Ed.), *Diagnosis of mental disorders: A handbook*. New York: Plenum Press.

Boll, T. J., & Barth, J. T. (1981). Neuropsychology of brain damage in children. In S. B. Filskov & T. J. Boll (Eds.), *Handbook of clinical neuropsychology*. New York: Wiley.

Bolter, J. F. (1982, October). *Neuropsychological correlates of the electroencephalogram in children with epilepsy. Caton Research Address*. Paper presented at the 35th annual meeting of the Southern Electroencephalographic Society, Williamsburg, VA.

Bolter, J. F. (1984). *Neuropsychological impairment and behavioral dysfunction in children with chronic epilepsy*. Unpublished doctoral dissertation, Memphis State University, Memphis, Tennessee.

Bolter, J. F., Berg, R. A., Ch'ien, L. T., & Cummins, J. (1984). A standardized assessment of emotionality in children suffering from epilepsy. *International Journal of Clinical Neuropsychology, 6*, 247–248.

Boshes, L. D., & Gibbs, F. A. (1972). *Epilepsy handbook*. Springfield, IL: Charles C. Thomas.

Bridge, E. M. (1949). *Epilepsy and convulsive disorders in children*. New York: McGraw-Hill.

Browne, T. R., & Feldman, R. G. (1983). Epilepsy: An overview. In T. R. Browne & R. G. Feldman (Eds.), *Epilepsy: Diagnosis and management*. Boston: Little, Brown.

Chadwick, D., Jenner, P., & Reynolds, E. H. (1977). Serotonin metabolism in human epilepsy: The influence of anticonvulsant drugs. *Annals of Neurology, 1*, 218–224.

Chadwick, D., Reynolds, E. H., & Marsden, C. D. (1976). Anticonvulsant-induced dyskinesias: A comparison with dyskinesias induced by neuroleptics. *Journal of Neurology, Neurosurgery and Psychiatry, 39*, 1210–1218.

Chaudhry, M. R., & Pond, D. A. (1961). Mental deterioration in epileptic children. *Journal of Neurology, Neurosurgery and Psychiatry, 24*, 213–219.

Chevrie, J., & Aicardi, J. (1978). Convulsive disorders in the first year of life: Neurological and mental outcome and mortality. *Epilepsia, 19*, 67–74.

Collins, A. L. (1951). Epileptic intelligence. *Journal of Consulting Psychology, 15*, 392–399.

Corbett, J. A., Harris, R., & Robinson, R. G. (1975). Epilepsy. In J. Wortis (Ed.), *Mental retardation and developmental disabilities* (Vol. 7). New York: Brunner/Matzel.

Corbett, J. A., & Trimble, M. (1977). *Neuropsychiatric aspects of anticonvulsant treatment in children with epilepsy*. Paper presented at the IVth World Congress of Psychiatry, Honolulu.

Corbett, J. A., & Trimble, M. R. (1983). Epilepsy and anticonvulsant medication. In M. Rutter (Ed.), *Developmental neuropsychiatry*. London: Guilford Press.

Dam, M. (1983). Chronic toxicity of antiepileptic drugs with respect to cerebellar and motor function. In J. Oxley, D. Jans, & H. Meinardi (Eds.), *Chronic toxicity of antiepileptic drugs*. New York: Raven Press.

DeHaas, A., & Magnus, O. (1958). In A. DeHaas (Ed.), *Lectures on epilepsy*. New York: Elsevier.

Dikmen, S. (1980). Neuropsychological aspects of epilepsy. In B. P. Hermann (Ed.), *A multidisciplinary handbook of epilepsy*. Springfield, IL: Charles C. Thomas.

Dikmen, S., Matthews, C. G., & Harley, J. P. (1975). The effect of early versus late onset of major motor epilepsy upon cognitive–intellectual performance. *Epilepsia, 16*, 73–81.

Dodrill, C. B. (1981). Neuropsychology of epilepsy. In S. B. Filskov & T. J. Boll (Eds.), *Handbook of clinical neuropsychology*. New York: Wiley.

Dodrill, C. B., & Wilkus, R. J. (1976). Neuropsychological correlates of the electroencephalogram in epileptics: II. The waking posterior rhythm and its interaction with epileptiform activity. *Epilepsia, 17,* 101–109.

Dodrill, C. B., & Wilkus, R. J. (1978). Neuropsychological correlates of the electroencephalogram in epileptics: III. Generalized non-epileptiform abnormalities. *Epilepsia, 19,* 453–462.

Dreisbach, M., Ballard, M., Russo, D. C., & Schain, R. J. (1982). Educational intervention for children with epilepsy: A challenge for collaborative service delivery. *Journal of Special Education, 16,* 111–121.

Epilepsy Foundation of America. (1975). *Basic statistics on the epilepsies.* Philadelphia: Davis.

Folsom, A. (1953). Psychological testing in epilepsy: I. Cognitive function. *Epilepsia, 2,* 23–26.

Forster, F. M., & Booker, H. E. (1984). The epilepsies and convulsive disorders. In A. B. Baker & L. H. Baker (Eds.), *Clinical neurology* (Vol. 3). Philadelphia: Harper & Row.

Gastaut, H. (1970). Clinical and electroencephalographical classifications of epileptic seizures. *Epilepsia, 2,* 102–113.

Glaser, G. H. (1979). The epilepsies. In P. B. Beeson, W. McDermott, & J. B. Wyngaarden (Eds.), *Cecil textbook of medicine.* Philadelphia: Saunders.

Golding, J., Perry, S. L., Margolin, R. J., Stotsky, B. A., & Foster, J. C. (1971). *The rehabilitation of the young epileptic: Dimensions and dynamic factors.* Lexington, MA: Lexington Books.

Green, J. R., & Hartlage, L. C. (1971). Comparative performance of epileptic and nonepileptic children and adolescents. *Diseases of the Nervous System, 32,* 418–421.

Green, J. R., & Sidell, A. D. (1982). Neurosurgical aspects of epilepsy in children and adolescents. In J. R. Youman (Ed.), *Neurological surgery: A comprehensive reference guide to the diagnosis and management of neurosurgical problems* (Vol. 6). Philadelphia: Saunders.

Grunberg, F., & Pond, D. A. (1957). Conduct disorders in epileptic children. *Journal of Neurology, Neurosurgery and Psychiatry, 20,* 65–68.

Gudmusson, G. (1966). Epilepsy in Iceland. *Acta Neurologica Scandinavica, 43* (Supplement 25).

Halstead, H. (1957). Abilities and behaviour of epileptic children. *Journal of Mental Science, 103,* 28–47.

Hartlage, L. C., & Green, J. B. (1972). The relation of parental attitudes to academic and social achievement in epileptic children. *Epilepsia, 13,* 21–26.

Henderson, P. (1953). Epilepsy in school children. *British Journal of Preventive and Social Medicine, 7,* 9–14.

Hermann, B. P. (1982). Neuropsychological functioning and psychopathology in children with epilepsy. *Epilepsia, 23,* 545–554.

Hoare, P. (1984a). The development of psychiatric disorder among school children with epilepsy. *Developmental Medicine and Child Neurology, 26,* 3–13.

Hoare, P. (1984b). Psychiatric disturbance in the families of epileptic children. *Developmental Medicine and Child Neurology, 26,* 14–19.

Hoare, P. (1984c). Does illness foster dependency? A study of epileptic and diabetic children. *Developmental Medicine and Child Neurology, 26,* 20–24.

Holdsworth, L., & Whitmore, K. (1974). A study of children with epilepsy attending ordinary schools. *Developmental Medicine and Child Neurology, 16,* 746–758.

Hudges, J. (1968). Electroencephalography and learning. In H. Myklebust (Ed.), *Progress in learning disabilities.* New York: Grune & Stratton.

Jackson, J. H. (1925). *Neurological fragments.* London: Oxford University Press.

Jackson, J. H. (1931). Lectures on the diagnosis of epilepsy. In J. Taylor (Ed.), *Selected writings of John Hughings Jackson* (Vol. 1). New York: Basic Books.

Kaufman, K. R., Harris, R., & Schaffer, R. D. (1980). Problems of categorization of child and adolescent EEGs. *Journal of Child Psychology and Psychiatry, 21,* 333–342.

Keating, L. E. (1960). A review of the literature on the relationship of epilepsy and intelligence in school children. *Journal of Mental Science, 106,* 1042–1059.

Keating, L. E. (1961). Epilepsy and behaviour disorder in school age children. *Journal of Mental Science, 107,* 161–180.

Klonoff, H., & Low, M. (1974). Disordered brain function in young children and early adolescence: Neuropsychological and electroencephalographic correlates. In R. M. Reitan & L. A. Davison (Eds.), *Clinical neuropsychology: Current status and applications.* Washington, DC: Hemisphere.

Klove, H., & Matthews, C. G. (1966). Psychometric and adaptive abilities in epilepsy with different etiology. *Epilepsia, 7,* 330–338.

Klove, H., & Matthews, C. G. (1974). Neuropsychological studies of patients with epilepsy. In R. M. Reitan & L. A. Davidson (Eds.), *Clinical neuropsychology: Current status and applications.* Washington, DC: Hemisphere.

Kurtzke, J. F., & Kurland, L. T. (1984). The epidemiology of neurologic disease. In A. B. Baker & L. H. Baker (Eds.), *Clinical neurology* (Vol. 4). Philadelphia: Harper & Row.

Lennox, W. (1942). Brain injury, drugs and environment as causes of mental decay in epilepsy. *American Journal of Psychiatry, 99,* 174–180.

Lennox, W. (1947). Sixty-six twin pairs affected by seizures. *Association for Research on Nervous and Mental Diseases, Proceedings, 26,* 11–33.

Lennox, W. (1951). The heredity of epilepsy as told by relatives and twins. *Journal of the American Medical Association, 146,* 529–536.

Lennox, W., & Lennox, M. (1960). *Epilepsy and related disorders.* Boston: Little, Brown.

Lindsay, J., Ounsted, C., & Richards, P. (1979a). Long-term outcome in children with temporal lobe seizures: I. Social outcome and childhood factors. *Developmental Medicine and Child Neurology, 21,* 285–298.

Lindsay, J., Ounsted, C., & Richards, P. (1979b). Long-term outcome in children with temporal lobe seizures: II. Marriage, parenthood and sexual indifference. *Developmental Medicine and Child Neurology, 21,* 433–440.

Lindsay, J., Ounsted, C., & Richards, P. (1979c). Long-term outcome in children with temporal lobe seizures: III. Psychiatric aspects in childhood and adult life. *Developmental Medicine and Child Neurology, 21,* 630–636.

Lishman, W. A. (1978). *Organic psychiatry: The psychological consequences of cerebral disorder.* Oxford: Blackwell.

London, D. R. (1980). Hormonal effects of anticonvulsant drugs. In R. Canger, F. Angeleri, & J. K. Penry (Eds.), *Advances in epileptology: The XIth Epilepsy International Symposium.* New York: Raven Press.

Long, C. G., & Moore, J. R. (1979). Parental expectations of their epileptic children. *Journal of Child Psychology and Psychiatry, 20,* 299–312.

Loveland, N., Smith, B., & Forster, F. (1957). Mental and emotional changes in epileptic patients on continuous anticonvulsant medication. *Neurology, 7,* 856–865.

Matthews, C. G., & Klove, H. (1967). Differential psychological performances in major motor, psychomotor and mixed seizure classifications of known and unknown etiology. *Epilepsia, 8,* 117–128.

Meighan, S. S., Queener, L., & Weitman, M. (1976). Prevalence of epilepsy in children of Multinomah County, Oregon. *Epilepsia, 17,* 245–256.

Mellor, D., Lowit, I., & Hall, D. (1974). Are epileptic children behaviorally different from other children? In P. Harris & C. Maudsley (Eds.), *Epilepsy: Proceedings of the Hans Berger Centenary Symposium.* Edinburgh: Churchill Livingstone.

Merritt, H. H. (1979). *A textbook of neurology.* Philadelphia: Lea & Febiger.

Mignone, R., Donnelly, E., & Sadowski, D. (1970). Psychological and neurological comparisons of psychomotor and nonpsychomotor epileptic patients. *Epilepsia, 11,* 345–359.

Mulder, H. C., & Sourmeijer, P. B. M. (1977). Families with a child with epilepsy: A sociological contribution. *Journal of Biosocial Science, 9,* 13–24.

Myklebust, H. R. (1978). Educational problems of the child with epilepsy. In *Report to the commission for the control of epilepsy and its consequences: Plan for nationwide action on epilepsy* (Vol. 2). Bethesda, MD: Department of Health, Education and Welfare.

Nuffield, E. J. A. (1961a). Electroclinical correlations in childhood epilepsy. *Epilepsia, 2,* 178–196.

Nuffield, E. J. A. (1961b). Neurophysiology and behavioural disorders in epileptic children. *Journal of Mental Science, 107,* 438–458.

Ounsted, C. (1969). Aggression and epilepsy: Rage in children with temporal lobe epilepsy. *Journal of Psychosomatic Research, 13,* 237–242.

Pazzaglia, P., & Frank-Pazzaglia, L. (1976). Records in grade school of pupils with epilepsy: An epidemiological study. *Epilepsia, 1,* 285–299.

Pond, D. A., & Bidwell, B. H. (1960). A survey of epilepsy in fourteen general practices: II. Social and psychological aspects. *Epilepsia, 1,* 285–299.

Pond, D. A., & Bidwell, B. H., & Stein, L. (1960). A survey of epilepsy in fourteen general practices: I. Demographic and medical data. *Psychiatria, Neurologia, Neurochirurgia, 63,* 217–236.

Price, J. C. (1950). The epileptic child in school. *Ohio State Journal of Medicine, 46,* 794.

Pritchard, P. B., Lombroso, C. T., & McIntyre, M. (1980). Psychological complications of temporal lobe epilepsy. *Neurology, 30,* 227–232.

Rayo, D., & Martin, F. (1959). Standardized psychometric tests applied to the analysis of the effects of anticonvulsant medication on the proficiency of young epileptics. *Epilepsia, 1,* 189–207.

Reynolds, E. H. (1976). Neurological aspects of folate and vitamin B12 metabolism. *Clinical Haematology, 5,* 661–696.

Reynolds, E. H. (1983). Mental effects of antiepileptic medication: A review. *Epilepsia, 24,* S85–S95.

Richman, N. (1964). *The prevalence of psychiatric disturbances in a hospital school for epileptics.* Unpublished D.P.M. thesis, University of London, London.

Ritvo, E., Arnitz, E. M., & Walter, R. D. (1970). Correlations of psychiatric disorders and EEG findings: A double blind study of 184 hospitalized children. *American Journal of Psychiatry, 126,* 988–996.

Rodin, E. (1968). *The prognosis of patients with epilepsy.* Springfield, IL: Charles C. Thomas.

Rose, S., Penry, J., Markush, R., Radloff, L., & Putman, P. (1973). Prevalence of epilepsy in children. *Epilepsia, 14,* 133–152.

Rutter, M., Graham, P., & Yule, W. (1970). *A neuropsychiatric study of childhood.* Philadelphia: Lippincott.

Rutter, M., Tizard, J., & Whitmore, K. (1970). *Education, health and behavior.* London: Longman.

Schain, R. J., Ward, J. N., & Guthrie, D. (1977). Carbamazepine as an anticonvulsant in children. *Neurology, 27,* 476–480.

Schmidt, R. P., & Wilder, B. J. (1968). *Epilepsy.* Philadelphia: Davis.

Schwartz, M. L., & Dennerll, R. D. (1970). Neuropsychological assessment of children with, without, and with questionable epileptogenic dysfunction. *Perceptual and Motor Skills, 30,* 111–121.

Shorvon, S. D., & Reynolds, E. H. (1982). Anticonvulsant peripheral neuropathy: A clinical and electrophysiological study of patients on single drug treatment with phenytoin, carbamazepine or barbiturates. *Journal of Neurology, Neurosurgery and Psychiatry, 45,* 620–626.

Stores, G. (1975). Behavioural effects of anticonvulsant drugs. *Developmental Medicine and Child Neurology, 17,* 647–658.

Stores, G. (1978). School children with epilepsy at risk for learning and behavior problems. *Developmental Medicine and Child Neurology, 20,* 502–508.

Stores, G. (1980). Children with epilepsy. In B. P. Hermann (Ed.), *A multidisciplinary handbook of epilepsy.* Springfield, IL: Charles C. Thomas.

Stores, G., & Hart, J. A. (1976). Reading skills in children with generalized or focal epilepsy attending ordinary school. *Developmental Medicine and Child Neurology, 18,* 705–716.

Stores, G., Hart, J. A., & Piran, N. (1978). Inattentiveness in school children with epilepsy. *Epilepsia, 19,* 169–175.

Stores, G., & Piran, N. (1978). Dependency of different types in school children with epilepsy. *Psychological Medicine, 8,* 441–445.

Tarter, R. E. (1972). Intellectual and adaptive functioning in epilepsy: A review of fifty years of research. *Diseases of the Nervous System, 33,* 763–770.

Tavriger, R. (1966). Some parental theories about causes of epilepsy. *Epilepsia, 7,* 339–343.

Tizard, B. (1962). The personality of epileptics: A discussion of the evidence. *Psychological Bulletin, 59,* 196–210.

Trimble, M. R., Chadwick, D., Reynolds, E. H., & Marsden, C. D. (1975). L-5-Hydroxytryptophan and mood. *Lancet, 1,* 583.

Trimble, M. R., Corbett, J. A., & Donaldson, D. (1980). Folic acid and mental symptoms in children with epilepsy. *Journal of Neurology, Neurosurgery and Psychiatry, 43,* 1030–1034.

Trimble, M. R., & Reynolds, E. H. (1976). Anticonvulsant drugs and mental symptoms. *Psychological Medicine, 6,* 169–174.

Trimble, M. R., & Thompson, P. J. (1983). Anticonvulsant drugs, cognitive function, and behavior. *Epilepsia, 24,* S55–S63.

Tymchuk, A. J., Knights, R. M., & Hinton, G. G. (1970). Neuropsychological test results of children with brain lesions, abnormal EEGs and normal EEGs. *Canadian Journal of Behavioral Science, 2,* 322–329.

Ward, A. A. (1969). The epileptic neuron: Chronic foci in animals and man. In H. H. Jasper, A. A. Ward, & A. Pope (Eds.), *Basic mechanisms of the epilepsies.* Boston: Little, Brown.

Wasterlain, C. G. (1974a). Inhibition of cerebral protein synthesis by epileptic seizures without motor manifestations. *Neurology, 24,* 175–180.

Wasterlain, C. G. (1974b). Mortality and morbidity from serial seizures: An experimental study. *Epilepsia, 15,* 155–176.

Wasterlain, C. G., & Plum, F. (1973a). Retardation of behavioral landmarks after neonatal seizures in rats. *Transactions of the American Neurological Association, 98,* 320–321.

Wasterlain, C. G., & Plum, F. (1973b). Vulnerability of developing rat brain to electrocon-vulsive seizures. *Archives of Neurology, 29,* 38–45.

Weinberg, W. (1972). Epilepsy: A study of school populations. In M. Alter & W. A. Hauser (Eds.), *The epidemiology of epilepsy* (NINCDS Monograph No. 14, DHEW Publi-cation, NIG 390).

Werry, J. S. (1979). Organic factors. In H. C. Quay & J. S. Werry (Eds.), *Psychopathologi-cal disorders of childhood.* New York: Wiley.

Whitehouse, D. (1976). Behavior and learning problems in epileptic children. *Behavioral Neuropsychiatry, 7,* 23–29.

Wilkus, R. J., & Dodrill, C. B. (1976). Neuropsychological correlates of the electroencepha-logram in epileptics: I. Topographic distribution and average rate of epileptiform activity. *Epilepsia, 17,* 89–100.

Yule, W. (1980). Educational achievement. In B. M. Kulig, M. Meinhardi, & G. Stores (Eds.), *Epilepsy and behaviour.* Lisse, The Netherlands: Swets & Zeitlinger.

Chapter 4

Neuropsychological Aspects of Psychiatric Disorders

RAYMOND S. DEAN

Neuropsychology Laboratory
Ball State University
Muncie, Indiana 47306
and
Indiana University School of Medicine
Muncie, Indiana 47306

INTRODUCTION

Children are not merely small adults. This statement is not as trite as it may seem when one examines continuous attempts to translate adult neuropsychological findings to children. Indeed, the sometimes naive application of neurological sequelae established in adult disorders (e.g., encephalitis) to childhood behavioral patterns (Strauss & Lehtinen, 1948) has been responsible for the premature rejection of a neuropsychological approach in the understanding of children's functioning (Dean, 1982a).

Neuropsychological assessment of children is a relatively recent pursuit. It grew out of the successes in defining brain–behavior relationships with adults (Boll, 1974). Clearly, greater numbers of adult referrals with documented neurological disorders and the opportunity to validate neuropsychological assessment procedures during surgery and autopsies are responsible for this research focus with adults (Dean, 1985).

CHILD NEUROPSYCHOLOGY, VOL. 2

Problems in translating adult neuropsychological research conclusions to children involves, in part, the ongoing anatomical changes in the child's brain (Boll, 1974). This point is emphasized with data showing that greater neuropsychological complexity is necessary to describe the within-subject variability on some 32 neuropsychological variables with increasing age (Crockett, Klonoff, & Bejerring, 1969). Although these results may represent invariant developmental trends or fluctuations between development levels, this hypothesis remains to be investigated. Developmental neuropsychology seems a most promising area in providing both advances in the understanding of the development of brain–behavior relationships and a base from which to interpret an individual child's performance from an individual difference quantitative approach. In fact, some research indicates that age-related differences in the psychological sequelae of childhood brain damage may be due to developmental changes in functional lateralization in children (Dean, 1982a).

Early successes in defining brain–behavior relationships (Broca, 1861/1960; Jackson, 1874/1932) led to the quest for localization of specific functions to microstructures of the cerebral cortex. Such a static approach to the localization of functions within the brain has been rejected by most neuroscientists. This is true because the locus, severity, and type of lesions interact with individual differences in biochemical, anatomical, and lateralization to make specific localization of functions a reactionary pursuit (Dean, 1985). From an interpretive point of view, premorbid history (e.g., education, occupation, demographics), time from onset to assessment, and the like serve to modify the neuropsychological test results with adults and children (Dean, 1982a).

The interpretation of children's performance on neuropsychological measures is further complicated by a number of potentially confounding variables more unique to children (Dean, 1986a). Moreover, the child's premorbid developmental history (Benton, 1974), developmental stage of the brain at onset (Boll, 1974), the acuteness of the disorder (Hartlage & Hartlage, 1977), and environmental history (Dean, 1983a) greatly complicate inferences about localization of brain functions with children. These factors emphasize the fact that similar lesions in mature and developing nervous systems may produce far different test patterns and expectations for the recovery of neuropsychological functioning (Dean, 1986a; Hartlage, 1981; Reed, Reitan, & Klove, 1965). Indeed, differential diagnosis of neurological disorders with children remains a more tenuous undertaking than that with adults.

Even when evidence of neurological insult exists, it often becomes difficult for the neuropsychologist to separate physiological changes of the brain from the frustration and stress associated with perceived changes in functioning as etiological factors in associated psychiatric disorders (Dean, 1985). Whatever the underlying mechanism, there appears to be a relationship between impairment and objective measures of psychopathology for neurological patients. Heaton and Crowley (1981) examined the relationship between an overall measure of neuropsychological impairment (average impairment ratings) and scales of the Minnesota Multiphasic Personality Inventory (MMPI) for both psychiatric and neurology patients. Although psychiatric patients were shown to exhibit more psychopathology, the relationship between the MMPI scales and impairment on the Halstead–Reitan Battery was minor. However, for neurological patients, the relationship between neuropsychological impairment and the MMPI was significant for 9 of the 12 scales examined. Similarly to prior research with other neurology patients (Lezak & Glaudin, 1969), impairment was most clearly associated with higher scores on the neurotic triad (hypochondriasis, depression, hysteria) and on the schizophrenia scale of the MMPI. It should be noted, however, while these associations were clear, each was rather modest ($> .35$). Thus, although it may be possible to cite neurological abnormality as a clear etiologic factor, from these data one is not able to argue in favor of psychiatric symptoms as a direct result of brain aberrations.

Although the preceding results are less than conclusive for adults, an even more confused picture exists for children. Moreover, numerous investigators who have examined psychiatric/emotional symptoms for brain-damaged children have failed to uncover specific symptoms or behaviors that may be seen as characteristic of neurologic abnormality (Ernhart, Graham, Eichman, Marshall, & Thurston, 1963; Rutter, 1977; Shaffer, 1974). This in no way, of course, lessens the six times greater risk of emotional disturbance for brain-damaged children than that found with normals (Rutter, 1977). Although overall low intellectual level and the presence of seizures increase the risk of emotional disturbance in brain-damaged children, there is less than a perfect relationship between these factors and diagnosable psychiatric disorders (Shaffer, 1974). Dean (1985) argues in favor of significant methodological difficulties that have limited research conclusions in this area. Specifically, greater sophistication in criteria definition with children has limited our ability to more fully understand and diagnose childhood psychiatric disorders. Thus, efforts to relate objective dimensions of behavior to levels of neuropsychological impairment may be a fruitful method to pursue the question of emotional disturbance in brain-damaged children.

NEUROPSYCHOLOGY OF
PSYCHIATRIC DISORDERS

The neuropsychological study of organic and functional psychiatric disorders has focused on differential diagnosis (Dean, 1985). In the past, neuropsychological impairment in psychiatric patients had been attributed to confusion in thought processes consistent with a psychosocial etiology. However, recent research suggests that many functional psychiatric disorders may have an underlying organic substrate that is reflected in neuropsychological assessment findings. With a review of early research that has attempted differential diagnoses of patients with mixed functional psychiatric and organic disorders, it becomes clear that standard neuropsychological test batteries suffered significant reduction in accuracy (Goldstein & Halperin, 1977). In the main, a tendency has been reported for measures of neuropsychological functioning to misdiagnose patients with functional mental disorders as brain damaged (Coolidge, 1976). However, more-recent research and a re-examination of early efforts indicates that the misdiagnosing of organic and functional mental disorders is directly proportional to the number of chronic or process schizophrenics included in groups of patients with functional psychiatric disorders (Dean, 1985; Heaton, Baade, & Johnson, 1978; Klonoff, Fibiger, & Hutton, 1970).

Indeed, the accuracy of diagnosing functional psychiatric and organic disorders using neuropsychological methods suffers when chronic schizophrenics are subsumed as a functional disorder. This conclusion is clearly portrayed by Heaton et al. (1978) in a metanalysis of the neuropsychological research of psychiatric disorders. In this investigation, Heaton et al. (1978) reported a media classification accuracy of functional and organic patients not significantly different than that most often reported between brain damaged and normals when chronic schizophrenics are eliminated from consideration. However, the accuracy in diagnosing functional and organic disorders with standard neuropsychological batteries approached the chance level (54%) when chronic schizophrenics are included in the analysis as a functional psychiatric disorder (Heaton et al., 1978). Research since Heaton et al.'s (1978) review substantiate their conclusions (Dean, 1985; Heaton & Crowley, 1981) concerning the neuropsychological similarities between process schizophrenics and patients with diffuse brain damage.

Research that has focused more specifically on childhood psychopathology further blurs the distinction between functional and organically related psychiatric disorders (Dean, 1985, 1986a). A number of investigators who have examined groups of children and adolescents with psychiatric disorders using neuropsychological measures cite brain dysfunction as a contributing factor in psychopathology (Hertzig & Birch, 1968; Seidel, Chadwick, & Rutter, 1975). Studying a group of adolescents with various psychiatric disorders, Hertzig and Birch (1968) reported that some 34% of these subjects were neurologically impaired. This finding stands in contrast to the rate of neurological dysfunction expected in the normal population (5%).

More recently, Tramontana, Sherrets, and Golden (1980), using the Halstead–Reitan Battery, reported that 60% of the child and adolescent (9–15 years) psychiatric patients examined had some form of neuropsychological abnormality. Interestingly, all of the children in this study had negative clinical neurological examinations when admitted to the psychiatric facility. Although generalizations are difficult, the areas of most severe impairment were tasks requiring complex cognitive–perceptual manipulation followed by sensory/sensory–motor deficits. These data are consistent with Rutter's (1977) earlier report, in that children with psychiatric disorders and normal neurological examinations, electroencephalograms, and histories were found to present with neuropsychological evidence of cerebral dysfunction.

Neuropsychological impairment found with child psychiatric patients seems related to the chronicity of the disorder. Indeed, a number of researchers have reported a higher probability of neuropsychological dysfunction when the duration of the presenting disorder exceeded 2 years (Tramontana, et al., 1980). As mentioned, a similar relationship between impairment and chronicity has been reported with schizophrenics (e.g., Wehler & Hoffman, 1978; Klonoff et al., 1970). Although any causative statement must be approached with care, neuropsychological impairment in the psychiatric patient increases the probability that one is dealing with a more-static disorder with a less-than-encouraging prognosis (Dean, 1985).

Cerebral Lateralization

Laboratory and clinical research over the past century suggest the hemispheres of the brain have specialized functions (Dean, 1986b). Empirical consideration of this phenomenon may be traced to clinical reports with individual brain-damaged patients of the late nineteenth century (Broca, 1861/1960; Dax, 1865; Jackson, 1874/1932). Since this time, rather convincing evidence has evolved favoring the functional lateralization of verbal–analytical or temporal processing to the left cerebral hemisphere in most normal right-handed individuals (e.g., Gazzaniga, 1970; Geschwind, 1974; Sperry, 1974; Dean & Hua, 1982). However, the right hemisphere has been portrayed as processing information in a more holistic, simultaneous, or visuospatial fashion (e.g., Milner, 1967, 1968; Sperry, 1974). Such research has provided neuropsychology a base from which localization inferences may be approached (Dean, 1986b; Hecaen, 1962). Although numerous variables confound the localization process so as to call into question highly specific, structural localization of functions, hemispheric differences remain of clinical utility in neuropsychological assessment (Dean, 1986b). Whereas consistent hemispheric differences are acknowledged by most neuroscientists, debate continues whether processing (Geschwind & Levitsky, 1968), attention (Kinsbourne, 1975), or storage (Hardyck, Tzeng, & Wang, 1978) are responsible for these observed differences.

The lack of, or incomplete, lateralization of functions to the hemispheres of the brain has frequently been cited as an etiological factor in a number of unadjusted behaviors (e.g., learning disorders, emotional disturbance, and the such) (e.g., Hicks and Pellegrini, 1978; Orton, 1937). Consistent with this point of view, investigators have reported significantly greater mixed lateralization in groups of psychotic patients than that seen with normals (Flor-Henry, 1977; Gur, 1977; Lishman & McMeekan, 1976; Nasrallah, McCalley-Whitters, & Kuperman, 1982; Walker & Birch, 1970). Luchins, Weinberger, and Wyatt (1979) for example, reported anomalous lateralization to occur more frequently in milder forms of schizophrenia than in other disorders.

However, at least one investigation has offered evidence favoring confused lateralization for schizoaffective psychotics, but not schizophrenics, as a distant disorder (Lishman & McMeekan, 1976). Dean, Schwartz, and Hua (in press) examined the motoric lateralization for three psychiatric groups formed using research diagnostic criteria. In this study, 30 schizophrenics were compared with like numbers of schizoaffectives and unipolar depressives on a multifactor measure of laterality. These data showed depressive and schizoaffective patients to be similar in laterality and significantly less mixed than schizophrenics on tasks requiring visual guided movement and visual preference. Interestingly, groups did not differ when summed across factors of dominance. Further, analyses of eye–hand patterns showed that schizophrenics had significantly more discrepant patterns than either depressives or schizoaffective patients. These data were interpreted as further support for considering schizoaffective illness as more of an affective disorder than schizophrenia. This finding of confused lateralization for schizophrenics seems robust when consistent criteria are used in diagnoses. Using DSM III criteria for schizophrenia, Piron, Bigler, and Cohen (1982) offer evidence favoring confused lateralization for schizophrenics with an early and gradual onset (process) of symptoms when compared to a general psychiatric control group.

Other research that has approached the question of confused lateralization and psychiatric symptoms for children and adolescents offers tentative data favoring the association of unadjusted behavior and more-confused patterns of lateralization (Blau, 1977; Dean & Smith, 1982; Hicks & Pellegrini, 1978; Orme, 1970). These data portray higher levels of anxiety as a concomitant of confused lateralization (Dean and Smith, 1982; Hicks & Pellegrini, 1978). Some evidence also suggests that inconsistency in patterns of peripheral activities in children may accompany objective measures of emotional instability and compromised frustration tolerance (Blau, 1977; Dean & Smith, 1982).

Although some rather interesting theories have been offered that cite confused cerebral dominance as an etiological factor in emotional disturbance (e.g., Blau, 1977), the basic correlational nature of the data in this area makes such conclusions tenuous. Indeed, while more symmetrical patterns of lateralization may be more preventative in some form of emotional disturbance, confused lateralization and aberrant behavior patterns may both have a common neurological cause (Dean, 1986b).

Such a hypothesis has been offered by Satz (1972) and seems as parsimonious with our present database as causative notions. Satz (1972) has suggested that incomplete dominance may be tied to early brain insult and with it the development of more functional symmetry than that found in normals. Congruent with Satz's theoretical formulation, Piran et al. (1982) suggest a shift in lateralization consistent with left-hemispheric dysfunction in many process schizophrenics. Clearly, the relationship between cerebral lateralization and psychiatric disorders remains to be fully explicated. At this point in time, confused or mixed cerebral lateralization should probably be a factor worthy of further investigation with the individual patient but is not pathological in isolation.

Psychoactive Medication

Although some authors have attributed neuropsychological impairment found with schizophrenics to extrapyramidal effects associated with neuroleptic medication, few systematic data substantiate this hypothesis. In a comprehensive review of the research in this area, Heaton and Crowley (1981) found little support for the hypothesis when confounding variables of severity of disturbance and length of hospitalization were controlled. In fact, some evidence suggests improved neuropsychological performance on measures of attention and cognitive functioning corresponding to a therapeutic response on neuroleptic medication following a 2- to 3-week stabilization period (Baker, 1968). It is important to note, one must ensure stabilization or be prepared to account for the confounding effect of extrapyramidal motor symptoms on neuropsychological performance most often seen in the initial phases of a neuroleptic drug regimen.

For various reasons, neuropsychological implications of medication in the treatment of affective disorders has received less attention. Nevertheless, from the evidence available, it seems that one may expect a significant, yet minor, neuropsychological performance deficit with a regimen of lithium carbonate (Judd, Hubbard, Janowsky, Huey, & Takahashi, 1977). While the research rarely shows levels indicative of brain damage, a relative deficit on measures associated with motor performance and abstract manipulation has been reported with lithium carbonate (Judd et al., 1977). Moreover, this deficit has been shown to exist even when blood lithium levels are in the therapeutic range (Small, Small, Milstein, & Moore, 1972). Similar to findings with lithium, research that has examined the neuropsychological effects of therapeutic levels of tricyclic antidepressants has failed to uncover any profound changes in neuropsychological findings concomitant with these medications (Liljequist, Linnoila, & Mattila, 1974); and, some studies have reported improvement (Sternberg & Jarvik, 1976). Interestingly, although consistent side effects have been reported for tricyclic drugs, the neuropsychological effects do not appear severe enough to misdiagnose individual performance as brain damaged (Covi, Lipman, Derocatis, Smith, & Pattison, 1974).

Level of Emotional Disturbance

From a review of the available research, it seems fair to conclude that the degree of emotional disturbance for mixed groups of psychiatric patients is not as closely related to performance on measures of neuropsychological functioning as once thought (Perkins, 1974; Spaulding, 1978; Squire & Chace, 1975). However, when chronic (process) schizophrenics are studied in isolation, the level of disturbance (measured by clinical and psychometric methods) is inversely related to performance on measures of neuropsychological functioning (Dean, 1983b; T. E. Smith & Boyce, 1962). These findings of impaired functioning concomitant with the acuteness of disturbance for schizophrenics are more similar to data with neurological patients who have suffered documented lesions than those with other psychiatric disorders. In both schizophrenics and brain-damaged patients, the level of emotional disturbance has been shown to be related to the degree of impairment. In psychiatric patients other than schizophrenics, the relationship between the degree of behavioral disturbance and neuropsychological impairment is not a robust finding (e.g., affective disorders, neurotic disturbances). Thus, chronic schizophrenics appear more similar to neurological patients than to patients with other psychiatric disorders when the relationship between the degree of emotional disturbance and neuropsychological assessment findings are examined. It seems clear that past difficulties in differentiating psychiatric groups from brain-damaged patients may well relate to an underlying neurological substrate for some functional mental disorders. The investigation of distinguishing neuropsychological patterns for specific functional mental disorders has only begun to be examined in a systematic fashion. Moreover, neuropsychological research interest in psychiatric disorders has been renewed with the continuing rigor of criteria for nosological inclusion. Dean (1985) argues that neuropsychology assessment in the psychiatric setting may begin to offer diagnostic markers of specific psychiatric disorders.

DIAGNOSTIC ISSUES

The diagnosis of psychiatric disorders has historically relied on clinical judgment. Although the subjectivity inherent in clinical judgment continues as an obstacle to reliable diagnosis, attempts have been made to develop objective diagnostic criteria (American Psychiatric Association [APA], 1980; Feighner, Robins, Guze, Woodruff, Winokur, & Munoz, 1972; Spitzer, Endicott, & Robins, 1978). This trend comes in response to the growing recognition of the importance of consistency in diagnosis for both clinical practice and research. Clearly, the continuing sophistication of somatic treatment approaches is predicated on an increasing nosological refinement. Dean, (1985) argues that the generalizability of research in the past has been hampered by diagnostic inconsistencies of the disorders under investigation. Indeed, the error variance inherent in diagnosis has been less than completely considered in psychiatric research of the recent past (Spitzer et al., 1978).

The refinement of nosological groups is an encouraging influence in research examining neuropsychological aspects of psychiatric disorders. Although the use of diagnostic criteria is generally seen as a positive direction in psychiatry, problems remain in comparing diagnoses that may employ different criteria. Indeed, while sets of diagnostic criteria have been shown to have similar reliability, patients diagnosed as schizophrenic by one system, for example, may receive an entirely different diagnosis when the criteria of another system are used (e.g., Endicott, Nee, Fleiss, Cohen, Williams, & Simon, 1982).

In any event, refinements in an agreed-upon diagnostic approach have

TABLE 1

Multiaxial diagnostic approach of DSM III

Axis	Features considered
I	Clinical syndromes
II	Personality and specific developmental disorders
III	Severity of psychosocial stresses
IV	Highest level of adaptive functioning in the past year

the potential for regularization in communication and treatment planning. In addition, the move toward objectifying diagnosis should promote a database useful for the future understanding of mental disorders (Feighner et al., 1972). It should be recognized that the use of diagnostic criteria represents an atheoretical–empirical approach to the psychopathological process. Viewing psychopathology as a complex interaction of biological, social, and psychological factors, the move toward diagnostic criteria is less concerned with etiology than other branches of clinical medicine. Thus, recent research has focused more on consistency in diagnosis than offering evidence necessary to substantiate individual diagnostic constructs (e.g., schizophrenia) (Dean, 1985).

With the publication of the *Diagnostic and Statistical Manual of Mental Disorders* (DSM III; APA, 1980), much of the subjectivity in the criteria for diagnosis was reduced. Although criticisms exist, the multiaxial approach taken by DSM III increases the likelihood that attention will be paid to aspects of the patient's environment that would be overlooked if a single diagnosis was maintained. As shown in Table 1, the multiaxial approach allows consideration of the patient's primary diagnosis and the etiological, physical, and environmental factors that may be contributing to the presenting symptomatology. From a research point of view, such efforts offer a promising direction in the reduction of error variance in the formation of psychiatric groups. Though this is an area of a good deal of research activity, criteria useful in diagnosing disorders with childhood onsets seem less precise than those presently available for adults (Dean, 1985).

Table 2 presents the major DSM III psychiatric disorders often seen first in infancy, childhood, or adolescence. Within this diagnostic scheme, the essential features of affective disorders and schizophrenia are portrayed as the same in both children and adults (APA, 1980). Therefore, the criteria for these disorders are purported to be similar across the life span. Although there is less than complete agreement as to the need for specific criteria for the diagnosis of affective disorders and schizophrenia in children and adolescents, the symptomatology necessary for diagnosis at present remains the same (Dean, 1985). Because of a potential social stigma and the prognosis associated with both these disorders, there seems to be a greater likelihood that children and adolescents will not receive such a diagnosis.

FUNCTIONAL PSYCHIATRIC DISORDERS

The majority of neuropsychological referrals in the psychiatric setting involve differential diagnostic questions where equivocal evidence exists favoring an organic base to a patient's psychiatric symptoms. In light of this fact, the functional–organic distinction made between psychiatric disorders deserves careful scrutiny. Indeed, the often-made distinction between functional (affective disorders, schizophrenia, and the like) and organic (organic brain syndrome, etc.) mental disorders is not as clear as once assumed. The assumption had been, of course, that functional disturbances were related less to abnormal brain functioning than to psychosocial influences. Although the terms hold a good deal of tradition in psychiatric literature, a recent database has accumulated that questions the biochemical and structural normality in the brains of patients with diagnosed psychiatric disorders hitherto assumed to have a functional locus. Neurological aspects of psychiatric disorders are examined in more depth later in this chapter. However, it suffices to say that the available evidence indicates rather clear that biochemical (Fish, 1977; Glassman, Perel, Shostak, Kantor, & Fleiss, 1977; Young, Taylor, & Holmstrom, 1977) and structural (Andreasen, Olsen, Dennert, & Smith, 1982; Johnstone, Crow, Frith, Husband, & Kreel, 1976) neurological abnormalities exist for a number of psychiatric disorders. In fact, neurochemical abnormalities have been identified for patients with both affective disorders (Glassman et al., 1977; Jarvik, 1977; Young et al., 1977) and some forms of schizophrenia (Fish, 1977; Goodman & Gilman, 1975). The force of these data are also supported by findings of aberrations in the brain structure and function for patients diagnosed as schizophrenic (Andreasen et al., 1982; Huag, 1963; Mirsky, 1969). It seems that for more debilitating forms of schizophrenia, a greater probability exists for both abnormal electrical activity (EEG) (Lester & Edwards, 1966) and enlargement of ventricular structures (Luchins, 1982). Similarly, patients diagnosed with primary affective disorders–depression have been shown to have an abnormal decrease in activity of the right hemisphere (d'Elia & Perris, 1974); and, more specifically, abnormal EEG findings have been reported in the area of the right temporal lobe (Flor-Henry, 1976). These data

TABLE 2

Major groups of DSM III psychiatric disorders often first seen in infancy, childhood, or adolescence

Behavior group by disorder

I. Intellectual
  Mental retardation (Mid–Unspecified)
II. Behavioral (Overt)
  Attention deficit disorder (with or without hyperactivity)
  Conduct disorder
    Undersocialized, aggressive
    Undersocialized, nonaggressive
    Socialized, aggressive
    Socialized, nonaggressive
    Atypical
III. Emotional
  Anxiety disorders
    Separation anxiety disorder
    Avoidant disorder
    Overanxious disorder
  Other disorders
    Reactive attachment—infancy
    Schizoid disorder
    Elective mutism
    Oppositional disorder
    Identity disorder
IV. Physical
  Eating disorders
    Anorexia nervosa
    Bulimia
    Pica
    Rumination disorder
  Stereotyped movement disorders
    Chronic motor tic
    Tourette's disorder
    Atypical stereotyped movement disorder
  Other disorders with physical manifestations
    Stuttering
    Functional enuresis
    Functional encopresis
    Sleepwalking disorders
    Sleep terror disorders
V. Development
  Pervasive developmental disorders
    Infantile autism
    Infantile autism—residual
    Childhood pervasive
      Developmental disorder

TABLE 2 (*Continued*)

Behavior group by disorder
Specific developmental disorder (axis II)
Developmental reading disorder
Arithmetic disorder
Language disorder (expressive & receptive)
Articulation disorder
Mixed specific disorder
Atypical specific

question the long-held distinction between organic and functional mental disorders. Dean (1985) argues that the organic–functional distinction for mental disorders would seem better understood as a continuum.

In sum, the available evidence cause one to question the traditional assumption that functional psychiatric disturbances (e.g., schizophrenia) are directly attributable to psychosocial influences. As just reviewed briefly, relatively recent research that examined neuropsychological aspects of psychiatric disorders has focused on differential diagnoses of functional, mixed, psychiatric, and organically related disorders (e.g., Golden, 1977; Klonoff et al., 1970; Matthews, Shaw, & Klove, 1966; Parsons & Klein, 1970; Reitan, 1976; Watson, Thomas, Anderson, & Felling, 1968). More-recent research, however, has begun to focus attention on the neuropsychological portrayal of specific functional mental disorders (Dean, 1982b; Flor-Henry, Fromm-Auch, Tappert, & Schoplocher, 1981; Rockford, Detre, Tucker, & Harrow, 1970; Taylor, Greenspan, & Abrams, 1979). Obviously, this research poses far more complex questions than the normal–brain-damaged distinction on which most neuropsychological measures were established (Dean, 1986a).

Intervening variables of medical history, age at onset, education developmental level, site of dysfunction, premorbid environment, and individual differences in anatomical structures are prominent factors in the evaluation of research in neuropsychology. Dean (1985) argues that a number of specialized variables need to be considered in neuropsychological research of psychiatric disorders. The most salient of these concern (1) the chronicity of the mental disorder; (2) secondary organic involvement in functional mental disorders; (3) treatment effects associated with somatic regimens (electroconvulsive treatment, medication, and the like); (4) length of hospitalization; (5) varying severity of individual symptoms; and, (6) contamination of results with the inclusion of patients referred for neuropsychological assessment and thus some clinical reason to suspect a neurological involvement.

Differential Diagnosis

The remainder of this section is devoted to an overview of research that has investigated neuropsychological differences between functional psychiatric disorders. The emphasis here is the identification of commonalities in the research as they may offer differential diagnostic information and directions in our understanding of specific psychiatric disorders.

Attempts to outline neuropsychological aspects of specific psychiatric disorders have grown geometrically since the mid-1970s (Dean, 1985). These efforts seem related quite closely to both the increasing objectivity of diagnostic criteria (e.g., Dean, 1982b; Rockford et al., 1970; Taylor & Abrams, 1984) and advances in the neurological understanding of functional mental disorders (Andreasen et al., 1982). The majority of the investigations in this area have focused on the relative differences in neuropsychological performance for schizophrenics and patients with affective disorders (Dean, 1985). Although often distinguishable from brain-damaged subjects, both groups have shown significant patterns on neuropsychological measures (Flor-Henry, 1976; Golden, Moses, Zelazowski, Graber, Zatz, Horvath, & Berger, 1980; Miller, 1975). In one early attempt to examine the neuropsychological differences between schizophrenic patients and those with affective disorders, Flor-Henry (1976) employed a multivariate design. Although methodological concerns exist, patients were correctly classified on the basis of neuropsychological performance with some 90% accuracy. In this study, both groups of patients were seen as having a relative frontal–temporal impairment. However, as a group, patients with affective disorders were relatively more deficient on right-hemispheric tasks than schizophrenics. These data, showing a relative deficit for patients with affective disorders, have been replicated and extended to include both unipolar and bipolar affective disorders (Abrams & Taylor, 1980; Taylor et al., 1979). Findings of right-hemispheric dysfunction for patients with affective disorders shown with neuropsychological methods are consistent with findings of aberrant right hemispheric electrical activity (EEG) (d'Elia & Perris, 1974).

Research efforts to isolate specific patterns of defects for schizophrenics have shown chronic schizophrenia to be more clearly related to an overall level of neuropsychological dysfunction than specific patterns of impairment (Taylor & Abrams, 1984). When neuropsychological protocol are evaluated blind to diagnosis, they are most likely to be interpreted as diffuse brain dysfunctioned when compared with the performance of individuals with documented brain damage (Dean, 1983b; Taylor & Abrams, 1984). Research that has compared the relationship between neuropsychological assessment findings and tests that require less overt responses from the patient (Electroencephalogram, computerized axial tomography [CAT] scan, and the like) support neuropsychological findings of rather diffuse abnormalities in the brains of schizophrenics (Andreasen et al., 1982; Shagass, Roemer, and Straumanis, 1982). Clearly, neurological dysfunction has been shown for schizophrenics in isolation and when compared with normals and other psychiatric disorders (Dean, 1983a; Joslyn & Hutzell, 1979; Piran et al., 1982).

Although schizophrenics have most often been reported to present neuropsychologically with a rather diffuse impairment (e.g., Flor-Henry, 1976; Rockford et al., 1970), some evidence suggests a relative left-hemispheric impairment for schizophrenics. Such inconsistent findings may well relate to differences in the degree to which chronic schizophrenics were included (Heaton & Crowley, 1981). Indeed, process schizophrenics (chronic) are most often found to be diffusely impaired on neuropsychological performance measures (Dean, 1985).

Apparently, the criteria used in diagnosing subjects may be another important factor in neuropsychological results. Although objective diagnostic criteria would seem preferable to clinical impressions, diagnosis has been shown to vary with the criteria used (Endicott et al., 1982). Moreover, the diagnosis of schizophrenia made by one set of diagnostic criteria (APA, 1980; Feighner et al., 1972; Spitzer, Endicott, & Robins, 1977, 1978) may not be substantiated by another diagnostic system (Endicott et al., 1982). Therefore, although such systems have similar interrater reliability, a good deal of research will be necessary to establish the construct validity of nosological schemes. However, each approach has utility in establishing more homogeneous groups than would be possible with clinical impressions. Obviously, such inconsistencies in forming groups of schizophrenics account in part for confusion in outlining the neuropsychological manifestations of this disorder.

Data favoring a spectrum of schizophrenic disorders are evident in research that has examined electroencephalographic data. For example, after evaluating a large number of schizophrenics, Hays (1977) discovered those subjects with a family history negative for psychosis to present with aberrant EEG results. Congruent with this finding, Hays also reported a higher frequency of head injuries for schizophrenics without such a family history. Klonoff et al. (1970), in examining neuropsychological patterns of performance for chronic schizophrenics, report a significant improvement in test performance related to a clinical improvement in psychiatric conditions. Although the research is less than conclusive, it seems clear that distinctions within schizophrenia such as the chronic–reactive dimension may hold promise in outlining distinctive neurological patterns. The more basic question, of course, relates to the heuristic value of schizophrenia as a single nosological category. It is also worth noting that these findings are based on adult patients. While most diagnostic schemes portray schizophrenia and affective disorders as essentially the same in adults and children, few data bear on this question.

Flor-Henry and associates (Flor-Henry et al., 1981; Flor-Henry, Yeudall, Koles, & Howorth, 1979) have reported initial data that the neuropsychological differences found with schizophrenics and patients with affective disorders may extend to other psychiatric disturbances. Although many of these findings are less striking and remain to be replicated across laboratories, they portray continuing efforts to examine the neuropsychological consequences of psychiatric disorders.

ORGANIC PSYCHIATRIC DISORDERS

Unsuccessful attempts to define the sequelae of a classic organic syndrome offers an appreciation for the complexity of brain–behavior relationships (Dean, 1985). The clinical notion of organicity as though it were a unitary entity seems related in part to the long standing functional–organic psychiatric distinction. The hypothesis itself would seem to have arisen from theories that portrayed the behavioral or emotional effects of brain damage as similar regardless of location of the lesion. The assumption underlying this hypothesis is that variations in the psychiatric symptoms of brain damage were seen to be less related to the type or location of a lesion than an interaction of the severity of cortical involvement and the patient's premorbid personality (Hughes, 1948; Piotrowski, 1937). Therefore, a classic syndrome of behavioral and psychogenic signs as being the archtype of organicity was sought. Although this notion continues to be exposed in some clinical settings, it has been successfully challenged with systematic investigations. These investigations have shown distinctly different, behavioral consequences can be attributed to focal lesions that differed in location (Reitan, 1955a, 1955b; Gazzaniga & Sperry, 1962). Indeed, research that has considered the patient's age, the acuteness of the lesion, and the length of the interval between brain damage and assessment interact in such a fashion as to seriously question the heuristic value of organicity as a unitary syndrome (Dean, 1985; Reitan, 1974).

The concentration of research on the neuropsychiatric aspects of specific neurological disorders has grown geometrically since the early 1960s. Early investigations attempted to validate neuropsychological predictions of brain damage for groups with rather heterogeneous lesions. Since these seminal efforts, researchers have begun to define distinct, emotional, cognitive, and psychomotor symptoms associated with a number of specific neurological disorders. Clearly, these data have significant implications in differential diagnosis and evaluating the success of medical interventions. Although differentiation of symptom constellations is compromised by factors such as the type, locus, age, and extent of the lesion, some consistencies remain. With this caveat in mind, the overriding criterion for the choice of areas that follow was the direct relevance to child neuropsychiatry.

Head Injuries

The relationship between psychiatric disturbance and head injury in children is complex. A number of investigators have reported significantly greater numbers of psychiatric symptoms for children with head injury than that found in normals (Shaffer, 1974). However, other research approaches indicate impaired neuropsychological functioning to occur more frequently in emotionally disturbed children than in normals (Reed & Reitan, 1963). Thus, difficulties often arise when attempts are made to consider the etiology of disorders.

Head injuries have been related to disturbances in cognitive and emotionally related behavior. While it is not possible to consider psychiatric symptomatology as a direct result of head trauma, certainly the data clearly favors a two-fold risk of psychiatric disorders (Dean, 1986b). The first risk factor relates to the actual physiological alteration in brain function, which may be the etiology of the psychiatric symptoms. A second, yet-related, factor concerns the patient's perceptions of changes in neuropsychological functioning, which offers sufficient psychosocial stress to account for the expression of psychiatric symptoms.

Common psychiatric symptoms reported following a head injury involve anxiety, depression, impulsivity, and distractibility (Boll, 1974; Dean, 1983b; Luria, 1966; Reitan, 1966). These symptoms may be present following head injuries even when physical diagnostic information is negative (e.g., CT Scan) (Schiffer, 1983). In such instances, when other diagnostic procedures are noncontributory, neuropsychological assessment procedures are useful in evaluating posttraumatic functional impairments. Moreover, neuropsychological data offer diagnostic information in the psychiatric setting relevant to the course of recovery and treatment approaches.

The interpretation of research that has examined the behavioral effects of localized lesions is often complicated by a failure to control for *contra-*

coup (Dean, 1985). This is to say, although measurable brain damage may be clear at the point of impact, the damage caused as the brain rebounds within the cranium is sometimes less obvious (Gardner, 1968). Although other methodological difficulties exist in this area of research, the majority of studies with patients who had suffered unilateral traumatic lesions report emotional disturbances that vary with the hemisphere involved. Gainotti (1972), for example, reports a significantly greater likelihood that damage to the right hemisphere will result in clinical levels of anxiety. Patients with lesions to the right hemisphere also are more likely to exhibit a general denial and rather inappropriate indifference to their medical condition. The emotional response to lesions of the left hemisphere seem most often expressed as depression–castastrophic reaction (Dikman & Reitan, 1977). In general, the research in this area has involved the documentation of lesions by physical means (surgery, CAT scan, and the like). Moreover, the relationship between new lines of neuropsychological functioning and emotional functioning is less well understood.

The patterns of neuropsychological dysfunction following head injury seem quite different for adults and children (Boll, 1974; Reed et al. 1965). That is to say, brain-injured children seem to have more-diffuse neuropsychological impairment than that seen in adults with similar lesions. Ernhart et al. (1963) report that following head injury, children are more likely to show impairment of those cognitive abilities (e.g., vocabulary) that are resistant to impairment in adults. Clearly, some of these differences may relate to the aforementioned factors (e.g., brain development at onset) that combine interactively to make reliable conclusions concerning the functioning of the child's brain a far more tentative undertaking than that with adults. At the same time, the work of Klonoff and his colleagues (Klonoff, Low, & Clark, 1977; Klonoff & Robinson, 1967; Klonoff & Thompson, 1969) suggests that the type of head injury children suffer may be responsible in part for the child–adult differences in neuropsychological impairment following head injury. Apparently, children are approximately three times more likely to present with brain damage resulting from falls than head injuries for adults. The extent to which the etiology of the brain damage interacts with neurodevelopmental factors in producing child–adult differences following head injury remains to be fully investigated.

Although clinical importance is often given to the duration of unconsciousness following trauma, neuropsychological and psychiatric data stress the importance of posttraumatic amnesia. Russell and Smith (1961) examined over 1700 adults who had suffered closed-head injuries. In this study, the duration of posttraumatic amnesia was the most salient index of the extent of cortical dysfunction. It is interesting to note this was true even in patients without identifiable structural lesions. Evidence since Russell and Smith's early report indicates that with both open- and closed-head injuries, the extent and duration of posttraumatic amnesia represent the most reliable measure of cortical damage and offers the best single predictor of neuropsychological and psychiatric impairment up to 5 years following injury (A. Smith, 1981; A. Smith & Sugar, 1975). Therefore, it would seem that initial neuropsychological assessment of the head-injured patient with a focus on objectifying the extent of memory loss would make good sense in differential diagnoses and generating a prognosis of continued neuropsychological and psychiatric impairment. Of interest here is the degree to which the clinician can attribute a given constellation of behaviors to actual cortical damage. Clearly, the coexistence of neuropsychological impairment and psychiatric symptomatology offer information relevant to diagnosis and treatment. Moreover, the extent of the patient's neuropsychological impairment and time since trauma are considered; statements may be approached that provide information relative to the prognosis of both the cognitive and psychiatric disturbances.

Seizure Disorders

The spectrum of disorders commonly referred to as epilepsy represents such a heterogeneous group so as to make generalizations difficult. However, certain psychiatric and neuropsychological aspects of functioning with these patients deserves mention. There is a large database portraying the heuristic value of considering the specific seizure type when examining neuropsychological functioning. As would be expected, patients with tonic–clonic seizures have been shown to have more generalized neuropsychological impairment than other seizure types. This stands in contrast to petit mal (generalized absence) attacks, in which these patients as a group do not differ significantly from normals on standardized measures of neuropsychological and emotional functioning. Across the spectrum of seizure disorders, epileptic patients have been shown to score lower on measures of cognitive ability than do normals or mixed psychiatric patients.

A number of factors serve to complicate the specific neuropsychological picture of a patient with a seizure disorder. Of primary importance in assessment must be the type and dosage of the anticonvulsant medication taken by the patient. The neuropsychological and emotional side effects of these drugs are not clear. High blood serum levels of phenytoin, for example, have been shown to relate to impaired motor performance. Therefore, for a given patient, test findings of impaired function may relate more to subcortical effects of phenytoin than cerebral dysfunction.

Although conclusions are somewhat hazardous in this area, it seems fair to say that seizure frequency and age at onset interactively relate to the extent of a patient's neuropsychological impairment (Dikman, Matthews, & Harley, 1977). Research in the area indicates overall greater neuropsychological impairment for adults with earlier onset of seizures. The frequency of seizures also seems important, with the bulk of research suggesting an inverse relationship between frequency and neuropsychological performance. Apparently, both onset age and frequency of seizures are important in predicting the extent of neuropsychological impairment with most forms of seizure disorders (Dean, 1983b; Keating, 1960).

Dean (1983b) has presented evidence that a clinical measure of total lifetime seizures is a better predictor of impaired functioning in children than when either age at onset or seizure frequency are considered separately. From these data, Dean (1983b) argued in favor of neuropsychological implications for the often cited kindling effect associated with total seizures. From this point of view, it seems there is neuropsychological support for biomedical data favoring the early diagnosis and administration of anticonvulsant medication.

Children with seizure disorders also present with a significantly greater number of psychiatric symptoms (anxiety, depression, and the like) than normals (Dean, 1985). Although convenient to assume a direct link between emotional symptoms and abnormal brain function, little data exist to establish such a causal relationship. Other than psychomotor (temporal lobe) attacks, a link between aberrant behavior and seizure disorders has not been established. Moreover, emotional disturbances in the seizure disorder patient may be related to psychosocial factors. The embarrassment and misunderstanding associated with seizure disorders may be as heuristically related to emotional disturbance as specific neurological aberrations. Clearly, neuropsychological assessment that examines both cognitive and emotional components can provide objective data of value in understanding the patient's overall level of functioning.

Specific Developmental Disorders

Children who exhibit learning problems in the absence of hard signs of neurological involvement have often been diagnosed as having a specific developmental disorder (APA, 1980). These children as a group represent an increasingly large proportion of the referrals to child neuropsychologists (Dean, 1982a). The inclusion of specific developmental disorders (i.e., learning disorders, etc.) as a psychiatric disorder (APA, 1980) (or as an organically related disorder for that matter) is not without controversy.

Moreover, children may receive such a diagnosis without specific signs of psychopathology or neurological involvement (APA, 1980). Indeed, children who present with symptoms that meet criterion for this disorder do so only in the educational environment. Although learning disorders are often considered as functional neurological disorders, childhood learning disabilities hold rather clear psychiatric implications. It is not the intent of this section to duplicate efforts concerning neuropsychological aspects of children's learning disorders found elsewhere in this volume (see Hopper and Boyd, Chapter 2 of this Volume) but rather to examine some of the emotional implications for children all with neuropsychological impairment who must interact with the educational system.

It is estimated that between 10 and 20% of primary school students (grades 1–6) do not learn adequately, despite normal intellectual capacity (IQ > 85) (Dean, 1982a). The long-term prognosis for competent social and emotional development is significantly less for these children than that for normal learners (Shaffer, 1972). Moreover, a number of childhood psychiatric diagnoses are significantly more prevalent with learning-disabled children than that found in the normal population (Shepard, Oppenheim, & Mitchell, 1966). At the same time, epidemiological investigations have pointed to an increased risk of psychiatric disorders in adulthood for individuals who were diagnosed as learning disabled as children (Shepard et al., 1966). In spite of such data, neuropsychological approaches to this disorder have focused on various underlying neurological processes, often to the exclusion of children's behavioral history and learned methods of coping with failure (Dean, 1983b; Fisk & Rourke, 1979).

It has been fairly well established that children diagnosed as learning disabled are more likely to display maladaptive emotional patterns in school than normals (Dean, 1982a). Indeed, a number of investigators have reported negative reactions to specific academic areas, and school in general, to exist in children with neuropsychological impairment (Dudek & Lester, 1968; Severson, 1970). Although researchers have pointed to significantly greater numbers of these behaviors (e.g., withdrawal, acting out) (e.g., Harris, 1947; Stott, 1970), few have correlated these behaviors directly with the child's attempt to cope with an educational environment that offers few positive features.

To study this issue, Dean (1983b) examined the ways learning disabled and normal learners coped with obvious failure. Groups of normal children and those with deficits in reading were presented extremely difficult words after they had read simple words. Unlike normal children, when very easy reading material was returned to, learning disabled children seemed unable to recover from the preceding failure. This finding was in contrast to the performance of a similar group of learning-disabled children who were given simple words throughout a session. Thus, it seems that at least some learning-disabled children may cope with classroom failure by withdrawal. In this same study, learning-problem children who experience failure often became reckless in their responses and presented behaviors that were rated less than appropriate for the setting.

Apparently, many children with learning disorders develop a pattern of behavior in the face of failure that is much what one would expect in the development of an aversive reaction to school-related material. From this point of view, these children may develop what could be likened to a phobic reaction in an attempt to cope with failure (Severson, 1970). Thus, it would seem that any intervention not only must focus on neuropsychological processing deficits, but also must examine the compounding effects of the child's personality patterns and methods of coping with failure. Aversive reactions are seen here as going beyond the immediate learning session to the creation of an emotional reaction to those subject areas where failure has occurred. What may begin as an early neuropsychological disorder may well lead to a paradigm of failure–aversion–failure as the child attempts to cope with the stress of failure.

Attempts have begun to isolate behavior constellations from neuropsychological measures, which may promote further understanding of categories of learning problems (Dean, 1978a, 1983b, 1985; Fisk & Rourke, 1979; Rourke, 1975, 1976, 1979). Few serious reviewers have considered learning disorders as a homogeneous diagnostic entity. Clearly, some forms of children's learning disorders relate to specific neurological dysfunction (Dean, 1982a). This conclusion is as obvious as the fact that many childhood learning problems may more heuristically be related to an interaction of environmental and developmental factors. Although a number of authors have argued in favor of a neuropsychological perspective that goes beyond the diagnosis of impaired neurological processes to the structuring of educational programs that maximize the child's assessed strengths (Dean, 1982a; Hartlage & Reynolds, 1981), future attempts to statistically segregate behaviors for children with learning problems hold considerable promise in our understanding and treatment of children's learning disorders.

In sum, although a large proportion of children's learning disorders may well have a neurological base, the child's ability to cope with negative feedback and related emotional factors should be considered simultaneously in establishing nosological classifications or treatment approaches. It seems clear that children with learning disorders cannot be approached simplistically from either a neuropsychological or a psychiatric point of view (Bryant, 1966; Dean, 1983b; Severson, 1970). Indeed, many of these children appear to have adapted methods of coping with failure that are as problematic as the child's original neurological difficulty in learning (Dudek & Lester, 1968). It has become apparent that children with histories of classroom failure retain an underlying aversive reaction to specific school tasks even after obvious success (Lang, 1969). Clearly, consideration of the child's learned pattern of coping with the psychosocial stress of classroom failure seems as important as identifying his or her neuropsychological difficulty. From a rehabilitation point of view, it would seem that children with learning disorders would benefit from an approach that offered academic remediation while attempting to modify negative emotional responses (Dean, 1983b).

SUMMARY

The intent of this chapter was to provide a neuropsychological examination of aspects of children's psychiatric disorders. Following an outline of the historical antecedents of our present understanding of psychiatric disorders, a review of advances in the use of diagnostic criteria was emphasized. Substantive issues in neuropsychological assessment relevant to the psychiatric setting were summarized. The utility of neuropsychological assessment in offering differential diagnostic information in functional and organic mental disorders was reviewed. In general, the rates of acute diagnoses between normals and brain-damaged patients were not seen as significantly different than the rates found when discriminating between organic and functional mental disorders if chronic schizophrenics were eliminated from consideration. Moreover, chronic schizophrenics were seen to more closely resemble patients with diffuse damage in terms of neuropsychological impairment than patients with other functional psychiatric disorders. The neuropsychological implications of more chronic childhood emotional disturbance were addressed. Relative neuropsychological functioning was reviewed for specific functional psychiatric disorders. The future of neuropsychological assessment as a tool to aid in differential diagnosis, treatment planning, and understanding of the etiology of mental disorders was emphasized.

REFERENCES

Abrams, R., & Taylor, M. A. (1980). A comparison of unipolar and bipolar depressive illness. *American Journal of Psychiatry, 137,* 1084.
American Psychiatric Association. (1980). *Diagnostic and statistical manual of mental disorders* (3rd ed.) Washington, DC: Author.

Andreasen, N. C., Olsen, S. A., Dennert, J. W., & Smith, M. R. (1982). Ventricular enlargement in schizophrenia: Relationship to positive and negative symptoms. *American Journal of Psychiatry, 139,* 297–302.

Baker, R. R. (1968). The effects of psychotropic drugs on psychological testing. *Psychological Bulletin, 69,* 77–87.

Benton, A. L. (1974). Clinical neuropsychology of childhood: An overview. In R. M. Reitan & L. A. Davison (Eds.), *Clinical neuropsychology: Current status and applications.* Washington, DC: Hemisphere.

Blau, T. H. (1977). Torque and schizophrenic vulnerability: As the world turns. *American Psychologist, 32,* 997–1005.

Boll, T. J. (1974). Behavioral correlates of cerebral damage in children aged 9 through 14. In R. M. Reitan & L. A. Davison (Eds.), *Clinical neuropsychology: Current status and applications.* Washington, DC: Hemisphere.

Broca, P. (1960). Remarks on the seat of the faculty of articulate language, followed by an observation of aphaesia. In G. von Bonin (Trans.), *Some papers on the cerebral cortex.* Springfield, IL: Charles C. Thomas. (Original work published 1861).

Bryant, N. D. (1966). Clinic inadequacies with learning disorders—The missing clinic educator. In J. Hellmuth (Ed.), *Learning disorders* (Vol. 2). Seattle: Special Child Publications.

Coolidge, F. L. (1976). Discriminant and factor analyses of the WAIS and the Satz–Mogel abbreviated WAIS in brain-damaged and psychiatric patients. *Journal of Consulting and Clinical Psychology, 44,* 153.

Covi, L., Lipman, R. S., Derocatis, L. R., Smith, J. E., & Pattison, J. A. (1974). Drugs and group psychotherapy in neurotic depression. *American Journal of Psychiatry, 131,* 191–198.

Crockett, D., Klonoff, H., & Bejerring, J. (1969). Factor analysis of neuropsychological tests. *Perceptual and Motor Skills, 29,* 791–802.

Dax, G. (1865). Lesions de la moitie gauche de l'encephale coincident avec l'oubli des signes de la pensee. *Gax. Hebrom. Med. Chir, 2,* 259–262.

Dean, R. S. (1978a). Cerebral laterality and reading comprehension. *Neuropsychologia, 16,* 633–636.

Dean, R. S. (1978b). *Laterality preference schedule.* Madison: University of Wisconsin Press.

Dean, R. S. (1982a). Neuropsychological assessment. In T. Kratochwill (Ed.), *Advances in school psychology* (Vol. 2). Hillsdale, NJ: Lawrence Erlbaum Associates.

Dean, R. S. (1982b). Cognitive neuropsychological differences in schizophrenia and primary affective depression. *Proceedings of the Society of Behavioral Medicine* (Vol. 2).

Dean, R. S. (1983a, February). *Dual processing of prose and cerebral laterality.* Paper presented at the annual meeting of the International Neuropsychological Society, Mexico City.

Dean, R. S. (1983b, August). *Integrating neuropsychological and emotional variables in the treatment of children's learning disorders.* Paper presented at the annual convention of the American Psychological Association, Los Angeles.

Dean, R. S. (1985). Neuropsychological assessment. In J. D. Cavenar, R. Michels, H. K. H. Brodie, A. M. Cooper, S. B. Guze, L. L. Judd, G. L. Klerman, & A. J. Solnit (Eds.), *Psychiatry.* Philadelphia: Lippincott.

Dean, R. S. (1986a). Foundation of rationale for neuropsychological bases of individual differences. In L. C. Hartlage & C. F. Telzrow (Eds.), *The neuropsychology of individual differences: A developmental perspective.* New York: Plenum Press.

Dean, R. S. (1986b). Perspectives on the future of neuropsychological assessment. In B. S.

Plake & J. C. Witt (Eds.), *Buros–Nebraska series on measurement and testing*. New York: Lawrence Erlbaum Associates.

Dean, R. S., & Hua, M. S. (1982). Laterality effects in cued auditory asymmetries. *Neuropsychologia, 20*, 685–690.

Dean, R. S., Schwartz, N. H., & Hua, M. S. (in press). Lateral preference patterns in schizophrenia and affective disorders. *Journal of Consulting and Clinical Psychology*.

Dean, R. S., & Smith, L. S. (1982). Personality and lateral preference patterns in children. *Clinical Neuropsychology, 3*, 22–28.

d'Elia, G., & Perris, C. (1974). Cerebral functional dominance and depression: An analysis of EEG amplitude in depressed patients. *Acta Psychiatrica Scandinavica, 49*, 191.

Dikman, S., Matthews, C. G., & Harley, J. P. (1977). Effect of early versus late onset of major motor epilepsy in cognitive–intellectual performance: Further considerations. *Epilepsia, 18*, 31–36.

Dikman, S., & Reitan, R. M. (1977). Emotional sequelae of head injury. *Annals of Neurology, 2*, 492.

Dudek, S., & Lester, E. P. (1968). The good child facade in chronic underachievers. *American Journal of Orthopsychiatry, 38*, 153–159.

Endicott, J., Nee, J., Fleiss, J., Cohen, J., Williams, J. B. W., & Simon, R. (1982). Diagnostic criteria for schizophrenia: Reliabilities and agreement between systems. *Archives of General Psychiatry, 39*, 884.

Ernhart, C. G., Graham, F. K., Eichman, P. L., Marshall, J. M., & Thurston, D. (1963). Brain injury in the preschool child: Some developmental considerations. *Psychological Monographs, 77*(11), 17–33.

Feighner, J. P., Robins, E., Guze, S., Woodruff, R. A., Winokur, G., & Munoz, R. (1972). Diagnostic criteria for use in psychiatric research. *Archives of General Psychiatry, 26*, 57–63.

Fish, B. (1977). Neurobiologic antecedents of schizophrenia in children; evidence for an inherited, congenital neurointegrative defect. *Archives of General Psychiatry, 34*, 1297–1313.

Fisk, J. L., & Rourke, B. P. (1979). Identification of subtypes of learning-disabled children at three age levels: A neuropsychological, multivariate approach. *Journal of Clinical Neuropsychology, 1*, 289–310.

Flor-Henry, P. (1976). Lateralized temporo-limbic dysfunction and psychopathology. *Annals of the New York Academy of Sciences, 280*, 777–797.

Flor-Henry, P. (1977). Progress and problems in psychosurgery. *Current Psychiatric Therapy, 17*, 283–298.

Flor-Henry, P., Fromm-Auch, D., Tappert, M., & Schopflocher, D. (1981). A neuropsychological study of the stable syndrome of hysteria. *Biological Psychiatry, 16*, 601–626.

Flor-Henry, P., Yeudall, L. T., Koles, Z. J., & Howorth, B. G. (1979). Neuropsychological and power spectral EEG investigations of the obsessive–compulsive syndrome. *Biological Psychiatry, 14*, 119–130.

Gainotti, G. (1972). Emotional behavior and hemispheric side of the lesion. *Cortex, 8*, 41.

Gardner, E. (1968). *Fundamentals of neurology* (5th ed.). Philadelphia: Saunders.

Gazzaniga, M. S. (1970). *The bisected brain*. New York: Appleton-Century-Crofts.

Gazzaniga, M. S., & Sperry, R. W. (1962). Language after section of the cerebral commissures. *Brain, 90*, 131–148.

Geschwind, N. (1974). The anatomical basis of hemispheric differentiation. In S. J. Dimond

& J. G. Beaumont (Eds.), *Hemispheric function in the human brain*. New York: Halsted Press.

Geschwind, N., & Levitsky, W. (1968). Human brain: left–right asymmetries in temporal speech region. *Science, 161,* 186–187.

Glassman, A. H., Perel, J. M., Shostak, M., Kantor, S. J., & Fleiss, J. L. (1977). Clinical implications of imipramine plasma levels for depressive illness. *Archives of General Psychiatry, 34,* 197–204.

Golden, C. J. (1977). Validity of the Halstead–Reitan neuropsychological battery in a mixed psychiatric and brain injured population. *Journal of Consulting and Clinical Psychology, 45,* 1043–1051.

Golden, C. J., Moses, J. A., Zelazowski, R., Graber, B., Zatz, L. M., Horvath, T. B., & Berger, P. A. (1980). Cerebral ventricular size and neuropsychological impairment in young chronic schizophrenics. *Archives of General Psychiatry, 37,* 619–623.

Goldstein, G., & Halperin, J. M. (1977). Neuropsychological differences among subtypes of schizophrenia. *Journal of Abnormal Psychology, 86,* 34–40.

Goodman, L. S., & Gilman, A. (1975). *The pharmacological basis of therapeutics.* New York: Macmillan.

Gur, R. E. (1977). Motoric laterality imbalance in schizophrenia. *Archives of General Psychiatry, 34,* 33–37.

Hardyck, C., Tzeng, O. J. L., & Wang, W. S. (1978). Lateralization of function and bilingual judgments: Is thinking lateralized? *Brain and Language, 5,* 56–71.

Harris, A. J. (1947). *Harris tests of lateral dominance.* New York: Psychological Corporation.

Hartlage, L. C. (1981). Neuropsychological assessment techniques. In C. R. Reynolds & T. Gutkin (Eds.), *Handbook of school psychology.* New York: Wiley.

Hartlage, L. C., & Hartlage, P. L. (1977). Psychological testing in neurological diagnosis. In J. Youman (Ed.), *Neurological surgery.* Philadelphia: Saunders.

Hartlage, L. C., & Reynolds, C. R. (1981). Neuropsychological assessment and individualization of instruction. In G. W. Hynd & J. E. Obrzut (Eds.), *Neuropsychological assessment and the school-age child.* New York: Grune & Stratton.

Haug, J. O. (1963). *Pneumoencephalographic studies in mental disease.* Oslo: Universitetsforlaget.

Hays, P. (1977). Electroencephalic variant and genetic predisposition to schizophrenia. *Journal of Neurology, Neurosurgery and Psychiatry, 40,* 753–755.

Heaton, R., Baade, L., & Johnson, K. (1978). Neuropsychological test results associated with psychiatric disorders in adults. *Psychological Bulletin, 85,* 141–163.

Heaton, R. K., & Crowley, T. J. (1981). Effects of psychiatric disorders and their somatic treatments on neuropsychological test results. In S. B. Filskov & T. J. Boll (Eds.), *Handbook of clinical neuropsychology.* New York: Wiley.

Hecaen, H. (1962). Clinical symptomatology in right and left hemisphere lesions. In V. B. Mountcastle (Ed.), *Interhemispheric relations and cerebral dominance.* Baltimore: Johns Hopkins University Press.

Hertzig, M. E., & Birch, H. G. (1968). Neurological organization in psychiatrically disturbed adolescents. *Archives of General Psychiatry, 19,* 528–537.

Hicks, R. A., & Pellegrini, R. J. (1978). Handedness and anxiety. *Cortex, 14,* 119–121.

Hughes, R. M. (1948). Rorschach signs in the diagnosis of organic pathology. *Rorschach Research Exchange, 12,* 165–167.

Jackson, J. H. (1874). On the duality of the brain. *Medical Press, 1,* 19. Reprinted in J.

Taylor (Ed.), *Selected writings of John Hughlings Jackson* (Vol. 1). London: Hodder & Stoughton, 1932.

Jarvik, M. E. (1977). *Psychopharmacology in the practice of medicine.* New York: Appleton-Century-Crofts.

Johnstone, E. C., Crow, T. J., Frith, C. D., Husband, J., & Kreel, L. (1976). Cerebral ventricular size and cognitive impairment in chronic schizophrenia. *Lancet, ii,* 924–926.

Joslyn, T., & Hutzell, P. A. (1979). Computed tomography in schizophrenics and normal volunteers. *Archives of General Psychiatry, 39,* 765–770.

Judd, L. L., Hubbard, B., Janowsky, D. S., Huey, L. Y., & Takahashi, K. I. (1977). The effect of lithium carbonate on the cognitive functions of normal subjects. *Archives of General Psychiatry, 34,* 355.

Keating, L. E. (1960). A review of the literature on the relationship of epilepsy and intelligence in school children. *Journal of Mental Science, 106,* 1042–1059.

Kinsbourne, M. (1975). Cerebral dominance, learning, and cognition. In H. R. Mylebust (Ed.), *Progress in learning disabilities.* New York: Grune & Stratton.

Klonoff, H., Fibiger, C., & Hutton, G. (1970). Neuropsychological patterns in chronic schizophrenia. *Journal of Nervous and Mental Disease, 150,* 291–300.

Klonoff, H., Low, M., & Clark, C. (1977). Head injuries in children, a prospective 5 year follow-up. *Journal of Neurosurgery and Psychiatry, 12,* 1211–1219.

Klonoff, H., & Robinson, G. (1967). Epidemiology of head injuries in children: A pilot study. *Canadian Medical Association Journal, 96,* 1308–1311.

Klonoff, H., & Thompson, G. (1969). Epidemiology of head injuries in adults: A pilot study. *Canadian Medical Association Journal, 100,* 235–241.

Lang, P. J. (1969). The mechanics of desensitization and laboratory study of human fear. In C. M. Franks (Ed.), *Behavior therapy.* New York: McGraw-Hill.

Lester, B. K., & Edwards, J. J. (1966). EEG fast activity in schizophrenics and control subjects. *International Journal of Neuropsychiatry, 2,* 143–156.

Lezak, M. D., & Glaudin, V. (1969). Differential effects of physical illness on MMPI profiles. *Newsletter for Research in Psychology, 11,* 27–28.

Liljequist, R., Linnoila, M., & Mattila, M. J. (1974). Effect of two weeks' treatment with chlovimipramine and nortriptyline, alone or in combination with alcohol, on learning and memory. *Psychopharmacologia, 39,* 181–186.

Lishman, W. A., & McMeekan, E. R. L. (1976). Hand preference patterns in psychiatric patients. *British Journal of Psychiatry, 129,* 158–166.

Luchins, D. J. (1982). Computed tomography in schizophrenia: Disparities in the prevalence of abnormalities. *Archives of General Psychiatry, 39,* 859–860.

Luchins, D. J., Weinberger, D. R., & Wyatt, R. J. (1979). Schizophrenia: Evidence of a subgroup with reversed cerebral asymmetry. *Archives of General Psychiatry, 36,* 1309–1311.

Luria, A. R. (1966). *Human brain and psychological processes.* New York: Harper & Row.

Matthews, C. G., Shaw, D. J., & Klove, H. (1966). Psychological test performances in neurologic and "pseudoneurologic" subjects. *Cortex, 2,* 244–253.

Miller, W. R. (1975). Psychological deficit in depression. *Psychological Bulletin, 82,* 238–260.

Milner, B. (1967). Brain mechanisms suggested by studies of temporal lobes. In C. H. Millikan & F. L. Darley (Eds.), *Brain mechanisms underlying speech and language.* New York: Grune & Stratton.

Milner, B. (1968). Visual recognition and recall after right temporal-lobe excision in man. *Neuropsychologia, 6,* 191–209.

Mirsky, A. F. (1969). Neuropsychological bases of schizophrenia. *Annual Review of Psychology, 20.*

Nasrallah, H. A., McCalley-Whitters, M., & Kuperman, S. (1982). Neurological differences between paranoid and non-paranoid schizophrenia: I. Sensory-motor lateralization. *Journal of Clinical Psychiatry, 43,* 305–306.

Orme, J. E. (1970). Left-handedness ability and emotional instability. *British Journal of Social and Clinical Psychology, 9,* 87–88.

Orton, S. T. (1937). Specific reading disability—strephosymbolia. *Journal of the American Medical Association, 90,* 1095–1099.

Parsons, O., & Klein,H. (1970). Concept of identification and practice in brain damaged and process reactive schizophrenic groups. *Journal of Consulting and Clinical Psychology, 35,* 317–323.

Perkins, C. W. (1974). Some correlates of category test scores for non-organic psychiatric patients. *Journal of Clinical Psychology, 30,* 176–178.

Piotrowski, Z. A. (1937). The Rorschach inkblot method in organic disturbances of the central nervous system. *Journal of Nervous and Mental Disease, 86,* 525–537.

Piran, N., Bigler, E. D., & Cohen, D. (1982). Motoric laterality and eye dominance suggest unique pattern of cerebral organization in schizophrenia. *Archives of General Psychiatry, 39,* 1006–1010.

Reed, H. B. C., & Reitan, R. M. (1963). Intelligence test performance of brain damaged subjects with lateralized motor deficits. *Journal of Consulting Psychology, 27,* 102–106.

Reed, H. B. C., & Reitan, R. M., & Klove, H. (1965). The influence of cerebral lesions on psychological test performance of older children. *Journal of Consulting Psychology, 29,* 247–251.

Reitan, R. M. (1955a). Certain differential effects of left and right cerebral lesions in human adults. *Journal of Comparative and Physiological Psychology, 48,* 474–477.

Reitan, R. M. (1955b). An investigation of the validity of Halstead's measures of biological intelligence. *Archives of Neurology and Psychiatry, 73,* 28–35.

Reitan, R. M. (1966). Problems and prospects in studying the psychological correlates of brain lesions. *Cortex, 2,* 127.

Reitan, R. M. (1974). Methodological problems in clinical neuropsychology. In R. M. Reitan & L. A. Davison (Eds.), *Clinical neuropsychology: Current status and applications.* Washington, DC: Hemisphere.

Reitan, R. M. (1976). Neurological and physiological bases of psychopathology. *Annual Review of Psychology, 27,* 189–216.

Rockford, J. M., Detre, T., Tucker, G. T., & Harrow, O. K. (1970). Neuropsychological impairments in functional psychiatric diseases. *Archives of General Psychiatry, 22,* 114–119.

Rourke, B. P. (1975). Brain–behavior relationships in children with learning disabilities: A research program. *American Psychologist, 30,* 911–920.

Rourke, B. P. (1976). Issues in the neuropsychological assessment of children with learning disabilities. *Canadian Psychological Review, 17*(2), 89–102.

Rourke, B. P. (1979). Conference overview. In R. M. Knights & D. J. Bakker (Eds.), *Treatment of hyperactive and learning disordered children.* Baltimore: University Park Press.

Russell, W. R., & Smith, A. (1961). Post-traumatic amnesia in closed head injury. *Archives of Neurology, 5,* 4.

Rutter, M. (1977). Brain damage syndromes in childhood: Concepts and findings. *Journal of Child Psychology and Psychiatry, 18,* 1–21.

Satz, P. (1972). Pathological left-handedness; An explanatory model. *Cortex, 8,* 121–135.

Schiffer, R. B. (1983). Psychiatric aspects of clinical neurology. *American Journal of Psychiatry, 140,* 205–207.

Seidel, U. P., Chadwick, O. F., & Rutter, M. (1975). Psychological disorders in crippled children: A comparative study of children with and without brain damage. *Developmental Medicine and Child Neurology, 17,* 563–575.

Severson, R. A. (1970). *Behavior therapy with severe learning disabilities.* Unpublished manuscript, University of Wisconsin, Madison.

Shaffer, D. (1972). Psychiatric aspects of brain injury in childhood: A review. In S. Chess & A. Thomas (Eds.), *Annual progress in child psychiatry and child development.* New York: Brunner/Mazel.

Shaffer, D. (1974). Psychiatric aspects of brain injury in childhood: A review. In S. Chess & A. Thomas (Eds.), *Annual progress in child psychiatry and child development.* New York: Brunner/Mazel.

Shagass, C., Roemer, R. A., & Straumanis, J. J. (1982). Relationships between psychiatric diagnosis and some quantitative EEG variables. *Archives of General Psychiatry, 39,* 1423–1428.

Shepard, M., Oppenheim, H., & Mitchell, S. (1966). Childhood behavior disorders and child guidance clinics: An epidemiological study. *Journal of Child Psychology and Psychiatry, 7,* 39–52.

Small, I. F., Small, J. G., Milstein, V., & Moore, J. E. (1972). Neuropsychological observations with psychosis and somatic treatment. *Journal of Nervous and Mental Disease, 155,* 6–13.

Smith, A. (1981). Principles underlying human brain functions in neuropsychological sequelae of different neuropathological processes. In S. B. Filskov & T. J. Boll (Eds.), *Handbook of clinical neuropsychology,* New York: Wiley.

Smith, A., & Sugar, O. (1975). Development of above normal language and intelligence 21 years after left hemispherectomy. *Neurology, 25,* 812–818.

Smith, T. E., & Boyce, E. M. (1962). The relationship of the Trail Making Test to psychiatric symptomatology. *Journal of Clinical Psychology, 18,* 450–454.

Spaulding, W. (1978). The relationships of some information-processing factors to severely disturbed behavior. *Journal of Nervous and Mental Disorders, 166,* 417.

Sperry, R. W. (1974). Lateral specialization in the surgically separated hemispheres. In F. O. Schmitt & F. G. Worden (Eds.), *The neurosciences: Third study program.* Cambridge, MA: MIT Press.

Spitzer, R. L., Endicott, J., & Robins, E. (1977). *Research diagnostic criteria (RDC) for a selected group of functional disorders (3rd ed.).* New York: New York State Psychiatric Institute, Biometries Research.

Spitzer, R. L., Endicott, J., & Robins, E. (1978). Research diagnostic criteria: Rationale and reliability. *Archives of General Psychiatry, 35,* 773–782.

Squire, L. R., & Chace, P. C. (1975). Memory functions six to nine months after electroconvulsive therapy. *Archives of General Psychiatry, 32,* 1557–1564.

Sternberg, D. E., & Jarvik, M. E. (1976). Memory functions in depression: Improvement with antidepressant medication. *Archives of General Psychiatry, 33,* 219–224.

Stott, D. H. (1970). Behavioral aspects of learning disabilities: Assessment and remediation. *Experimental Publication System, 2.* (Ms No. 400-36).

Strauss, A. A., & Lehtinen, L. E. (1948). *Psychopathology and education of the brain-injured child* (Vol. 1). New York: Grune & Stratton.

Taylor, M. A., & Abrams, R. (1984). Cognitive impairment in schizophrenia. *American Journal of Psychiatry, 141,* 196–201.

Taylor, M. A., Greenspan, B., & Abrams, R. (1979). Lateralized neuropsychological dysfunction in affective disorder and schizophrenia. *American Journal of Psychiatry, 136,* 1031–1034.

Tramontana, M. G., Sherrets, S. D., & Golden, C. J. (1980). Brain dysfunction in youngsters with psychiatric disorders: Application of Selz–Reitan rules for neuropsychological diagnosis. *Clinical Neuropsychology, 2,* 118–123.

Walker, H. A., & Birch, H. G. (1970). Lateral preference and right–left awareness in schizophrenic children. *Journal of Nervous and Mental Disease, 151,* 341–351.

Watson, C. G., Thomas, R. W., Anderson, D., & Felling, J. (1968). Differentiation of organics from schizophrenics at two chronicity levels by use of the Reitan–Halstead organic test battery. *Journal of Consulting and Clinical Psychology, 32,* 679–684.

Wehler, R., & Hoffman, H. (1978). Intellectual functioning in lobotomized and non-lobotomized chronic schizophrenic patients. *Journal of Clinical Psychology, 34,* 449–451.

Young, L. D., Taylor, I., & Holmstrom, V. (1977). Lithium treatment of patients with affective illness associated with organic brain symptoms. *American Journal of Psychiatry, 134,* 1405–1407.

Chapter 5

Neuropsychological Effects of Closed-Head Injury in Children

RICHARD A. BERG*

Psychiatry/Psychology Division
St. Jude Children's Research Hospital
Memphis, Tennessee 38101

INTRODUCTION

Trauma to the skull resulting in brain injury is one of the more common neurological disorders in children. It has been estimated that over 1 million children sustain head injuries each year (Young, 1969). Head injury, of course, can occur at any time in life, but the infant and young child are at especially high risk, particularly for nonpenetrating, closed-head injury (Spreen, Tupper, Risser, Tuokko, & Edgell, 1984). Closed-head injuries may occur due to any number of factors, such as when toddlers fall down a flight of stairs or out of a window or when unrestrained infants in vehicles that stop quickly or collide are thrown up against the dashboard or windshield.

The behavioral sequelae of head trauma are reportedly less severe in children than in adults (Heiskanen & Sipponen, 1970). However, the presence, nature, and degree of deficits following head injury are so widely varied depending on severity, age at the time of the trauma, and even the type of outcome assessment that this general statement offers little in the way of meaningful information. For example, the occurrence

* Present Address: Department of Behavioral Medicine, West Virginia University Medical Center, Charleston, West Virginia 25330.

113

of an easily identifiable consequence of head injury such as seizure activity has been shown to vary tremendously with the age of the child in patients with mild to moderate trauma. In a study of head-injured children aged birth to 15 years, Black, Shepard, and Walker (1975) found that the total incidence of early seizures (i.e., 1 week or less posttrauma) was higher than that in adults, while late-occurring seizures were less frequent in children than in adults. Interestingly, two differing patterns were noted. Children aged 2 through 15 years showed a high incidence of early seizures and a low rate of late seizures. However, infants between birth and 2 years of age showed an unusually low incidence of early seizures and a high incidence after 1 week. Thus, even among children, the effects of brain trauma may vary considerably with age.

This chapter focuses on that which is known about the effects of closed-head injury in children. In addition, an attempt is made to identify areas in which the sequelae of head trauma differ from that seen with adults. Finally, significant discrepancies between what is known and what clinical tradition and common practice assume about the effects of closed-head injuries is identified. (Throughout the chapter, the reader may note the use of the terms closed-head injury, brain trauma, head injury, etc. These terms are used as being synonymous.)

MECHANISMS OF CLOSED-HEAD INJURY

A discussion of the neuropsychological effects of closed-head injury begins with understanding how such injury to the brain occurs, especially given the extent to which the brain is protected. A head injury can occur in any number of ways—a blow to the head with a baseball, a fall while running, an accident while riding a bicycle, and so on. What becomes important here, however, is that the mechanics of the head injury always occur in the same general way. The head injury is the result of the forces of *compression* (pushing tissues together), *tension* (tearing tissues apart), and *shear* (sliding portions of tissues over other portions of tissues). Compression, tension, and shear operate either simultaneously or in succession, resulting in damage to brain tissue (Gurdijian, Thomas, Hodgson, & Patrick, 1968).

Skull Deformation

A blow to the head results in a temporary deformation of the cranial vault, which is greater in the relatively fixed head than in the freely moving head (Gilroy & Meyer, 1975). This deformation leads to a decrease in volume and a temporary rise in cerebrospinal fluid pressure. If the velocity of the impacting force is high enough, a depressed fracture or skull perforation occurs. Slightly less velocity results in a linear fracture of the skull while a bit less force leads to the closed-head injury. The actual brain injury occurs in one of three ways.

Acceleration

In acceleration injuries, which are the result of linear or angular acceleration, the slower-moving contents of the brain are damaged by the sudden impact with the bony protuberances of the skull or the edge of the dural membranes. An example of this form of injury would be getting hit in the head with a thrown baseball. As the ball hits the head, the skull is forced to move in a direction opposite the impact. The brain, moving more slowly, impacts initially against the inner table of the skull at the point where the baseball hit. There may be bruising or contusion of the brainstem or the undersurface of the occipital lobes or on the superior surface of the cerebellum against the edge of the tentorium cerebelli. The upper surface of the corpus callosum can be easily damaged by the free edge of the falx. The tips of the frontal and temporal lobes are particularly vulnerable to damage as they move in anterior to posterior and inferior to superior directions, hitting the bony ridges dividing the anterior and middle sections of the skull.

An additional factor in acceleration-type injuries is the effect of the pressure waves that traverse the skull and brain from the point of impact. The highest pressure occurs at this point with the lowest pressure, often negative, at the point directly opposite (contrecoup) the point of impact. Theoretically, if the negative pressure reaches the pressure of vapor, a partial vacuum occurs, resulting in the tearing of tissues, and thus, a contrecoup injury occurs. The contrecoup injury is often more severe than that at the point of impact because of the tissue tearing as well as the fact that the pressure wave spreads out from the impact point and effects a larger area opposite from the impact (Gilroy & Meyer, 1975).

Deceleration

When the moving head strikes a fixed and solid object (as in an automobile accident where the head hits the dashboard), there is a rapid deceleration of the skull and results in damage at both the point of impact and at the contrecoup site. A fall on the back of the head results in contusion of the frontal and temporal areas, probably resulting from the inertia of the brain. The development of a pressure wave with negative pressure in the area of injury and rotation of the brain so that the frontal and temporal lobes abut against bony prominences are also important factors in this type of injury (Ommaya, Grubbs, & Naumann, 1971). The midbrain may be damaged by striking the clivus as a result of the same type of injury. Blows over the lateral aspect of the freely moving head generally lead to a contusion in the opposite temporal lobe. A fall on the frontal region has a somewhat different effect and, therefore, contrecoup injuries to the occipital regions are rare. This is probably because of the smooth contours and absence of bony projections in the occipital region of the skull (Ommaya, Grubbs, & Naumann, 1970). Both acceleration and deceleration injuries can result in the rupture of both superficial and deep blood vessels, with the formation of hemorrhages as a consequence.

Rotation

When energy impacts on the head, distortion of the skull is produced. Linear movement of the head (acceleration or deceleration) and rotation of the head occurs. Rotation occurs as a result of hyperflexion, hyperextension, lateral flexion, and turning movements of the head on the neck, which produces shearing forces in the brain and tearing of cerebral tissue. This mechanism is probably the major cause of contrecoup injuries to the brain (Ommaya et al., 1970). An occipital impact of sufficient severity to produce a concussion can result in a contrecoup injury to the frontal and temporal lobes.

It should be noted that the effects of closed-head injury in childhood, especially infancy and early childhood, differ in some respects from those in adult life (Cummins & Potter, 1970). The skull of a child is less rigid than that of an adult, so that there is greater cushioning and less-frequent contrecoup damage (Courville, 1965). On the other hand, there is likely to be greater distortion of the brain and, thus, more-marked generalized damage due to shearing forces (Rutter, Chadwick, & Shaffer, 1983).

AGE AT ONSET

Of great importance when discussing the effects of closed-head injury in children (as well as in child neuropsychology as a whole) are the effects of brain trauma across the age range. The consequences of failing to appreciate the complexity of brain–behavior interactions can be particularly severe when dealing with children (Boll & Barth, 1981). Not only must the clinician consider all those variables normally a part of the assessment of brain integrity, but he or she must also take into account the role of development. The brain does not develop completely prior to birth. Rather, there is a large degree of development that occurs postnatally. The complexity and fullness of dendritic connections as well as synaptic organization are subject to influence by a wide variety of factors, ranging from general physical health to environmental adequacy and opportunity (Dreifuss, 1975). Trauma at an early age effects an incompletely developed brain and an incomplete repertoire of behaviors.

Perinatal Head Injuries

Despite the obvious importance of understanding the consequences of closed-head injuries in the child's first 2 years, studies of the consequences of injury during this period are relatively rare (Spreen et al., 1984). Generally, the examination of early life head trauma is limited to perinatal injuries. Otherwise, children with head injuries are included in broader studies of head injury which cover the entire period of childhood and early adolescence without a systematic evaluation of age either at the time of injury or at the age of testing. For this reason, some time is spent discussing perinatal head trauma.

The perinatal period is a time of increased risk for central nervous system (CNS) injury due to mechanical causes arising from the passage of the fetus through the birth canal and the final emergence of the fetus from the mother. During the course of this passage, a variety of head injuries can occur as a result of the extreme forces to which the head of the fetus is subjected. Additionally, the use of forceps to extract the neonate may result in damage to brain tissue.

Forced bleeding from intracranial blood vessels can occur due to perinatal mechanical injury. A subdural hemorrhage can be particularly damaging. Such a hemorrhage is usually a result of trauma during delivery caused by excessive molding of the head (Oxorn, 1980). The molding increases stress and strain on the meningeal structures. Blood from this form of hemorrhage does not readily reabsorb in the bloodstream. Towbin (1970) reported that a cerebral subdural hemorrhage results in a thin layer of blood over the entire cerebrum with 30 to 50% of the survivors of such damage likely to left with focal cerebral signs and hydrocephalus (Volpe, 1977). In contrast, a hemorrhage in the posterior fossa region of the brain may either be fatal or leave the individual with severely limited cognitive capabilities.

The overall prognosis following a subdural hemorrhage is poor. Natelson and Sayers (1973) reported that of 13 survivors of such perinatal damage, only three had normal IQs 8 to 13 years later, and all 13 suffered from seizure disorders.

Perhaps the most common form of intracranial hemorrhage is the subarachnoid variety (Volpe, 1977). With subarachnoid hemorrhages, the bleeding is usually bilateral and occurs largely over the temporal regions, with the major result being hydrocephalus. Volpe (1977) has identified three syndromes of subarachnoid hemorrhage (1) primarily preterm infants with minor bleeding without significant behavioral–cognitive sequelae; (2) full-term infants in whom the hemorrhage results in very early seizure activity; and (3) those infants with massive hemorrhages for whom the outcome is generally fatal, largely due to both severe anoxia and the traumatic injury itself.

Structural Injuries

Brain structures are very much subject to direct damage from perinatal mechanical influences. Damage such as lacerations, transections, and contusions can be directly attributable to mechanical influences. Other forms of damage such as brainstem compression are likely to occur as a result of hemorrhaging.

Cerebral damage that is not secondary to anoxia or hemorrhage, while not common, does occur. Excessive forceps pressure in delivery may lead to localized skull depressions in the parietotemporal areas. The skull depressions may result in cortical or meningeal lacerations. These areas of the brain are particularly vulnerable to damage (Spreen et al., 1984), and early damage may lead to serious later dysfunction as the parietotemporal region subserves a variety of important later-developing cognitive functions.

Later-Occurring Injury

As the child gets older, closed-head injuries are more likely to be the result of some form of trauma. The effects of the trauma are likely to vary considerably with the age at the time of the injury. Brink, Garrett, Hale, Woo-Sam, and Nickel (1970), for instance, found a direct relationship between the length of coma following head injury and IQ at follow-up. Younger children (2–8 years of age) demonstrated more-severe deficiencies in intellectual functioning than an older group of brain-injured children (aged 9–10 years) despite a shorter coma duration.

Woods and Teuber (1974) reported that, in a group of children whose injuries occurred from infancy through the preschool years, when the injury was in the left hemisphere, deficits were evident in both verbal and nonverbal skills relative to healthy children. However, unlike that which is typically seen in adults with left-hemisphere damage, dysphasia was not prevalent.

From a neuropsychological perspective, the effect of the age at which the head injury occurs depends heavily on the type of ability being assessed (Boll, 1973; Teuber & Rudel, 1962). At birth, both hemispheres appear to have the capacity to subserve the entire range of human abilities; however, individually, neither hemisphere is capable of performing tasks as well as when both sides of the brain work together. Alajouanine and Lhermitte (1965) found that severe damage to either hemisphere leads to a temporary disruption of langauge functioning. Around the age of 5 years, damage to the right hemisphere no longer has much of a disruptive effect on language (Boll & Barth, 1981). Between ages 5 and 12 years, a left-hemisphere injury produces aphasia, albeit generally milder and more transitory than that found with similar injury later in life. It is only after about age 16–18 that adult-like aphasia is seen with left-hemisphere injuries.

Woo-Sam, Zimmerman, Brink, Uyehara, and Miller (1970) found that intellectual impairment several years after head trauma was more frequent in children younger than 8 years of age at the time of the injury than in those over 10 years of age. It may be that although younger children recover more rapidly, they do so less completely. Alternatively, the effects of age are greater in the first few years of life than they are during the school-age years, or the age at injury may bear directly on the type of cognitive deficit found later. Woods (1980) found that lesions occurring in the child's first year tended to be associated with somewhat greater intellectual deficits that involved both verbal and nonverbal skills, whereas the effects of injury sustained after the first year depended on the side of the lesion. The later left-hemisphere lesions were found to lead to decreased verbal and nonverbal test scores, whereas right hemisphere lesions were found to be associated with impaired nonverbal skills.

The literature to date concerning the effects of age is really too limited and too contradictory for any firm conclusions. It can be tentatively stated that the main distinction appears to lie between the effects of trauma in infancy and those later in childhood, with only comparatively minimal effects noted during the school-age years. It also would seem that the effects of age differ with regard to speed of recovery, pattern of dysfunction, and extent of impairment. The short-term and long-term sequelae may not be the same, and the ultimate consequences of head injury may reflect changes in intellectual requirements and developmental alterations in cerebral plasticity. Hebb (1942) found that brain damage has its greatest effect on new learning. Thus, greater impairment in younger children may be seen as they have less accumulated knowledge and established skills on which to rely and more new learning to accomplish (Rutter, 1981). Intellectual deficiencies may be more apparent in later childhood because the demands and need for autonomy and cognitive flexibility on the older child are greater than that on the younger child.

The impact of early closed-head injury cannot be meaningfully described as less than or greater than that of later-occurring damage. Most authors concur that the long-term effects of closed-head injury in children can be understood only by systematic longitudinal research that accounts for not only the age at injury and age at testing, but also the location, focal specificity, extent of lesion, and developmental complexity of the behavior under investigation (Boll & Barth, 1981; Levin, Benton, & Grossman, 1982).

ADULTS VERSUS CHILDREN

At one time, there was a general consensus that the findings of the effects of head injury in adults could be readily generalized to children. And, to a limited extent, there is some validity in this notion. The areas of apparent differences between adults and children may be needlessly exaggerated by a misunderstanding of the functions being assessed and compared. There are, however, major differences neurologically, neuropathologically, and psychologically between the child and the adult that must be understood.

Anatomically, children are not born with a fully developed CNS, as mentioned earlier. At birth, certain structures are present, such as the enlarged superior surface of the left temporal lobe, which suggests the predisposition of that area to subserve future language functions (Boll & Barth, 1981). In contrast, the fibers of the corpus callosum, which facilitates interhemispheric communication, are not functional at birth (Gazzaniga, 1970), and the dendritic connections and organization of connections continue to develop long after birth (Dreifuss, 1975). The effects of childhood injuries tend to be far more generalized than focal and are usually not subject to strict anatomic localization.

Adults have a far greater history of functioning and accomplishment that allows much greater ease in establishing premorbid functional status and, thus, determining deficits that result from head injury. Those readily available pieces of baseline information so useful in the evaluation of an adult's functional status, such as level of education, functional literacy, and occupation, cannot be used in establishing a child's premorbid capabilities. Academic records can offer some insight into the child's premorbid level but, more often than not, school records are poor and, at best, imprecise. Further, there are tremendously large differences in both quantitative and qualitative psychological capacity and accomplishment that are so characteristic of a child's development in at least the first 10–12 years, whereas changes in an adult's capabilities occur far less on a

year-to-year basis (Alpern & Boll, 1972; Flavel, 1963). Essentially, for a head-injured child, an assessment of the amount and type of ability lost is required at a time when prediction of current abilities is the most difficult. Despite the lack of significant or permanent loss of function, the subsequent damage to the order, rate, and level of future development and learning capability may significantly alter the child's neuropsychological course.

Thus, it could be argued that the neuropsychological effects of head injury in children and adults bear little resemblance to each other. It has been demonstrated that adult head injury leads to poor performance on tests of learning, recent memory, abstraction, and problem-solving skills, while a lesser impact is observed on fund of general information, remote memory, and overlearned skills (Golden, 1981a). Psychometrically, this can be seen in the performance differences obtained by brain-injured adults on the measures included in formal neuropsychological batteries, as well as those specialized tests that have been designed to identify specific forms of dysfunction (Boll, 1981; Golden, 1981b; Parsons, 1970). Of note though, are those brain-injured individuals who may score normally on the Wechsler Intelligence Scales for a variety of reasons. By contrast, head-injured children are far more likely to perform poorly on the Wechsler scales (Boll, 1978). Adults, therefore, may experience cognitive changes resulting from brain damage that are qualitatively different from those experienced by children. One must keep in mind that, although the possibility exists that these differences reflect differences in the type of intellectual processes measured, seemingly similar neuropsychological tests may actually be assessing different functions at different ages (Boll, 1978). The majority of neuropsychological tests for children have not been designed with neuropsychological development in mind. Rather, these instruments are simplified adult tests with tasks tapping cognitive functions that have likely not yet developed in the child.

TYPES OF CLOSED-HEAD INJURY

The effects of head trauma may vary tremendously, depending on the strength of the trauma, the resilience of the injured individual, and, as noted earlier, the relative movements of the head and impacting object. Not all head trauma will produce significant neuropsychological deficits, whereas some trauma can cause permanent and severe deficits. The degree to which the trauma affects functioning depends, in some measure, on the type of head injury incurred by the child. Basically, there are four types of head injuries to be considered—concussion, contusion, laceration, and hematoma.

Concussion

A concussion occurs when the child loses consciousness due to a blow to the head. If the trauma is limited to a concussion, there tends to be minor neuropsychological deficits (Golden, 1981a). These deficits tend to be limited to the focus of the injury and the opposite side of the head as a result of contrecoup.

The effects of the concussion are generally focal in the injured hemisphere and more diffuse in the area of contrecoup. The severity of the deficit has been related to the length of time the patient was unconscious (Klonoff & Paris, 1974; Dailey, 1956). The focal dysfunction rarely takes on the character of a highly limited disorder. Generally, the overall impairment is less. The amount of impairment depends on the length of the unconsciousness and immediately after consciousness is regained, there may be generalized losses in cognitive skills (Becker, 1975) and in memory abilities. (Brooks, 1974). The focal symptomatology will only appear after the child regains awareness and is able to show sustained awareness, attention, and effort. Early evaluation of a child with a head injury may, thus, serve to establish a baseline against which recovery of function may be measured.

In a mild concussion, recovery is rapid and typically occurs within a few minutes. Recovery from moderate and severe head trauma can be divided into five stages. In stage one (coma), the posttraumatic unconsciousness can be of short duration but can also range upward to several months or years, depending on the degree of damage. With a coma, there is a complete paralysis of all cerebral functions with the exception of life-maintaining activities such as pulse, blood pressure, and respiration. While the pupils of the child's eye react to light, and reflex eye movements in response to head movements are preserved, there is no response to other stimulation, even painful stimuli.

In the second stage of recovery (semicoma), response to painful stimulation can be seen, as can other purposeful movements. Stage three (stupor) is characterized by appropriate response to simple commands. During stage four (obtundity), the patient is quietly confused. While the child may respond to the examiner, he or she will likely be disoriented and a good deal of confabulation may be seen. The fifth and final stage (full consciousness) generally occurs over a period of hours or days and usually begins with the recovery of orientation, followed by the ability to retain information and remember recent events (Gilroy & Meyer, 1975).

Contusions

Two types of contusions resulting from head injury have been identified (Robbins, 1974). A small object hitting against the head may cause bleeding in the brain directly under the site of impact; however, when a large object impacts with the head, the skull will tend to move away from the object faster than the brain. This will result in a separation between the brain and the skull at the point opposite the point of impact. A tearing of blood vessels interconnecting the brain and the meninges may occur. This tearing causes the major effects of contusion in the contrecoup area.

The neuropsychological deficits resulting from the contusion will generally be more severe than that from concussion in the area of bleeding, causing a stronger focal deficit (Golden, 1981a). It will be accompanied by a less-focal deficit opposite the contusion. Here again, the amount of injury will vary greatly. Milder contusions tend to leave more cognitive functions and behaviors intact, whereas more-severe contusions may result in a relatively widespread depression of ability (Rourke, Bakker, Fisk, & Strang, 1983). These dysfunctions generally involve higher cognitive functions more so than basic sensorimotor functioning (Reitan & Fitzhugh, 1971).

Lacerations

A laceration occurs when there is an interruption in the continuity of brain tissue (Robbins, 1974). This can happen in severe contrecoup injuries or in open-head trauma. The type of neuropsychological deficits that may be associated with a closed-head laceration tend to be similar to those already noted for contusions. These deficits, however, may be greater in severity and may demonstrate a more precise localization (Levin & Eisenberg, 1979b). Usually there are also secondary deficits opposite the laceration.

Whether an injury is a contusion or a laceration, it can result in permanent damage to the brain and cause the formation of scar tissue. These scars are highly irritative and may result in a seizure disorder secondary to the original injury. There may be long-term dysfunction, usually those that are dependent on the area of the injury. As a general rule of thumb, the more severe the initial laceration, the more obvious and severe the behavioral sequelae (Pendse, Sran, Dandia, & Narula, 1971).

Hematoma

As a result of a closed-head injury, blood vessels may be disrupted, producing pools of blood within and between the meninges. Of greatest interest to the practicing neuropsychologist is the subdural hematoma. The acute form arises as a result of a laceration that allows blood and cerebrospinal fluid to accumulate in the subdural space. This follows head injury directly and is usually dealt with during the child's overall medical treatment following head trauma. Consequently, it is rare that the acute form is seen in clinical practice.

The chronic form of hematoma is that which is likely to be seen by neuropsychologists and is the variety most frequently associated with closed-head injury (Golden, 1981a). It is caused by a rupture of smaller blood vessels either at the site of injury or contrecoup. These vessels slowly leak blood into the subdural space, accumulating over time into a significant encapsulated mass (Auld, Aronson, & Gargans, 1965). This has the effect of compressing the brain on the side of the hematoma and shifting the midline cerebral structures. Because a hematoma can take several months to form, observable deficits may not be present initially. When deficits do finally appear, a tumor may often be misdiagnosed if the child's history is not carefully examined.

NEUROPSYCHOLOGICAL IMPLICATIONS

The neuropsychological sequelae of closed-head injuries in children have, perhaps, their greatest relevance for educational and overall adjustment (Levin & Eisenberg, 1979b). Not only must the clinician assess and deal with the cognitive disorders resulting from the head injury, but also a variety of other etiological factors bear upon the outcome of any injury to the brain.

A head-injured child may demonstrate changes in personality (Levin & Eisenberg, 1979a). Klonoff and Paris (1974) have reported a variety of sequelae to head injury, including declines in academic achievement and deterioration of relationships both at home and with peers. In addition, they found that, particularly with younger children ages 3 to 8 years, parents demonstrated significant increases in protectiveness, to the point where the children became virtually isolated from their environment during the first year posttrauma. _parental overprojection_

Unlike a variety of brain disorders, closed-head injuries can result in deficits in parts of the brain remote from the point of the most obvious deficit. Therefore, the clinician cannot search only for certain syndromes or deficits, as the obvious deficits may conceal other dysfunction that can affect the child's potential for recovery, as well as his or her subjective complaints (Golden, Moses, Coffman, Miller, & Strider, 1983). It is important to note, however, that patients and families may not be aware of these deficits and may not complain of problems. A major difficulty in treating a head-injured child lies in the fact that, to parents and educators, the child looks well long before recovery is completed. As a result of the lack of awareness of deficits, test batteries chosen only to evaluate those specific areas of complaint are likely to miss highly important aspects of the child's performance. Moreover, in comparison to tumors and cerebrovascular disorders, the effects of head trauma are far more difficult to localize to specific brain areas using neuroradiologic and neurodiagnostic techniques. Such measures are often normal in head trauma or may reflect only a portion of the actual injury (Golden et al., 1983). As a consequence, medical referral sources may not be aware of the actual extent and effects of the trauma insofar as neuropsychological testing is concerned.

In many cases of closed-head injury, there is a high likelihood of damage to the frontal lobes of the brain because of the tendency of these areas to absorb many blows that occur at the back of the head. Such damage is quite common in automobile accidents. Frontal-lobe damage is important because the effects of such damage may be so substantial as to make the clinician think that there is diffuse, widespread damage, or alternatively, damage that is so subtle that it likely to be missed completely or mistaken for another deficit. This becomes more important when one considers the notion that this region of the brain continues to develop in terms of functional capacity long after birth, frequently continuing into adulthood (Wilkening & Golden, 1983).

The frontal region is largely responsible for the control of most human behavior (Luria, 1966). With more-severe injuries, damage in this area may result in a complete loss of ability to inhibit and control behavior in older children. In the young child, injury to the frontal regions may likely impede or completely arrest development of these functions that are critical to adequate functioning as an adult. Children with frontal lobe dysfunction may have difficulty in taking standardized tests because of an inability to follow instructions or deal with any level of complexity (Golden et al., 1983).

Psychological Reactions to Trauma

In an extensive study of the effects of head trauma in children, Klonoff and Paris (1974) uncovered a variety of psychological sequelae to head injury. They found that for children aged 2 to 8 years, denial or a lack of concern about the injury was the most common reaction, followed by a change in response to potential dangers. There was a negligible occurrence of changes in relationships with others, greater dependence, and changes in self-concept. In older children (9–15 years), Klonoff and Low

(1974) noted a significant change in self-concept. These authors also noted that parental reactions to the child after injury were important. Parents of younger children initially became more protective and concerned about the possibility of another accident, whereas parents of older children exhibited more denial of past or current concern about the effects of the injury on the child.

Brown, Chadwick, Shaffer, Rutter, and Traub (1981) examined the incidence and type of psychiatric disturbance after head injury in two groups of children—a severe- and a mild-injury group. Twenty-eight children were placed in the severe group, defined by the presence of posttraumatic amnesia of 1 week or more following the head injury. The mild head-injury group included 29 children with post-traumatic amnesia of at least 1 hour and less than 1 week. Assessments were conducted immediately after the injury as well as at 4, 12, and 28 months. The severe-injury group had more psychiatric disorder than either the mild-injury group or a group of 28 age-matched and psychosocially matched orthopedic controls. Fifty percent of the severe head-injured group developed new psychiatric disorders postinjury, three times as often as the mild injury or control groups. The most prominent disturbance of the severe-injury group directly attributable to the injury was disinhibition, characterized by socially inappropriate behavior, social insensitivity, failure to follow social conventions, performing embarrassing actions, and making inappropriate personal comments. Lack of reserve, overtalkativeness, poor hygiene, forgetfullness, and impulsiveness were also signs of the disinhibited state. The symptom pattern is similar to that seen in adults with frontal lobe lesions.

Overeating was found to be a problem for these children with severe head injury at 2 years postinjury; however, the authors did not attempt to directly attribute overeating to the injury, due to the time span between the injury and the noted overeating. The variety of emotional and behavioral problems noted were consistent with those found with children in general (Spreen et al., 1984). Brown et al. (1981) also explored whether any preinjury groups within the severe-injury group were predisposed to new psychiatric disorders. They found that preinjury disorders tended to be exacerbated postinjury, while children with no preinjury history of disorder were less likely to demonstrate new disorders. Thus, increases in new psychiatric disturbances were found to be a function not only of the head injury, but also of the preinjury personality and adjustment of the child. Mild head injury was not found to be related to psychiatric outcome.

In studies of children with brain damage due to factors other than closed-head injury, it has been reported that psychiatric disorders are more frequent in those with either a low level of general intellectual functioning or severe reading difficulties. There has been a similar trend in studies of children with head injuries, although the relationship has been neither as strong nor as consistent (Brown et al., 1981; Shaffer, Bijur, Chadwick, & Rutter, 1980). In a prospective study of head-injured children, Brown et al. (1981) noted a trend for children with psychiatric disorders emerging after the trauma to have somewhat lower nonverbal IQ scores. However, these authors reported that this was most prominent in relation to the IQ scores obtained soon after the trauma. These results suggest that the relationship between psychiatric disturbances and IQ was strongest when the IQ reflects the results of brain trauma. It was further found that the posttrauma IQ predicted psychiatric disorder only during the first year of follow-up.

Although there is good evidence that closed-head injury can be a contributing factor in the posttraumatic development of psychiatric disturbance, its effects are less direct and less consistent than is the case with cognitive sequelae. A number of other factors also contribute, such as family reactions, pretrauma behavior, and personality (Rutter et al., 1983). The etiology of psychiatric disturbances after head injury is extremely complex. Brain injury per se certainly plays an important role, but it constitutes only one element in a complex multidetermined phenomenon involving both neurological and nonneurological variables.

Cognitive Impairment

In general, neuropsychological deficits found in children with closed-head injuries tend to be pervasive during the first 6 months following the injury (Levin and Eisenberg, 1979a). Memory deficits appear to be the most prominent of the residual effects of closed-head injury. Levin and Eisenberg (1979a) found that nearly one-half of 64 children studied demonstrated impaired verbal learning and memory and/or continuous recognition memory. Visual–spatial dysfunction was another key deficit noted. The presence of memory and visuospatial deficits was found to be directly related to the severity of acute neurological impairment at the time of hospital admission. However, these authors also found that even those children with a relatively brief coma duration or no loss of consciousness at all frequently exhibited measurable neuropsychological impairment. This finding is in accord with those of earlier studies (e.g., Klonoff, Low, & Clark, 1977). Levin and Eisenberg (1979a) also found that a test of selective reminding by Buschke (1974) was particularly sensitive to the effects of closed-head injury. Children with left temporal lesions demonstrated a particularly severe impairment of storage and retrieval in verbal learning and memory. Visual–motor abilities were also vulnerable to the effects of head injury in this study. Intellectual abilities at 6 months post-injury were found to be within the normal range in all but the most severe cases; however, Levin and Eisenberg (1979a) noted that comparison with estimates of premorbid ability suggested that only partial recovery on intellectual functioning was generally achieved.

In another study, Levin and Eisenberg (1979b) found that approximately one-third of patients studied demonstrated a language deficit, as compared to the adult figure of 50%. These findings are in agreement with those reported in previous studies of acquired aphasia (Hecaen, 1976) which have shown more rapid and complete recovery and language functions in children as compared to adults. Hecaen (1976) has written that, based on his and others' work, the developing brain of a child has a greater potential of intrahemispheric reorganization among the regions of the brain that subserve language—thus, the more rapid recovery of language in children with acquired aphasia.

Mutism is characteristic of acquired aphasia on children with closed-head injuries but is less common in adults with head injuries (Hecaen, 1976). De Mol and Deleval (1979) described five young patients with head injuries and posttraumatic mutism. These authors characterized *mutism* as a condition of total abolition of speech in which the patient could communicate by writing, head nodding, or using block letters. No consistent finding regarding the presence or localization of a mass lesion was evident using a variety of neuroradiologic and neurodiagnostic techniques. The persistence of the mutism appeared to be related to coma duration, although the authors did not describe the acute impairment of consciousness in detail.

In a series of prospective studies, a number of authors found that timed visuospatial and visuomotor tests tended to show more impairment than verbal tests did, as reflected in Wechsler Intelligence Scale scores (Chadwick, Rutter, Brown, Shaffer, & Traub, 1981; Chadwick, Rutter, Shaffer, & Shrout, 1981). Mandleberg and Brooks (1975) have reported similar findings in adults. That aside, however, no deficit pattern specific to head injury was noted. Chadwick et al. (1981) administered a wide range of specialized tests dealing with measures of paired-associate learning, immediate and delayed recall, attentiveness, distractibility, verbal fluency, and speed of information processing to attempt to isolate subtle or specific deficits in children without global intellectual impairment. Apart from a tendency for the speed of visuomotor and visuospatial functioning to be impaired, no other distinct deficits were evident. These authors felt this to be partially a result of cognitive patterns varying among children, as well as a consequence of finding it to be rather unusual to get marked deficits on specific tests of narrowly defined functions, unless some degree of global intellectual impairment was also demonstrated. A wide-range intelligence test such as the Wechsler Scales identifies most intellectual deficits that result from head injury, and, based on these results, it would appear that extensive neuropsychological test batteries do not do much better.

It is accepted that the pattern of cognitive deficits after unilateral cerebral lesions in adults tends to differ in relation to which hemisphere is damaged (Chadwick, Rutter, Thompson, & Shaffer, 1981; Lishman, 1978; McFie, 1975a). In general, verbal impairment is most characteristic of left-hemisphere lesions and visuospatial impairment of right-hemisphere lesions. This differential pattern can be seen even when there is no general intellectual loss. Overall decreases in IQ are likely to be in evidence after left parietotemporal injury and, occasionally, after frontal lesions on either side. The effects of laterality are generally most marked in the immediate posttrauma period (Fitzhugh, Fitzhugh, and Reitan, 1962); however, they have been found to last as long as 20 years afterward (Rutter et al., 1983).

The findings with regard to children have been far less clear-cut, although there has been a slight tendency in the same direction noted. McFie (1961) reported that memory for designs was poorer with right-sided trauma but that there was only a mild tendency for verbal deficits to be worse with left-hemisphere damage. The results of a later study with a larger sample of children (McFie, 1975b) showed essentially the same results. No consistent trend for decreased verbal IQ was noted with left-hemisphere lesions, although new-word learning was more impaired. Laterality effects appear to be more pronounced in older rather than in younger children.

When considered as a whole, the literature concerning the cognitive sequelae of head trauma in children suggests that cognitive deficits are somewhat similar to those associated with adult injuries. However, the effects tend to be less specific and less differentiated in children. For all practical purposes, therefore, the pattern of cognitive dysfunction noted in children following head injuries offers no useful information as to the location of the injury in the individual child. This notion has been borne out by Chadwick et al. (1981), who found no significant laterality or localization effects with respect to cognitive functioning either on the Wechsler Intelligence Scale for Children (WISC) or on more-specific tests in children with lesions of known location. Rather, diffuse dysfunction was noted. It should be further noted, however, that there is a slight but consistent tendency for all tests of academic ahievement to show greater impairment with left-hemisphere injury. This tendency was somewhat more pronounced in children who were under age 5 years at the time of injury.

Long-Term Sequelae of Head Injuries

Despite the fact that a good deal of research investigating the acute and comparatively short-term effects of closed-head injuries in children has been conducted, surprisingly few authors have investigated the long-term sequelae of head injury. Fuld and Fisher (1977) have reported that children with closed-head injuries demonstrate serious posttraumatic intellectual impairment long after EEG's and neurological evaluations are normal. These changes, while not apparent to parents, physicians, or educators, were such that school placement in special classes was necessary for several years after the injury.

Vignolo (1980) was able to find and evaluate 21 individuals who had sustained head trauma 9 to 10 years earlier. All participants in the study had incurred a closed-head injury at approximately 11 years of age. The results of the study suggested that the long-term neuropsychological prognosis of closed-head injury sustained at school age is generally good. Of the 21 participants, only three were seriously impaired as adults. One case demonstrated deficits in writing, calculation skills, and verbal memory. The second impaired individual evidenced difficulties in writing, comprehension of written material, and recall memory. The third individual had performance decrements on tasks measuring verbal comprehension, auditory short-term memory for unrelated information, and word recall. Although the sample size of this study was relatively small, the authors felt the findings to be encouraging.

Klonoff et al. (1977) studied children hospitalized with head injuries ranging from mild to moderate in severity. These patients were matched to controls and evaluated at annual intervals for 5 years. A comprehensive battery of neuropsychological procedures was administered in standard fashion at each interval. The results from this set of studies appears to be the most ambitious and comprehensive picture of children's recovery from closed-head trauma conducted to date (Klonoff, 1971; Klonoff & Low, 1974; Klonoff et al., 1977; Klonoff & Paris, 1974; Klonoff, Robinson, & Thompson, 1969).

Klonoff et al. (1977) obtained data concerning (1) antecedent factors such as age, sex, environmental hazards, and premorbid personalities; (2) circumstances at the time of the trauma; and (3) consequential factors, including effect on the family and education, development of seizures, and general posttraumatic adaptation. Patients were divided into two groups: those injured prior to age 9 years and those who were injured after the age of 9.

General clinical belief suggests that the majority of recovery from closed-head injury in adults occurs during the first year. Brink et al. (1970) also found that children made the most recovery in the first 12 months postinjury. Klonoff et al. (1977) found that young children differed significantly from their matched controls at the time of discharge from the hospital on 28 of 32 neuropsychological measures, and the older children varied on 42 of 48 measures. At 1 year postinjury, impairment on 20 and 31 variables was found for younger and older children, respectively. A continuing decrease in impairment was found on subsequent annual evaluations during years 2–5.

Within what appeared to be a course of steady improvement, two differing patterns of recovery emerged. One group of 114 children demonstrated no discernible neuropsychological dysfunction while the other group (87) continued to evidence significant measureable impairment. At the fifth-year evaluation, the normal matched controls and the recovered head trauma group did not differ in terms of neuropsychological functioning, while the residual deficit group was significantly different from both the control and recovered groups. For approximately 76% of those children who returned to a normal level of functioning despite initial deficits, recovery continued over the 5-year period.

The best predictors of sequelae from injury at ages 4 and 5 were found to be the initial post-head-injury full-scale IQ and coma duration. The significance of the 23–24% with what appeared to be permanent residual dysfunction is exemplified by the data from those children whose head trauma occurred prior to beginning school. One-quarter of these children either failed one or more grades or required special education placement. The size of the group who are at risk for permanent deficiences from such a frequent cause of brain injury in children indicates the need for a careful initial as well as repeated evaluation of the child's functional capabilities to provide information needed for both appropriate reassurance and recommendations for remediation–rehabilitation during the recovery process (Boll & Barth, 1981).

CONCLUSION

As was noted at the outset of this chapter, closed-head injury in children is one of the most common injuries sustained during childhood, with over 1 million cases reported annually. Despite the lack of research in this area to date (when compared to the existing adult literature concerning closed-head trauma), it appears that the effects of brain trauma in children depend on a multitude of factors, not the least of which is the stage of neuropsychological development of the child at the time of the injury. One common thread that appears throughout the available literature is that recovery from closed-head injury is a lengthy process, which can take up to several years. As Levin and Eisenberg (1979a) have so correctly noted, the physical capability of a closed-head-injured child to attend school and perform a variety of common social activities does not necessarily imply a complete or good recovery, as a wide range of cognitive problems may be overlooked. Consultation with parents, teachers, and other related professionals concerning the child's neuropsychological status can greatly assist in planning the resumption of academic activities and determining the need for special education and rehabilitation services.

The study of the neuropsychological effects of closed-head injuries is a relatively new and dynamic area of study. Clearly, there is a great deal to be learned about normal cortical development and the related effects of brain trauma on cerebral and cognitive development. Although, as was pointed out in an earlier chapter, the plasticity of the human cortex and options for the development of unusual functional systems is acknowledged, the limits of such adaptability are not, as yet, known. Continued research with a variety of neuropsychological instruments, especially in conjunction with the newer, more revealing forms of physiological measures (e.g., computerized tomography [CT] scan, positron emission tomography [PET] scan, nuclear magnetic resonance) will assist in the investigation of these questions. This information, in turn, can then be used to help in understanding the short- and long-term results of closed-head trauma.

REFERENCES

Alajouanine, T., & Lhermitte, F. (1965). Acquired aphasia in children. *Brain, 88,* 653–662.
Alpern, G., & Boll, T. J. (1972). *Developmental profile.* Aspen, CO: Psychological Development Publications.
Auld, A. W., Aronson, H. A., & Gargans, F. (1965). Aneurysm of the middle meningeal artery. *Archives of Neurology, 13,* 369–374.
Becker, B. (1975). Intellectual changes after closed head injury. *Journal of Clinical Psychology, 31,* 307–313.
Black, P., Shepard, R. H., & Walker, A. E. (1975). Outcome of head trauma: Age and post-traumatic seizures. In R. Porter & D. FitzSimmons (Eds.), *Outcome of severe damage to the central nervous system* (Ciba Foundation Symposium, Vol. 34). Amsterdam: Elsevier, Excerpta Medica.
Boll, T. J. (1973). *The effect of age and onset of brain damage in adaptive abilities in*

children. Paper presented at the meeting of the American Psychological Association, Montreal.

Boll, T. J. (1978). Diagnosing brain impairment. In B. Wolman (Ed.), *Diagnosis of mental disorders: A handbook*. New York: Plenum Press.

Boll, T. J. (1981). The Halstead–Reitan Neuropsychological Battery. In S. B. Filskov & T. J. Boll (Eds.), *Handbook of clinical neuropsychology*. New York: Wiley.

Boll, T. J., & Barth, J. T. (1981). Neuropsychology of brain damage in children. In S. B. Filskov & T. J. Boll (Eds.), *Handbook of clinical neuropsychology*. New York: Wiley.

Brink, J., Garrett, A., Hale, W., Woo-Sam, J., & Nickel, V. (1970). Recovery of motor and intellectual function in children sustaining severe head injuries. *Developmental Medicine and Child Neurology, 12*, 565–571.

Brooks, D. N. (1974). Recognition memory and head injury. *Journal of Neurology, Neurosurgery and Psychiatry, 39*, 593–600.

Brown, G., Chadwick, O., Shaffer, D., Rutter, M., & Traub, M. (1981). A prospective study of children with head injuries: III. Psychiatric sequelae. *Psychological Medicine, 11*, 67–74.

Buschke, H. (1974). Components of verbal learning in children: Analysis by selective reminding. *Journal of Experimental Child Psychology, 18*, 488–496.

Chadwick, O., Rutter, M., Brown, G., Shaffer, D., & Traub, M. (1981). A prospective study of children with head injuries: II. Cognitive sequelae. *Psychological Medicine, 11*, 49–61.

Chadwick, O., Rutter, M., Shaffer, D., & Shrout, P. (1981). A prospective study of children with head injuries: IV. Specific cognitive deficits. *Journal of Clinical Neuropsychology, 3*, 101–120.

Chadwick, O., Rutter, M., Thompson, J., & Shaffer, D. (1981). Intellectual performance and reading skills after localized head injury in childhood. *Journal of Child Psychology and Psychiatry, 22*, 117–139.

Courville, C. B. (1965). Contrecoup injuries of the brain in injuries. *Archives of Surgery, 90*, 157–165.

Cummins, B. H., & Potter, J. M. (1970). Head injury due to falls from heights. *Injury, 2*, 61–64.

Dailey, C. A. (1956). Psychological findings 5 years after head injury. *Journal of Clinical Psychology, 12*, 349–352.

De Mol, J., & Deleval, J. (1979). Le mutisme post-traumatique: À propos de cinq cas. *Acta Neurologie Belgique, 79*, 369–383. (English abstract)

Dreifuss, F. P. (1975). The pathology of central communicative disorders in children. In D. B. Tower (Ed.), *The nervous system: Human communication and its disorders* (Vol. 3). New York: Raven Press.

Fitzhugh, K. B., Fitzhugh, L. C., & Reitan, R. M. (1962). Wechsler–Bellevue comparison in groups with "chronic" and "current" lateralized and diffuse brain lesions. *Journal of Consulting and Clinical Psychology, 26*, 306–310.

Flavell, J. (1963). *The developmental psychology of Jean Piaget*. Princeton, NJ: Van Nostrand.

Fuld, P. A., & Fisher, P. (1977). Recovery of intellectual ability after closed head-injury. *Development Medicine and Child Neurology, 19*, 495–502.

Gazzaniga, M. S. (1970). *The bisected brain*. New York: Appleton-Century-Crofts.

Gilroy, J., & Meyer, J. S. (1975). *Medical neurology*, (2nd ed.). New York: Macmillan.

Golden, C. J. (1981a). *Diagnosis and rehabilitation of clinical neuropsychology* (2nd ed.). Springfield, IL: Charles C. Thomas.

Golden, C. J. (1981b). A standardized version of Luria's neuropsychological tests: A quantitative and qualitative approach to neuropsychological evaluation. In S. B. Filskov
& T. J. Boll (Eds.), *Handbook of clinical neuropsychology*. New York: Wiley.

Golden, C. J., Moses, J. A., Jr., Coffman, J. A., Miller, W. R., & Strider, F. D. (1983).
Clinical neuropsychology: Interface with neurologic and psychiatric disorders.
New York: Grune & Stratton.

Gurdijian, E. S., Thomas, L. M., Hodgson, V. R., & Patrick, L. M. (1968). Impact head
injury. *General Practice, 37,* 78–87.

Hebb, D. O. (1942). The effect of early and late brain injury on test scores, and the nature of
normal adult intelligence. *Proceedings of the American Philosophical Society, 85,*
275–292.

Hacaen, H. (1976). Acquired aphasia in children and the ontogenesis of hemispheric functional specialization. *Brain and Language, 3,* 114–134.

Heiskanen, O., & Sipponen, P. (1970). Prognosis of severe head injury. *Acta Neurologica
Scandinavica, 46,* 343–350.

Klonoff, H. (1971). Head injuries in children: Predisposing factors, accident conditions,
accident proneness, and sequelae. *American Journal of Public Health, 61,* 2405–
2417.

Klonoff, H., & Low, M. (1974). Disordered brain function in young children and early
adolescents: Neuropsychological and electroencephalographic correlates. In R.
M. Reitan & L. A. Davison (Eds.), *Clinical neuropsychology: Current status and
applications*. Washington, DC: Hemisphere.

Klonoff, H., Low, M. D., & Clark, C. (1977). Head injuries in children with a prospective 5-
year follow-up. *Journal of Neurology, Neurosurgery and Psychiatry, 40,* 1211–
1219.

Klonoff, H., & Paris, R. (1974). Immediate, short term and residual effects of acute head
injuries in children: Neuropsychological and neurological correlates. In R. M.
Reitan & L. A. Davison (Eds.), *Clinical neuropsychology: Current status and
applications*. Washington, DC: Hemisphere.

Klonoff, H., Robinson, G. C., & Thompson, G. (1969). Acute and chronic brain syndromes
in children. *Developmental Medicine and Child Neurology, 11,* 198–213.

Levin, H. S., Benton, A. L., & Grossman, R. G. (1982). *Neurobehavioral consequences of
closed head injury*. New York: Oxford University Press.

Levin, H. S., & Eisenberg, H. M. (1979a). Neuropsychological impairment after closed
head injury in children and adolescents. *Journal of Pediatric Psychology, 4,* 389–
402.

Levin, H. S., & Eisenberg, H. M. (1979b). Neuropsychological outcome of closed head
injury in children and adolescents. *Child's Brain, 5,* 281–292.

Lishman, W. A. (1978). *Organic psychiatry*. Oxford: Blackwell.

Luria, A. R. (1966). *The working brain*. New York: Basic Books.

Mandleberg, I. A., & Brooks, D. N. (1975). Cognitive recovery after severe head injury: I.
Serial testing on the Wechsler Adult Intelligence Scale. *Journal of Neurology,
Neurosurgery and Psychiatry, 38,* 1121–1126.

McFie, J. (1961). Intellectual impairment in children with localized postinfantile cerebral
lesions. *Journal of Neurology, Neurosurgery and Psychiatry, 24,* 361–365.

McFie, J. (1975a). *Assessment of organic impairment*. New York: Academic Press.

McFie, J. (1975b). Brain injury in childhood and language development. In N. O'Connor
(Ed.), *Language, cognitive deficits, and retardation*. Washington, DC: But-
terworth.

Natelson, S., & Sayers, M. (1973). The fate of children sustaining severe head trauma during birth. *Pediatrics, 51,* 169–180.

Ommaya, A. K., Grubbs, R. L., & Naumann, R. A. (1970). Coup and contrecoup cerebral contusions. An experimental analysis. *Neurology, 20,* 388–389.

Ommaya, A. K., Grubbs, R. L., & Naumann, R. (1971). Coup and contrecoup injury: Observations on the mechanics of visible injuries in the rhesus monkey. *Journal of Neurosurgery, 35,* 503–516.

Oxorn, H. (1980). *Human labor and birth* (4th ed.). New York: Appleton-Century-Crofts.

Parsons, O. A. (1970). *Neuropsychology: Current topics in clinical and community psychology.* New York: Academic Press.

Pendse, A. K., Sran, H. S., Dandia, S. D., & Narula, I. M. S. (1971). Cloused pediatric head injury. A study of 100 cases. *Indian Journal of Pediatrics, 38,* 385–388.

Reitan, R. M., & Fitzhugh, K. B. (1971). Behavioral deficits in groups with cerebrovascular lesions. *Journal of Consulting and Clinical Psychology, 37,* 215–222.

Robbins, S. L. (1974). *Pathologic basis of disease.* Philadelphia: Saunders.

Rourke, B. P., Bakker, D. J., Fisk, J. L., & Strang, J. D. (1983). *Child neuropsychology: An introduction to theory, research, and clinical practice.* New York: Guilford Press.

Rutter, M. (1981). Psychological sequelae of brain damage in children. *American Journal of Psychiatry, 138,* 1533–1544.

Rutter, M., Chadwick, O., & Shaffer, D. (1983). Head injury. In M. Rutter (Ed.), *Developmental neuropsychiatry.* New York: Guilford Press.

Shaffer, D., Bijur, P., Chadwick, O., & Rutter, M. (1980). Head injury and later reading disability. *Journal of the American Academy of Child Psychiatry, 19,* 592–610.

Spreen, O., Tupper, D., Risser, A., Tuokko, H., & Edgell, D. (1984). *Human developmental neuropsychology.* New York: Oxford University Press.

Teuber, H. L., & Rudel, R. G. (1962). Behavior after cerebral lesions in children and adults. *Developmental Medicine and Child Neurology, 4,* 3–20.

Towbin, A. (1970). Central nervous system damage in the human fetus and newborn infant. *American Journal of the Disabled Child, 119,* 529–535.

Vignolo, G. E. (1980). Closed head injuries of school-age children: Neuropsychological sequelae in early adulthood. *Italian Journal of Neurological Sciences, 1*(2), 65–73.

Volpe, J. J. (1977). Neonatal intracranial hemorrhage: Pathophysiology, neuropathology, and clincial features. *Clinics in Perinatology, 4*(1), 77–82.

Wilkening, G. N., & Golden, C. J. (1983). Pediatric neuropsychology: Status, theory, and research. In P. Karyoly, J. Steffens, & D. O'Grady (Eds.), *Child health psychology: Concepts and issues.* New York: Pergamon Press.

Woods, B. T. (1980). The restricted effects of right-hemisphere lesions after age one: Wechsler test data. *Neuropsychologia, 18,* 65–70.

Woods, B. T., & Teuber, H. L. (1974). Mirror movements after childhood hemiparesis. *Neurology, 3,* 273–279.

Woo-Sam, J., Zimmerman, I. L., Brink, J. A., Uyehara, K., & Miller, A. R. (1970). Socioeconomic status and post-traumatic intelligence in children with severe head injuries. *Psychological Reports, 27,* 147–153.

Young, W. M. (1969). Poverty, intelligence, and life in the inner city. *Mental Retardation, 7,* 24–29.

Part II

Neuropsychological Evaluation: Perspectives

Chapter 6

Neuropsychological Screening and Soft Signs

DAVID E. TUPPER

Cognitive Rehabilitation Department
LIFEstyle Institute
Edison, New Jersey 08820

INTRODUCTION

The neuropsychological assessment of children is truly in its beginning stages. Not only are there few well-developed testing procedures available to adequately evaluate the child suspected of central nervous system (CNS) dysfunction, but there is as yet a small formal theoretical or research base from which to fully develop such measures. Nevertheless, the neuropsychological approach is considered by many (e.g., Gaddes, 1981) to represent an advanced, comprehensive state of understanding or way to view impairments of the CNS. This approach will ultimately lead to the development of valid test instruments and the considered, thoughtful application of those instruments to individual children. Fortunately, with the current explosion of interest in the neuropsychological endeavor, not only by neuropsychologists but also by clinical child psychologists, school psychologists, and educators, the promise of future advancement in child neuropsychology is great, and it signals many growing opportunities for the brain-injured child. Neuropsychological assessment of children therefore, while in its beginning stages, shows promise for full-blown theoretical and applied development (as the current volumes certainly attest).

CHILD NEUROPSYCHOLOGY, VOL. 2

One area within child neuropsychology that holds both the pitfalls and the promises of any newly developing area is that of the neuropsychological screening of children with suspected CNS damage. This is especially true for those children with minimal or difficult-to-assess impairments who have been regarded as showing minor CNS damage on measures of neurological function (so-called *soft* neurological *signs*), and who, in the future, many evidence devastating neuropsychological difficulties in coordination, reading, spelling, writing, et cetera because of these CNS impairments. Neuropsychological assessment of children, and screening in particular, is beset with myths and false beliefs (Boll, 1983). Many of these beliefs have arisen not on the basis of empirical work, but on the basis of unwarranted assumptions from the past concerning the nature of brain injury in children and the ways to measure it (as though it were a unitary matter).

Examples of some of the beliefs include the idea that brain damage is a unitary phenomenon; that a *single* test can assess organicity; that there are characteristic patterns of behavioral disturbance attributable to brain damage; and that questionable (borderline) performances on tests means that the status of the brain is also questionable. These myths are hard to shake, partly because so many people believe them (or operate as though they believe them), and partly because some components of them are true. While this chapter does not confront all (or most) of these beliefs, it is necessary to address them within their appropriate context.

The chapter does, at the same time, provide a rather comprehensive survey of the existing literature and available techniques for assessing neurological dysfunctions in children for the purpose of early detection. Screening techniques for neuropsychological deficits in children have as yet to be fully exploited, in spite of their widespread appeal, their efficiency, especially at a time when neuropsychological screening is predicted to gain both in general popularity (Jones & Butters, 1983), and in their popularity among related educational disciplines (Hynd, Quackenbush, & Obrzut, 1980). Screening for neuropsychological dysfunctions can involve brief, select forms of traditional assessment batteries emphasizing definite signs of brain damage. Examinations oriented toward screening are covered later in this chapter. The assessment of soft neurological signs is a second focus of this chapter. *Soft signs* are those manifestations of neurological dysfunction that have been called unreliable, irreproducible, or minor by some authors but that have generally served diagnostic, explanatory, or classificatory functions in child neuropsychological assessment.

To cover both of these topics, it is necessary to begin with a perspective. The perspective is that of a typical two-sided coin, the coin representing the neuropsychological assessment of children: neuropsychological screening represents one side of the coin, and assessment of soft signs is on the flip side. Thus, one can view several complementary situations when one looks at the coin. Soft signs generally deal with diagnosis, more specifically from a neurological vantage point. Screening techniques, on the other side, are concerned more with early detection and secondary prevention of behavioral and neurological disorders. Thus, this coin represents the neurobehavioral assessment of children from a neuropsychological perspective in terms both of diagnosis and early detection and of related neurological and behavioral correlates of performance. Before discussing each of these flip sides, it is necessary to present several crucial theoretical and practical concerns that have impact on the practice of neuropsychological screening and measurement of soft signs. These concerns have to do with the nature of CNS dysfunction in children and its manifestations.

SIGNS AND MANIFESTATIONS OF CNS
DYSFUNCTION IN CHILDREN

In the area of neuropsychological screening and soft signs, one comes face to face with some of the most difficult-to-answer questions confronting both clinicians and researchers in neuropsychological assessment. Myths are especially pervasive here, and there is as-yet little firm evidence to counter them. First of all, as scientists, we need to consider whether brain damage or brain dysfunction represents a unitary phenomenon that can be assessed or screened for easily. If this is not the case, then we have to decide what it means for our screening or measurement techniques. Second, the issue arises as to whether brain damage can vary in degree; whether it is possible to have minor or minimal brain damage, and to consider what minor degrees of brain damage may mean for the assessment. Finally, it needs to be considered whether neurobehavioral assessment measures (vs. neurodiagnostic procedures) are really the most effective and informative ways to screen for more-subtle CNS disturbances, or whether the neurobehavioral measurement of soft signs even makes any sense.

Numerous investigators, especially in the 1930s and 1940s, made the assumption that brain damage was a unitary quantity that was either present or absent in a given individual. Such beliefs have persisted into the present and have led to the development of assessment devices that ignore the now well-known complexity of brain–behavior relationships. For example, the use of the Bender–Gestalt as a test for organicity was quite frequent in the past and still enjoys a fairly great popularity, although there have been recent attempts to update its use (Lacks, 1984). Needless to say, there are significant difficulties associated with assuming that brain damage is an all-or-none phenomenon that, when present, produces a characteristic pattern of behavioral disturbance that can be assessed with a single test. It should be noted that this is as true for adults as it is for children. As Boll (1983) has pointed out, the major problem with positing an all-or-none effect for brain damage in children is that diagnosis of brain damage tends to turn into an end in itself and does not lead to further clinical action (Herbert, 1964). We are far enough along in our clinical and scientific wisdom that this state of affairs should no longer exist. Therefore, the assumption that underlies this chapter is that screening of children for CNS dysfunction is *not* an end in itself but rather just the beginning of appropriate service delivery.

As is shown later, there has been a tremendous interest in that large group of children who have been said to show minimal brain damage, on the basis of only slightly inferior performance on neuropsychological or neurological assessment measures. Assessment of minor variations in performance poses difficulties for both clinicians and researchers alike in our present state of knowledge because there has been little direct evidence, and few well-designed studies, available to show strong support for the direct connection between minor cerebral damage and borderline test performances (H. G. Taylor, 1983; H. G. Taylor & Fletcher, 1983), although the evidence available is attractive and does suggest some kind of connection.

Finally, the issue of screening children for neuropsychological impairments makes sense when one considers the large numbers of children who currently are suspected of showing significant learning or behavioral disabilities and who are now mandated by PL (Public Law) 94-142 to receive some form of remedial intervention. Neuropsychological screening, if carefully considered and implemented, may prove to be as cost-effective as other methods of examining children for learning impairments. It also may more easily be carried out in schools or other places where it can catch as many children as possible.

Diagnostic and Theoretical Concerns

Three areas of concern in child neuropsychological assessment require further consideration before addressing the measurement of soft signs and neuropsychological screening for clinical purposes. These areas represent not only areas of diagnostic and theoretical confusion but also related categories of children who are likely to benefit from neuropsychological

assessment. It is not the aim of this chapter to cover these topics extensively or to present alternative views; the aim is only to identify areas of
concern for those intending to conduct assessments of soft signs or to
screen these children. The three areas to be presented are (1) the concept
of minimal brain dysfunction, (2) the question of identifying patterns of
neuropsychological disability in children, and (3) the identification of
those children at risk for neuropsychological impairment.

Minimal Brain Dysfunction

Minimal brain dysfunction (MBD) is almost by definition a broad category. It has been called a wastebasket category (Ross, 1973), and the use
of the term has been considered to be not a diagnosis but an escape from
making one (Ingram, 1973; Touwen, 1978). MBD children have often
included children that have been otherwise labeled learning disabled, dyslexic, hyperkinetic, attention-deficit disorder, or specific developmental
disorder. Clements (1966) has, in fact, presented a list of 99 (!) different
signs and symptoms of MBD in children, and more recently, Small (1982)
has listed almost as many (or so it seems) symptoms that are attributed to
MBD of unspecified origin. It is this overinclusiveness of signs and symptoms that has clouded the issue of the diagnosis of MBD and has led to
the uncritical diagnostic use of the label MBD (Weiss, 1980). Much of the
sloppiness can be encompassed in the phrase "minimal cerebral damage
(maximal neurologic confusion)" proposed by Gomez (1967, p. 589).

To look more critically at this area, as Gomez, one is easily confused.
Nevertheless, it is clinically apparent that there is a large group of children out there who show minor deviations from the norm on neuropsychological or neurological measures, and who show no other signs of
definite brain damage. The use of the category MBD has more traditionally been made on the basis of behavioral, not neurological criteria (Benton, 1973; MacKeith & Bax, 1963) and this has undoubtedly also contributed to the confusion. However, one fact that is often ignored is the
heterogeneity of this group of children (see Shaffer, 1980, for a discussion
of this issue with hyperkinesis). In more recent years, there has been an
increased awareness of this heterogeneity, and the term MBD has become
modified to minimal brain dysfunctions to somehow include all these
diverse children (H. E. Rie & Rie, 1980; Small, 1982). The term still,
however, more commonly refers to groups of *behavioral* not neurological
disorders, and the presumption of minimal damage to neurological structures is only an assumption (H. G. Taylor, 1983).

The possible etiologies of MBD using the term as a *neurological,* not a
behavioral concept, can be varied (Spreen, Tupper, Risser, Tuokko, &
Edgell, 1984), adding to the confusion. They could range through prena-

tal, perinatal, and postnatal factors and could lead to brain damage (unfortunately, it is difficult to stay away from using this unitary-sounding term) varying in severity from mild to severe. Using this more restricted definition of MBD helps us more adequately describe these children and to see that the children require more adequate diagnosis than is implied by just the label MBD. If we restrict discussion of MBD children to those children shown to have *proven* evidence of slight damage to the nervous system, we obviate many of the behavioral classification problems and see that MBD is not a primary diagnosis of a unitary disorder at all, but at best, an accessory diagnosis—one that is of limited value.

Neuropsychological Patterns of Disability

A better approach to look at brain–behavior correlations in children is to use a multivariate perspective where neurological factors are only one possible influence on behavioral performance (H. G. Taylor, Fletcher, & Satz, 1984) and where neuropsychological patterns of performance (both intact capabilities and disabilities) are evaluated in their own right. Heterogeneity is explicitly acknowledged in this approach. Thus, a researcher using this approach would look at subtypes of neuropsychological abilities (see Rourke, 1981; Rourke, Bakker, Fisk, & Strang, 1983) and compare groups of children (e.g., spelling or reading disabled) with an eye toward the more complete description of their basic competencies and abilities, and any neurological limits to these competencies. A clinician also would use the approach in a clinical neuropsychological evaluation to emphasize the *behavioral* capacities of the child rather than the neurological workings of the child's brain, although neurological evidence is useful for hypothesis generation about the child's abilities. In this way, brain–behavior relationships as assessed by neuropsychological test performance emphasize not the *confirmatory* role (although sometimes this is useful) but the *descriptive–prescriptive* role of the clinician. It is beyond the scope of this chapter to delve into the evidence supporting this function of the child neuropsychologist, and the reader is referred elsewhere (Rourke et al., 1983; Satz & Fletcher, 1980; Taylor et al., 1984; Gaddes, 1981; Boll, 1983; Boll & Barth, 1981). It is sufficient to say here that while "confirmation" of brain dysfunction is often a goal of neuropsychological evaluation, it is not the only or best goal of such an evaluation. In terms of screening, neuropsychological screening examinations will have to be sufficiently broad-based to provide power to detect subtle neuropsychological problems.

Children at Risk for Neuropsychological Impairment

It is the identification of children with subtle neuropsychological deficits that is the main focus of this chapter. Neuropsychological screening techniques are seen as attempting to identify those children at risk for future neuropsychological impairment and to refer such children for more comprehensive evaluation. CNS dysfunction is presumed to be the factor that makes the children *vulnerable* to this increased risk of neuropsychological difficulty (Tarter, 1983). The assessment of vulnerability to CNS dysfunction, however, is itself a complex process (Tarter, 1983) and has yet to receive the widespread attention that is necessary for us to be secure in our screening devices. Few longitudinal studies of children at risk for neuropsychological impairment based on neurological evidence have been performed (see the Florida Longitudinal Project; Fletcher, Satz, & Morris, 1982; Spreen, 1981). Therefore, little direct evidence is available concerning the *outcome* of children with minor CNS impairments. Some authors, like Rutter (1981, 1982; Rutter, Chadwick, & Schacher, 1983), have discussed the possibility of a *threshold* for risk after brain injury. Thus, investigators have to consider not only the presence or absence of neurological damage as risk factors, but also the degree or type of damage in order for the risk to be present or increased. Screening examinations therefore have to become very elaborate indeed, which affects their cost-effectiveness.

Most often, pathognomonic (hard or soft) signs have been used in screening exams as *markers* for the identification of children at risk for later neuropsychological difficulties resulting from suspected minor neurological dysfunction. As the section on soft signs discusses, however, the use of such signs is questionable to diagnose cerebral impairment. However, they may be useful as indicators of specific neurobehavioral disturbances, such as incoordination, in their own right. The development of screening techniques to detect at-risk children is a very fruitful area for further research and deserves much study.

Definitions

Before discussing in more detail neuropsychological assessment techniques designed for screening or measuring children with subtle CNS disturbances, it is useful to provide some relatively standard definitions of terms that have tended to be misused in the past.

A *sign* (neurological or otherwise) is traditionally defined as "any *objective* evidence or manifestation of an illness or disordered function of the body. Signs are more or less definitive and obvious . . . in contrast to *symptoms* which are subjective'' *(Taber's cyclopedic medical dictionary,* 1973, p. S-46) (italics added).

The term *screening,* as used in a neuropsychological context, refers to a procedure that will designate positive instances of a category (the category here referring to organicity or MBD). It identifies "those individuals in need of further assessment in order to determine if they are 'positive' with respect to the characteristic in question" (Rourke et al., 1983, p. 114). Thus, the aim is to make some type of decision regarding appropriate referral of the child for a diagnosis, not to make a diagnosis by itself. *Taber's* adds further information to understand the screening process, as it defines *screening* as, "Testing or examining an individual or large groups of people by utilizing only a portion of the usual examining procedures" (1973, p. S-24). Therefore, the traditional definitions of screening emphasize the process of decision-making with cost-effective examining procedures.

SOFT NEUROLOGICAL SIGNS

Clinical Manifestations

As was indicated, the identification of a sign of neurological dysfunction is based on objective evidence of the underlying disturbance. Such is the case for obvious or hard signs of neurological disturbance, such as an abnormal Babinski (extensor plantar) reflex, which indicates significant corticospinal disease. These traditional signs of neurological disturbance are considered *pathognomonic* of (i.e., invariably associated with) CNS dysfunction and are an important method of inference-making used in comprehensive neuropsychological assessment (Boll, 1978). Pathognomonic signs include such signs as a markedly asymmetric motor or sensory pattern on half of the body (e.g., hemiplegia), dysarthria, abnormal reflexes, changes in pupillary size, and some visual field deficits. Evidence for these pathognomonic signs has accumulated over the years and has been extensively documented (see any current neurology text).

In the neurological assessment of MBD children with minor behavioral disturbances, or children with learning disabilities and without obvious neurological impairment, however, there has been some variability or uncertainty about these traditional hard signs. Clearly, these signs are not found with the frequency or severity that could be found in children with definite brain damage, although *some* findings are apparent on the neurological exam. Not willing to give up the notion altogether that they reflect something about the status of the brain, clinicians and researchers have called these uncertain signs *soft neurological signs* to distinguish them from the *hard* or *pathognomonic signs*. They have also been called minor signs by some authors (Touwen, 1979). These soft signs include such signs as associated movements, motor incoordination, right–left confusion, mild hemiparesis, and so forth, and are described in more detail.

Bender (1947) was the first to use the term *soft neurological signs* in her description of 100 schizophrenic children whom she tested on neurological examination. Prior to that time, beginning at about the turn of the century, the existence of these soft signs were known (Kennard, 1960), and they were frequently considered to be equivocal, emphasizing the fact that the early clinicians did not know how to fully interpret these signs. However, it was Bender's use of the term *soft signs* and the growing climate of interest in neuropsychological disorders in children in general due in large part to A. Strauss and colleagues (Strauss & Lehtinen, 1947; Strauss & Kephart, 1955), that catapulted soft neurological signs into a position of importance in the diagnosis of MBD (also called the Strauss syndrome). It was this historical background that has led to the situation where now soft signs have become a common means for documenting MBD or other neurologically based learning disorders (Gaddes, 1981; Small, 1982).

The acceptance of soft signs as evidence for MBD is not without contention, however. At the time of the Oxford International Study Group on Child Neurology in 1962, it was realized that the inference of brain damage from an essentially behavioral description of the child formed a logical error, and the term *minimal brain dysfunction* was proposed as a substitute (MacKeith & Bax, 1963). At approximately the same time in the United States, a national task force was formed to clarify the concept of MBD, which in retrospect it did not do, but it did criticize the diagnostic use of soft signs (Clements, 1966). One of the most outspoken critics of the use of soft signs was Ingram (1973), who stated that reference to soft signs was "diagnostic of soft thinking" (p. 529). Thus, Ingram stated what many clinicians and researchers had felt all along: that use of soft neurological signs as direct evidence of minimal cerebral damage was faulty.

Because of Ingram's statement in the early 1970s, and because our understanding of the meaning of soft signs was (and is) fuzzy, many researchers have since then taken a more critical look at the measurement, diagnostic utility, and meaning of these signs. One of the earliest attempts to decipher the meaning of soft signs was made by Rutter, Graham, and Yule (1970), in their Isle of Wight study. They proposed that we are dealing not with equally valid signs of disturbance but rather with three different groups of soft signs:

1. Signs that indicate developmental delay and disappear with age.

2. Signs that are difficult to elicit and have poor reliability in the neurological examination—these are generally considered difficult to test, irreproducible, or unreliable signs. They are the ones typically considered soft signs and suggest the presence of minor degrees of CNS damage, as contrasted with hard signs suggesting definite presence of brain damage.

3. Signs that result not from pathological neurological conditions but from causes other than neurological damage; for example, symptoms such as nystagmus or strabismus.

Recently, many investigators have followed Rutter et al.'s (1970) lead and have begun subgrouping soft signs. Subgrouping does have several advantages, even though at present there is little empirical justification for subgrouping of soft signs. The major advantage of subgrouping is for the exclusion of signs that are unreliable or due to nonneurological factors. A second advantage is that at present, due to our lack of research knowledge concerning soft signs, it may be useful to investigate the classes of soft signs separately; for example, signs that would indicate developmental delay might be correlated with developmental disorders; signs that indicate abnormality might be examined in other abnormal populations; et cetera. Thus, on the research side, it may be useful to investigate the subgroups of soft signs.

On the clinical side, subgroups of soft signs seem to make sense, at least on the surface. Most clinicians currently divide soft signs into two categories: One category consists of those signs that would be considered normal in a younger child and that, because they persist, are abnormal in the older child. This category has been called *developmental-only* by Denckla (1978) and the *soft-developmental type* of soft sign by Gardner (1979). It corresponds to Rutter et al.'s (1970) Category 1. The second category of soft signs are those signs that are pathological at any age, but which are more-subtle manifestations of the hard signs. These are Rutter et al.'s (1970) Category 2 and are what Denckla (1978) has referred to as "pastel classics" from the neurological exam or what Gardner (1979) has called the "soft neurological type" of soft sign. Unfortunately, not everyone interested in soft signs has made such a division, and the literature is replete with many studies and tests that lump all soft signs together. This chapter makes this division of soft signs, using the terms *developmental soft signs* and *soft signs of abnormality*.

Developmental Soft Signs

This type of soft sign consists of those signs that are considered abnormal only if they persist beyond the age that they are traditionally seen.

This category makes the assumption that there are certain behaviors that the child outgrows, and that are only problems when they continue. A second type of developmental soft sign is the delayed appearance of a developmental milestone. Two examples illustrate these types. The first example is of the late suppression of a primitive sign like the Babinski reflex; the Babinski reflex generally is present soon after birth and disappears early in development, usually by about 1 year of age. It would be abnormal for a 3-, 4-, or 5-year-old child to show a positive Babinski sign (even asymmetric) and thus it is generally taken as evidence of some type of neurological dysfunction when it persists (usually along with accompanying evidence). A second example, this time of the delayed appearance of a developmental milestone, would be the child who at 2 years of age had not yet begun to walk. Because most children walk between 10 and 14 months of age and most neurologists would consider a child not walking by about 19 to 20 months of age as showing a developmental lag, late appearance of walking would be a developmental soft sign and suggest some type of neurological disturbance.

A further point needs to be made concerning developmental soft signs. Because these signs are related to the child's development, it is expected that they can outgrow the problem, and thus the difficulty represents a delay rather than a deficit, which would occur if the delay persisted indefinitely. Hence, if a child not walking at 24 months were still not walking at 6 years of age, one would probably consider the child motorically impaired, cerebral palsied, or some other diagnostic term. Thus, it is possible for a child's developmental soft sign to turn into a hard sign just by persisting as the child gets older. Even though authors like Kinsbourne (1973), and Friedlander, Pothier, Morrison, and Herman, (1982) consider MBD to represent a delay or maturational lag, there is no guarantee that the child will outgrow the problem. Unfortunately, there are all too few longitudinal studies that have tested this assertion. The longitudinal studies available do suggest, however, that the difficulties evidenced by the MBD child (including so-called developmental soft signs) do not go away but rather change form as the child grows older (Peter & Spreen, 1979; Satz, Taylor, Friel, & Fletcher, 1978); it is beyond the scope of the chapter to review all this evidence.

Table 1 lists most of the developmental soft signs that have been described in the literature. They include such traditional neurological signs as associated or overflow movements, motor impersistence, and others, as well as such vague developmental changes as maturity of pencil grasp, clumsiness, and difficulty on constructional tasks. Clearly, this table has been generated based mostly on clinical anecdotal experience. It is unfortunate that more-refined measures are unavailable (see the following section on measurement).

TABLE 1

Developmental soft signs[a]

Associated movements (overflow or mirror movements)
Difficulty building with blocks
Immature grasp of pencil
Inability to catch a ball
Latness in developmental milestones (e.g., standing, talking, walking)
Lateness in suppressing primitive signs (e.g., Babinski, tonic neck reflexes)
Motor awkwardness; clumsiness for age
Motor impersistence
Poor gait, posture, stance
Slowness of gait, hand movements, opposing the fingers to the thumb, tapping
Speech articulation problems
Tactile extinction on double simultaneous stimulation

[a] Taken from Denckla (1978), Gardner (1979), Rapin (1982), H. G. Taylor & Fletcher (1983), and others.

Finally, another point needs to be made concerning the assessment of developmental soft signs. There are as yet few research reports that evaluate soft signs with regard to developmental differences (Rudel, Healy, & Denckla, 1984; Fog & Fog, 1963; Connolly & Stratton, 1968). Thus, it would be expected that different developmental soft signs would be more applicable at different ages, but no one has made that differentiation. Developmental norms are sorely needed in this area of clinical assessment if one is to make valid inferences concerning "delays" or "lags" (Spreen & Gaddes, 1969).

Soft Signs of Abnormality

Soft signs of abnormality are those soft signs whose appearance at any age would be considered abnormal, although they are minor in degree with respect to hard signs. Table 2 presents a fairly comprehensive listing of these signs. Soft signs of abnormality are Denckla's (1978) "pastel classics" or Gardner's (1979) "soft neurological type" of soft neurological sign. These are mild abnormalities that one would find when conducting a traditional neurological examination, and they include such abnormalities as reflex asymmetries, hypo- and hyperreflexia, nystagmus, dysarthria, tremors, or hypokinesis. An example of a child with such signs would be the right-handed, average IQ child with significant reading disability (independently assessed) who showed some asymmetric, right-sided incoordination, bilateral associated movements, very mild word-finding difficulty, and who had an EEG record of diffuse, nonlocalizing

TABLE 2

Soft signs of abnormality[a]

Astereognosis
Asymmetries of associated movements
Auditory-visual integration difficulties
Choreiform movements
Diffuse EEG abnormalities
Dysarthria
Dysdiadochokinesis
Dysgraphesthesia
Hypokinesis
Labile affect
Motor impersistence
Nystagmus
Oromotor apraxia, drooling, active jaw jerk
Pathological reflex
Postural and gait abnormalities
Posturing of hands while walking
Reflex asymmetries
Reflex increase or decrease from normal
Significant incoordination
Tone increase or decrease from normal
Tremors
Word-finding difficulty

[a] Taken from various authors

abnormalities, judged as borderline by the electroencephalographer. The child may be diagnosed as MBD or dyslexia.

These soft signs of abnormality are not the usual pathognomonic signs that the neurologist encounters; they are also typically not found in the same type of child as other hard signs. The etiological or localizing significance of these signs is most often not apparent, either. Thus, some authors have referred to these signs as nonfocal neurologic signs, as compared to soft or equivocal signs (Hertzig & Shapiro, in press; Shapiro, Burkes, Petti, & Ranz, 1978).

Measurement of Soft Signs

Both types of soft signs, developmental and abnormal, suffer many methodological and measurement problems. Aside from general measurement concerns, which are important for any assessment measure, such as reliability and validity (American Psychological Association [APA],

1974), E. Taylor (1983) and Shafer, Shaffer, O'Connor, and Stokman (1983) have pointed out specific methodological and measurement problems related to soft signs. E. Taylor (1983), for example, emphasizes the necessity of demonstrating several types of validity for soft signs. Construct validity is crucial because any neuropsychological or neurological assessment technique needs to be demonstrated to be specifically related to other measures of neural functioning, such as tests of the structural integrity of the brain (radiological measures like the CT scan), indexes of insults to the brain such as an abnormal perinatal history or postnatal head trauma, or the presence of other minor congenital abnormalities (Paulsen and O'Donnell, 1980). E. Taylor (1983) also suggests the use of criterion-referenced tests that emphasize discriminant as well as convergent validation; thus, a good evaluation for soft signs not only does show relations to abnormality in brain functioning, but also does not show associations to other factors that confound the assessment, such as social class, parental education, or even low IQ.

Shafer et al. (1983) have taken a hard look at the methodological difficulties with soft-sign measurement. These researchers conclude that, while there are a multitude of methodological concerns in soft-sign measurement, many measures of soft signs are in fact reliable. It is useful to summarize some of their methodological concerns here. The first issue they deal with is the reliability of the measures in terms of interrater agreement. In their review of past indices of interrater agreement, they found a fair amount of agreement, ranging from about 57% to greater than 80%. These authors cite past reports that include Rutter et al. (1970), Werry, Minde, Guzman, Weiss, Dogan, and Hoy (1972), Nichols and Chen (1981) and Quitkin, Rifkin, and Klein (1976). Some studies have obviated the interrater agreement difficulty by using only one examiner (Kennard, 1960; Peters, Romine, & Dykman, 1975). Therefore, Shafer et al. (1983) find fairly good support to suggest that, at this state of knowledge, interrater agreement for soft-sign measures is adequate.

The next methodological issue that they address is the stability of measures of soft signs over time: measures of intra-observer variability. Conflicting reports on this issue are found in the literature: Denckla (1973) found high levels of agreement for fine motor coordination items when retesting the same subjects at 3 weeks; Peters et al. (1975) found adequate agreement up to 6 months later, and Shapiro et al. (1978), although without statistical evidence, demonstrated consistency of their nonfocal neurological signs on follow-up at either 1, 2, or 7 days. Quitkin et al. (1976) also showed a test–retest correlation of .96 on retesting within 2 days of the initial examination. McMahon and Greenberg (1977), on the other hand, reported repeat examinations over an 8-week period, but with only

12 of 44 subjects receiving consistent scores on their soft-signs measure. However, in total, the majority of studies that have addressed the issue of short-term stability of soft-signs measures have reported adequate stability (Shafer et al., 1983). Such is also the case for the only study available reporting an assessment of long-term stability (Hertzig, 1982), measured after 4 years. Measures of soft-sign reliability therefore have received some attention in the past and generally support the idea that soft signs can be reliably measured.

Other methodological concerns that Shafer et al. (1983) raise include possible confounding effects of including subjects with evidence of a focal neuroanatomical abnormality or lowered cognitive ability in a study. Past research is mixed on this issue: Hertzig, Bortner, and Birch (1969) separated their children into groups with and without focal abnormality, while Kennard (1960) did not. Most researchers, however, do not define specifically any exclusionary criteria for neurological conditions, although some indicate use of them (Lerer & Lerer, 1976; Owen, Adams, Forrest, Stolz, & Fisher, 1971; Peters et al., 1975; Prechtl & Stemmer, 1962; Werry et al., 1972). Clearly, presence of focal neurological deficit is a potentially confounding problem in measurement of soft signs (Shafer et al., 1983), can affect construct validation, and needs to be accorded appropriate attention. Other confounding effects in soft-sign studies include errors of inference due to inappropriate multiple statistical comparisions, selection bias—also referred to as Berkson's paradox—operating in clinical settings, and examiner bias (Shafer et al., 1983).

There are other measurement issues that have not been addressed as well in the past literature and that more directly affect clinical practice. Such issues as the reliability of individual soft signs, as compared to aggregate measures or batteries, has yet to be addressed directly, although it could potentially be useful in eliminating unreliable or problematic items (Werry & Aman, 1976). The development of reliable *items* would most likely increase the likelihood that individual investigators would adopt the item as part of their battery, thereby increasing the comparability and communication of results across studies.

A second issue, thus far alluded to but not addressed adequately, is the lack of normative—especially age-related—data to support the items themselves. Only Gardner (1979) has made a concerted attempt to provide normative data on measures used for neurological soft-sign measurement. Data such as these are especially crucial for the measurement of developmental soft signs, as it may provide the only criteria against which to base the interpretation. Finally, scaling of soft-sign measures also deserves attention. Many soft-sign items are scored on an all-or-none basis (presence–absence) (for example, the Neurological Dysfunctions of Chil-

TABLE 3

Soft sign examinations

Examination	Ages tested	Source
Examination of the Child with Minor Nervous Dysfunction (2nd ed.)	All ages	Touwen (1979)
Extended Neurological Examination	Not noted, presumably a wide range	Voeller (1981)
Gardner's Soft Neurological Sign Examination	Approximately 5–15 yrs.	Gardner (1979)
Neurological Dysfunctions of Children (NDOC)	3–10 yrs.	Kuhns (1979)
Peters' "Special" Neurological Examination for School-Age Children	6–14 yrs.	Peters, Davis, Goolsby, Clements, & Hicks (1973)
Physical and Neurological Examination for Soft Signs (PANESS)	Not noted, presumably a wide range	Guy (1976)
Quick Neurological Screening Test (Rev. ed.) (QNST)	Wide range	Mutti, Sterling, & Spalding (1978)

dren [NDOC]) but some, like the items in Gardner's (1979) series of tests, or the items on the Physical and Neurological Examination for Soft Signs (PANESS) or Quick Neurological Screening Test (QNST) are items with graded responses. It is unclear exactly what are the differences among some of these measures, except for test developers' preferences, and thus this issue needs further clarification and research.

Representative Soft-Sign Examinations

Investigators have typically chosen and developed their own items and examinations in research and clinical application of soft signs. This makes integration of information from various studies difficult, and it can lead the clinician to wonder how to select a reliable soft-sign measure to use in practice. Nevertheless, there have been several soft-sign examinations that have been used more frequently by researchers and that, in general, are more accessible to the clinician. These exams are discussed briefly in this section, with no specific recommendations to be made: At this point, no one exam can be clearly recommended over others, and only a few have reported reliability. Table 3 lists the exams to be discussed with the ages that they cover and their sources.

Touwen's (1979) *Examination of the Child with Minor Neurological Dysfunction* is more of a traditional neurological examination than some of the others. It is a rather comprehensive examination including (1) assessment of sitting, standing, walking, lying; (2) examination of the motor system and reflexes and the functioning of various parts of the body including the trunk and the head; and (3) specific tests for coordination, involuntary and associated movements, as well as a consideration of general data about the child. It is not specified in the manual what ages are appropriate for the examination, although it can be concluded from the variety of items included that the examination (or some parts) are appropriate for almost any age child. There is a rather unique feature to Touwen's (1979) examination (see also Touwen, 1978). Each item is defined in terms of an optimal response—this is the best response obtainable, rather than a normal response. The responses are scored numerically in terms of the optimal score. Thus, the presence of a strong optimal response is scored 3, a weak response is scored 2, and the absence of a response is scored 0. (This holds for items requiring the presence of an optimal response; some items are scored in the opposite direction to indicate that sometimes the optimal response will be 0 when the item should typically be absent.) No data is reported regarding either reliability or validity of the examination, although Touwen (1979) describes the interpretation of various clusters of items into hemisyndromes so that it is meant to be primarily a clinically useful examination.

The proposed Extended Neurological Examination described by Voeller (1981) is a much more flexible incorporation of neuropsychological assessment techniques into a standard neurological examination. Voeller (1981) has provided an extensive list of follow-up procedures for the neurological examination, including measures of hand preference, fine-motor functioning, language processing, body image, visuospatial processing and constructional abilities, receptive language, and academic skills. The chosen tests are generally well standardized and reliable and can be used to follow up more closely minor difficulties noted during the standard neurological exam. Thus, Voeller (1981) suggests careful, systematic diagnostic follow-up of individual children with suspected neurological dysfunction.

Gardner (1979), in his book on the objective diagnosis of MBD, devotes a chapter to the assessment of soft neurological signs, both developmental soft signs and soft signs of abnormality. The author also recommends a selective choice of test procedures to follow up the suspicion of MBD in a child, and hence also does not have a battery per se. However, the author does provide useful tests for the measurement of both types of soft signs and demonstrates a major preoccupation with objective standard, well-designed measures of soft signs. Only a few examples of the tests are provided here; readers wanting more information should consult Gardner, 1979, which also provides normative data on many of the measures. Gardner describes several measurement examples of the soft developmental type of soft neurological sign, including examples of primitive reflexes, developmental milestones (emphasizing speech development), articulation, and pencil grasp. Gardner (1979) went to the trouble of collecting quantitative and qualitative data on types of pencil grasp and gives data concerning pencil grasp in both normal and MBD children. The data are particularly interesting in identifying a neurodevelopmental lag in grasp for MBD children and suggesting that a mature grasp is expected in normal children by about age 12. The soft neurological type of soft-sign exam includes measures of tremors and choreiform movements, motor impersistence, and motor overflow. Standardized tests suggested here include subtests of the Lincoln-Oseretsky Scale (Sloan, 1955), the Denver Developmental Screening Test (Frankenburg & Dodds, 1971), Garfield's (1964) motor impersistence tests, Kinsbourne's (1973) Finger-Stick test for associated movements, and tests of motor overflow from Abercrombie, Lindon, and Tyson (1964) and Cohen, Taft, Mahadeviah, and Birch (1967). Each of these references need to be consulted for further reliability and validity information.

Kuhns's (1979) NDOC is an 18-item screening evaluation for soft neurological signs, designed to be used by psychologists, physicians, school psychologists, or other professionals. It has the restricted goals of aiding the examiner in the diagnosis of neurologically based learning disorders, and identifying children to be referred for further neurological evaluation. The NDOC consists of 16 tasks that the child is asked to perform, including items such as fingertip touching, visual pursuit, standing on one leg, walking along a straight line, and tongue movements. Item 17 is a measurement of the child's head circumference and Item 18 consists of a structured parental interview, used to collect information on the child's developmental history. Each item is scored either *yes* (indicating mild to moderate impairment) or *no* (normal functioning), and all items are considered in terms of developmental age. The age range covered for the NDOC is 3–10 years of age. Interpretation from the NDOC is done not from separate item ratings but from 13 interpretation clusters of items described well in the manual. Referral recommendations are made based on the clusters evidenced by the child. The NDOC has much to offer the inexperienced clinician in the interpretation of soft signs. The manual includes not only a complete description of the administration of each item but also a theoretical interpretation of each item and the clusters.

Adequate reliability (test–retest and interrater) over a 3-week period, as well as some validity data, are provided in the manual.

Peters, Davis, Goolsby, Clements, and Hicks (1973), in the *Physician's Handbook: Screening for MBD,* provide a Special Neurological Examination for School-Age Children (ages 6–14 years), which has been used to investigate soft signs in children with learning disabilities (Peters et al., 1975). The examination consists of nine items, rated mild, moderate, or severe (abnormality). The items include hopping on one foot, skipping, touching thumb to fingers, alternating hand movements, tapping index finger on thumb, associated movements, right–left confusion, eye tracking, and writing to dictation. No reliability or validity data are provided, but qualitative observations are provided to assist interpretation.

The PANESS (Guy, 1976) was developed at the National Institute of Mental Health's (NIMH) Department of Health, Education, and Welfare as part of a comprehensive drug evaluation program. It is now one of the most widely used soft-sign exams in existence. The PANESS consists of two parts: the first part is a 15-item exam for the assessment of physical status including such items as the child's height, weight, pulse, and head circumference. The second part is the 43-item exam for the assessment of neurological soft signs. The items are scored from 1 (performed correctly) to 4 (unsuccessful), and they include items for finger-nose touching, touching a heel to a leg, identifying figures traced in the hand, hopping on one foot, finger tapping, motor persistence, and others.

Werry and Aman (1976) have examined the interrater reliability of the PANESS with two different examiners over variable periods of time. These authors report that although examiners did achieve a high level of agreement about global neurological status, many of the signs, though reliable, did not occur in the majority of children, thus leading to the conclusion that the PANESS may contain a substantial number of noncontributory items. Mikkelsen, Brown, Minichiello, Millican, and Rapoport (1982), however, have found adequate reliability for the exam as a whole and suggest that it may serve as a valid measure of developmental neurological maturity not necessarily specific to diagnostic category. Camp, Bialer, Snerd, and Winsberg (1978) and Holden, Tarnowski, and Prinz (1982) came to a similar conclusion though, as Werry and Aman (1976) suggested, Camp et al. (1978) caution against the routine acceptance of the PANESS as the definitive exam for soft signs.

The final soft-sign exam reviewed here is the QNST (Mutti, Sterling, & Spalding, 1978). This soft-sign screening test is also designed to be used by nonneurologists. It is appropriate to a wide age range of children and consists of 15 items testing hand skill, figure recognition and production, eye tracking, double simultaneous stimulation, tandem walking, left–right discrimination, repetitive hand movement, finger to nose touching, and other soft-sign items. Each item is given a numerical score, but the most informative aspect of the test for the individual child is the qualitative information gained on each item. The manual includes several interpretive and medical considerations for the items, and there is a section on educational implications of the results. A final section of the manual describes limited past research done with the QNST, mostly by the authors (H. M. Sterling & Sterling, 1977a,b; P. J. Sterling & Sterling, 1980), but there is no reliability information presented, and the main usefulness of the test is the qualitative descriptive data generated.

Past Research and Clinical Applications

If one assumes that soft signs can be reliably assessed, then one is still left with the question of whether soft signs bear any direct relationship to neurological status or if they can be used to identify neurobehavioral difficulties during routine clinical examination. Unfortunately, Ingram's (1973) statement about soft signs being diagnostic of soft thinking is especially applicable when one reviews this literature. Except for the association reported between increased incidence of soft signs in children with MBD, the evidence to provide a direct relationship between soft signs and neurological status is nonexistent (Schmitt, 1975; Touwen & Sporrel, 1979). One is therefore left with only presumptive evidence (H. G. Taylor, 1983; H. G. Taylor & Fletcher, 1983) regarding the association. The investigation of soft-signs–neurological-status correlations in a well-designed study is the major research necessity in the soft-sign area.

Investigators supportive of soft-sign research who have searched for the indirect evidence suggestive of biological factors in behavioral disorders contend that children with behavioral or learning disorders tend to have a greater number of soft signs than do normal children. Thus, a great many studies have compared normal children with hyperactive, learning disabled, language disordered, or motor disordered children, all in search of the indirect link between neurological and behavioral status. One of the overlooked factors in this association, however, is that even if there is an increased frequency of soft signs in developmentally or neurologically impaired children, it is unclear what exactly this increase would imply or whether it would aid in distinguishing neurologically impaired children from the broader classification of other childhood behavioral disorders (Satz & Fletcher, 1980; H. G. Taylor & Fletcher, 1983). Soft signs, therefore, would be another nonspecific factor in assessment of these children.

An early investigation into this area, aside from the work of Bender

(1947) and Kennard (1960, 1969), was that of Hertzig et al. (1969), who compared 90 learning disabled children with controls and found that 69% of the learning-disabled children showed soft signs while only 6% of the controls showed soft signs. It should be noted though that admission to the facility that these children were in was based on a confirmed diagnosis of brain damage (see also Copple & Isom, 1968; Bortner, Hertzig, & Birch, 1972). Kenny and Clemmens (1971), on the other hand, concluded on the basis of evaluations of 100 children with learning and/or behavioral problems that there was no significant relation between neurological examination (including soft signs) and final diagnosis. Nevertheless Page-El and Grossman (1973), at about the same time, were arguing that involvement of the CNS is a common denominator in learning disabilities and MBD, and they recommended neurological examination as a prime assessment procedure.

Adams, Kocsis, and Estes (1974), in a screening of 368 children, compared 9- and 10-year old learning-disabled and normal control children with soft signs and found that graphesthesia and diadochokinesia were lower in the disabled group than the controls, but that the magnitude of the differences was not sufficient for clinical usefulness. Hart, Rennick, Klinge, and Schwartz (1974) found a similar increased incidence of soft signs in learning-disabled children. Peters et al. (1975) compared two groups of boys, learning disabled and normal controls, on 80 special neurological signs. They report statistical significance for 44 of the signs; these were mostly motor coordination items. On this basis, these authors argued for the validity of the neurological examination of children with minimal CNS deviations and have developed their special neurological examination with this in mind. More recently, E. D. Rie, Rie, Stewart, and Rettemnier (1978) have identified, in a group of 80 children with learning difficulties, six different factors in a soft-sign battery. The factors included a general broad-range ability factor, verbal–motor and visuomotor integration factors, and age, sex, and hyperactivity factors. It is one of the only studies that has looked more specifically at the individual items.

Similar results have been obtained for children with other developmental neurological abnormalities, specifically hyperactivity, language or reading disorders, or others, including psychosis (Tucker, 1979) and other psychiatric disorders (Shaffer, 1978). In an early classic investigation, Prechtl and Stemmer (1962) found a high incidence of reading difficulties in children with excessive clumsiness and choreiform movements. Wolff and Hurwitz (1973) also compared a group of normal boys with boys who showed choreiform movements and found that the choreiform group (measured with soft signs) showed more reading, spelling and behavioral difficulties than the control children. These authors argue that the neurological examination can be a powerful tool in clinical diagnosis. Werry et al. (1972) have also found a greater frequency of soft signs in a group of hyperactive children compared to a group of neurotic children without hyperactivity. The most differentiating signs included those reflecting sensorimotor incoordination. Further studies in this area include those of Kenny, Clemmens, Cicci, Lentz, Nair, and Hudson (1972) and Stine, Saratsiotis, and Mosser (1975), who report, in a large-scale study of children, that neurological signs are not predictive of any particular form of behavior. Hertzig (1981) has also studied a group of low-birthweight children and has found an increased incidence of soft (nonfocal) signs in that abnormal group.

Clearly, then, most studies have been able to find an increased incidence of soft signs among a variety of exceptional children, although there have been some conflicting reports. Still, this does not leave one with concrete information regarding the utility or meaning of soft signs (Shaffer, O'Connor, Shafer, & Prupis, 1983). One is left with presumptive evidence of the soft-signs–neurological-status and soft-signs–behavioral-status relationships, and soft signs become another nonspecific measure of neuropsychological functioning. Barlow (1974) questions especially the usefulness of soft signs for the prediction of individual performance (diagnosis) and raises the issue of guilt by statistical association. The overlap of soft signs in both abnormal and normal groups is also a significant cause for concern (Helper, 1980).

What then is the clinician to conclude for clinical practice? First of all, the measurement of soft signs can be done reliably. Therefore, for a clinical examination the examiner can be confident (depending on the exam used) that the signs measured have reliability. Second, there are a host of soft sign exams available. It is recommended that the clinician wishing to assess for soft signs choose a manageable examination that has been shown to be reliable. Third, as the validity of soft signs, except for face validity, is currently questionable, it is suggested that measurement of soft signs be used as only *part* of a more extensive evaluation of suspect children (as it should be anyway; see H. G. Taylor et al., 1984) and that diagnostic statements, particularly about brain status, be avoided. Finally, as is so often true of clinical practice, it is the examiner's knowledge and expertise more than any other factor that can consider the presence of soft signs in an individual case and give them their proper weight and interpretation, in the context of other information about the child, to be truly useful for long-term management or planning. Until more research is available, this is the most that can be said about the relationship of soft signs and neurological status in clinical practice.

NEUROPSYCHOLOGICAL SCREENING IN CHILDREN

Screening techniques are enjoying an increasing popularity in neuro-psychology in general (Jones & Butters, 1983) and in child neuropsychology in particular (Hynd et al., 1980). Screening was noted earlier to have three general characteristics:

1. Screening was said to be used to make a decision, typically about the possible presence of CNS dysfunction in children, and to lead to a further diagnostic evaluation.
2. In making decisions about children requiring further neuropsychological evaluations, screening would cut down on the number of children referred on.
3. Thus screening would ultimately be more cost-effective than complete neuropsychological evaluations being administered to every child who was remotely suspected of CNS or neuropsychological difficulties.

Screening techniques could also be learned by nonneuropsychologists (e.g., school psychologists) and could provide more readily available initial identification of suspect children. Screening would thus *not* be useful for children with obvious evidence of neuropathology (e.g., the mentally retarded), nor would it be needed for cases already referred for complete neuropsychological assessment because it would duplicate services. Hence, screening children suspected of (at risk) CNS abnormalities provides an early warning system (Lezak, 1983) for the detection of subtle neuropsychological abnormalities.

The main purpose, ultimately, of screening children is to serve as a form of *prevention* (Stangler, Huber, & Routh, 1980) because the goal of screening is to identify deviations from normality and to provide appropriate services earlier (it is hoped) than they might otherwise be provided. Commonly, prevention is discussed in terms of three levels related to the natural history of disease progression (Stangler et al., 1980): Primary prevention is the prevention of disease occurrence, usually taking place at the prepathogenic stage of disease development. Few neuropsychological instruments have been designed to address directly this stage of symptom manifestation, although primary prevention is a major focus of much medical research.

Secondary prevention occurs at the preclinical stage when there are not yet obvious symptoms of the disorder and before help is sought spontaneously. The most common example of medical screening at the secondary prevention level is the screening of children suspected to have phenylketonuria (PKU). Early detection can result in substantially improved prospects for the PKU child's life. Another example of routine neurodevelopmental screening is that of Bax and Whitmore's (1973) screening in the school-entrant medical examination in Britain. Secondary prevention is most commonly used in neuropsychology as the early warning system for detecting those children at risk for neuropsychological impairment. Silver (1978) has also called this form of assessment "scanning," although he more generally means the scanning (or screening) of *entire populations* to detect abnormality (and he rightly emphasizes the predictive validity that needs to be demonstrated for such instruments).

Tertiary prevention consists of the identification and treatment of a problem after there are readily recognizable symptoms and when the disease is manifesting obvious clinical symptomatology. Diagnosis typically takes place during this stage, and in child neuropsychology, this is the time of most comprehensive neuropsychological evaluations.

Screening serves as an introductory level procedure into more formalized methods of neuropsychological interpretation, such as pattern analysis or integrated interpretation (Lezak, 1983), and it should never be seen as a substitute for more-detailed neuropsychological examination. Unfortunately, at least two myths are common in the neuropsychological screening of children. The first myth is that screening somehow tests for organicity (Delaney, 1982). It is obvious from all that has been stated that screening cannot serve such an omnibus function, as the concept of organicity is far too outdated. Screening can test for abnormality, however.

The second myth is that tests used to screen in adults can be just as valid when applied to children (e.g., the Memory for Designs, Benton Visual Retention test, and others). In fact, few tests or batteries can be shifted down the age range so easily without significant modification and substantial research. It is probably more beneficial to develop tests specifically for the purpose of neuropsychological assessment of children (Telzrow, 1983).

Before describing neuropsychological screening techniques used to assess children, it is necessary to review the characteristics of screening examinations in general. This will be done with the idea of screening for disturbances of neurobehavioral functioning in mind.

What Makes a Screening Examination?

As described, screening tests are generally intended to be administered to relatively large groups of children with suspected CNS impairment. As such, the tests are designed to differentiate between those children who actually do manifest neurobehavioral disturbance and those children who are probably normal; therefore, even though screening tests are not meant to be diagnostic, they must be sensitive and capable of detecting the problem they were designed to identify. In the medical realm, as the list of conditions for which one must screen has grown, so has the number of screening tests (Frankenburg & Camp, 1975). This could conceivably occur also in neuropsychology as the heterogeneity of clinical disorders in children becomes more readily apparent. Thus, in the future we could see more screening tests for visual disorders, spelling disorders, reading disorders, and so forth.

In fact, one of the current controversies regarding screening examinations is whether single tests of organicity are sufficient to screen for neurobehavioral disturbance, or whether groups of tests carefully selected to show high hit rates are the method of choice. It is the present author's opinion that, unlike some other areas of life, screening operates under a more-is-better rule, as long as the tests themselves are carefully chosen for the problem at hand.

Lezak (1983) recommends using a combination of tests for screening purposes, including some tests that are very sensitive to specific impairment (e.g., tests that narrowly evaluate perseveration, which may not be seen often but which is highly pathognomonic of brain dysfunction) and some tests that are sensitive to conditions of general neural dysfunction (e.g., tests that evaluate general symptoms like impaired immediate memory or attentional difficulties). Thus, she recommends a balanced approach to neuropsychological screening that attempts to provide a good hit-rate; with few false positive and false negative errors. This general approach has much to recommend it (but few screening techniques are planned this way a priori).

Another alternative, particularly useful for identifying a specific disorder, is to stack the deck with highly sensitive specific tests that, used together as a screening measure, have high probability to catch in their screen the disorder in question (few false positive errors). For example, one might want to use several measures of language functioning together to screen for language disorders. The major potential disadvantage to this method is that its high specificity is limited in general neuropsychological screening, as it will let many children with other disorders slip through the screen.

General Requirements

There are some basic requirements that can be stated for defining a *good* neuropsychological screening instrument (see Table 4). Practically, a screening device should be appropriate to the purpose of the evaluation; be appropriate for the age and abilities of the child being screened; be acceptable to those who will be affected by its results, including parents

TABLE 4

Requirements for a neuropsychological screening examination[a]

A *good* neuropsychological screening examination should

1. Be appropriate for the age and abilities of the child being screened
2. Be acceptable to the professionals who will be doing follow-up evaluations
3. Be simple—to learn, to teach, and to give
4. Be reliable
5. Be valid
6. Have a good *hit rate;* that is, be sensitive (select "true" abnormals), and be specific (identify "true" normals)
7. Consider and correct for the *base rates* of the disorder in the population
8. Be *cost-effective* in relation to the benefits of early detection of the problem (the "cost" of false positives and false negative should be low)

[a] Adapted from Frankenburg & Camp (1975), Lichenstein & Ireton (1984), Stangler, Huber, & Routh (1980), and others.

and professionals; be simple to administer; and show low cost (Frankenburg & Camp, 1975; Stangler et al., 1980). Therefore, neuropsychological screening tests must, in terms of their general acceptability, be useful to the children screened by identifying them at the level of secondary prevention and assisting them to find further diagnostic and remedial services. They must be able to make appropriate referrals to neuropsychologists for full evaluations when necessary, and they must be sensitive enough to detect the problem that was screened and provide the appropriate decision.

A major criteria for neuropsychological screening tests in children is that they must be appropriate to the age of the child screened. This may mean in some cases that tests need to be devised that reflect developmental progressions and that provide sufficient normative data for decision making. Screening tests should also be analyzed for their ease of administration, simplicity of learning, and cost in terms of the equipment involved, the personnel involved in doing the testing, personal costs to the individual—especially of inaccurate results, and the total cost of the test in relation to the benefits of early identification. These are only some of the practical considerations that are involved when assessing a screening device, although they are all very crucial. For example, it would be a waste of time, money, and personnel to have an expensive neuropsychologist administer a 2-hour screening battery to a child, when possibly the same information (i.e., the need for a more comprehensive evaluation) could be gained from a 1-hour screening test administered by a school psychologist right in the child's school.

In addition, another set of criteria are necessary to ensure a good neuropsychological screening device. These include several statistical or methodological criteria related to test construction, such as the reliability and validity of the test instrument (APA, 1974), the test's hit rate or ability to select true normal individuals and to identify those children at risk for impairment. The test (and tester) also needs to consider and correct for the base rates of the disorder in the local population; that is, to consider the prevalence of the disorder because it influences the number of cases likely to be discovered through screening (Meehl & Rosen, 1955). Reliability, both test–retest and interrater, as well as validity, have been discussed in reference to soft signs. The same problems hold for neuropsychological tests designed to be used as screening devices. Nevertheless, it is expected that basic standards of reliability and validity are to be achieved before use of a screening test or any other assessment device (APA, 1974). Finally, the cost-effectiveness of the screening technique needs to be addressed in terms of the broader context of the benefits to the community of early detection of the problem.

Hit Rates

The *hit rate* of an assessment procedure refers to the ability of that test to identify to which of two predetermined clinical groups (normal/abnormal) an individual belongs. The percentage of cases that the test correctly classifies is termed its hit rate. Neuropsychology has had a major preoccupation with hit rates (Spreen & Benton, 1965), yet few child screening tests have been judged by the criterion of the hit rate. The relationship between screening test results, hit rates, and diagnostic findings from further comprehensive evaluations are indicated in Table 5. This table compares the classifications (normal/abnormal) made by a screening test and by a diagnostic examination. Each test can classify an individual either normal or abnormal, resulting in a 2×2 classification table. Classification by the screening test that would result in correct referrals are listed as the valid positives (a) and valid negatives (d). These correct referrals are a measure of the screening test's *sensitivity,* that is its ability to identify abnormal cases as abnormal, and its *specificity,* its ability to identify true normal cases. It also provides the test's hit rate ($a + d$) in reflecting the test's ability to classify correctly. Incorrect classifications (over- and underreferrals) are calculated as ($b + c$).

Hit rates should not be applied uncritically as the only criteria on which to judge a test (Lezak, 1983), although they are important. In fact, two further issues are important to consider, particularly when evaluating screening tests for early detection purposes. These are the consideration of *base rates* of the disorder in the population, and the issue of *predictive*

TABLE 5

Relationship between screening test results and diagnostic findings[a,b]

	Classification by diagnostic exam		
Classification by screening test	Abnormal (positive)	Normal (negative)	Total[c]
Abnormal (positive)	Correct referrals (valid positives) a	Overreferrals (false positives) b	$a + b$
Normal (negative)	Underreferrals (false negatives) c	Correct referrals (valid negatives) d	$c + d$
Total (with actual diagnosis)	Total positives $a + c = 1.00$	Total negatives $b + d = 1.00$	

[a] Adapted from Frankenburg & Camp (1975), Satz & Fletcher (1979), and Stangler, Huber, & Routh (1980).

[b] a = proportion of valid positives (positives called positive); b = proportion of false positives (negatives called positive); c = proportion of false negatives (positives called negative); d = proportion of valid negatives (negatives called negative).

[c] Marginal totals $(a + b)$ and $(c + d)$ do not sum to 1.00 and are meaningless in ignorance of the base rates.

utility (Satz & Fletcher, 1979). The concept of predictive utility, as used by Satz and Fletcher, implies that the detection signs (valid positives and negatives—hit rate) should be evaluated within the broader context of the prevalence estimates of the disorder that is predicted. This is especially crucial in early detection of learning disorders with a predictive model. Satz and Fletcher (1979) caution that early detection may not be possible in cases where base rates are not considered, because confoundings of high-risk children (false negatives) and low-risk children (false positives) occur. Briefly, this refers to the incidence or base rate of the disorder in question. Base rates, because they represent the general incidence of the disorder in the population (and represent prior probability estimates) influence the conditional probability values for each of the predictive test signs (see also Meehl & Rosen, 1955; Rimm, 1963). Although this type of information is rare, Berger and Berger-Margulies (1978), for instance, provide estimates of the base rates or frequency of minor neurological dysfunction in school-age children. By using Bayesian statistics, it is possible to calculate each of the conditional probability values for the signs, hence considering the base rates. These are often markedly different from those values determined without the base rates. Further discussion of this issue is beyond the scope of this chapter; the reader is referred to Satz and Fletcher (1979) or Meehl and Rosen (1955) for more complete discussions of this issue.

However, the conclusions to be drawn here for application to screening evaluations are not only that these tests need to be evaluated for their overall classification or hit rate, but also that prior probability estimates (base rates) need to be considered in the evaluation of the screening test's predictive utility.

Cost-Effectiveness

Determining the cost-effectiveness of a neuropsychological screening technique is a complex process. Aside from practical considerations, such as considering monetary and personal cost and appropriateness of screening techniques already discussed, several further issues need to be addressed in evaluating the broader costs and utility of screening techniques. This is especially the case because the costs of an individual screening test must always be measured against the cost of not having the disorder identified early.

Because deviations from normality do not *always* mean a problem is present, and because screening for all types of neurodevelopmental problems is not feasible (Dawson, Cohns, Eversole, Frankenburg, & Roth, 1979), several criteria affect cost-effectiveness decisions in neuropsychological screening. This includes considering the seriousness of the disorder to the general public (which is usually only a concern for infectious neurological diseases that would not require screening). However, because childhood disorders have a major impact on public health in general, screening is necessary for some of the more serious ones; an example of this is PKU, where the potential consequences are so serious to the individual and the family that screening is usually justified despite its low prevalence. Presumably, screening of more subtle symptoms of CNS dysfunction would have a somewhat lower cost to the public (although with intervention available, that is debatable) and the effectiveness of screening examinations for MBD would also have to be questioned. Thus, cost-effectiveness when considering the screening of neuropsychological deviations is an uncertain issue, although in terms of its effectiveness in saving time and effort, it certainly has many potential benefits. Other criteria that affect consideration for a cost-effectiveness analysis of neuropsychological screening include (1) whether there are definable diagnostic criteria available, (2) whether the disorder is treatable or controllable (it makes no sense to screen for a disorder for which nothing can be done to alleviate its effects), (3) whether further diagnostic services are available for follow-up, and (4) whether the total cost for screening for the problem (including diagnosis and treatment) is justified by the benefits of the early detection (Stangler et al., 1980). These are only some of the considerations that neuropsychologists should use to evaluate the cost-effectiveness of their screening techniques.

The following sections provide general considerations for three categories of screening tests in children and describe the status of some selected screening tests for each category. The categories are formed largely on the basis of the age of the child being screened and on the purposes of the evaluation, (e.g., general or specific screening). This chapter distinguishes between developmental screening and screening of preschool and school-age children on the basis of the purpose of the evaluation; developmental screening is used for screening general developmental delays, whereas the other types of screening are more specific to neuropsychological impairment.

Developmental Screening

Screening for general developmental delays is a fairly common practice. Such tests of general development provide important information about the overall well-being of the child and can identify the possible presence of specific impairments as well. Developmental screening tests not only can identify early developmental abnormalities, but also can be useful to judge developmental milestones and to teach parents what to expect about their children if done within a comprehensive screening, diagnostic, and remedial program. They can also provide important information about the natural history of neurological diseases. Because delays in general development can have serious consequences for the future (whatever the cause), it is beneficial to try to catch the high-risk children as early as possible, and thus, developmental screening tests have a prominent position in the neurological and psychological assessment of children.

Although it is usually impossible to cure the problems causing developmental delay (except for the PKU child), it is usually possible to provide treatment to alleviate the impact of the problem. Prognosis of children with developmental disabilities is usually improved with early detection. Thus, with the presence of early intervention programs, identification of developmental delays is desirable at any age. Early identification of developmental disabilities is also usually economically justified because the cost of most tests for screening general development of young children is comparatively low, while the cost of unidentified developmental disability may be great.

There are many developmental screening tests available. They usually screen for many parameters of development rather than having a specific focus, like language or motor development, although the content of the exams typically varies depending on the age of the child being screened. Developmental screening tests tend to be, therefore, multifaceted tests, assessing in a brief manner many aspects of the child's functioning. Because developmental screening is useful at any age, the exams available usually assess a range of ages, typically within the early developmental years. Frankenburg and Camp (1975), however, suggest that the optimum ages for developmental screening occur at three points; the first when the child is between 1 and $2\frac{1}{2}$ years of age (after onset of walking); next, at 3 years of age, when speech is well developed; and at 5 years of age, prior to school entrance. Developmental screening exams place high priority on availability of normative observations for the different ages, and, more often than not, normative interpretation relative to an expected age standard is the main method of inference-making for these tests. The exams reviewed here are selected to be a representative, not a comprehensive, sample of the available screening exams. They cover the age range from about birth to age 6 years. These exams, along with the preschool and school-age screening exams discussed here later, are listed in Table 6. The developmental screening exams presented are the Denver Developmental Screening test, the Developmental Profile, and the Developmental Screening Inventory. Readers wanting further information should consult the sources cited, Frankenburg and Camp (1975), or Stangler et al. (1980).

The Denver Developmental Screening Test (DDST) is a general developmental screening device designed for the identification of developmental deviations in children from birth through 6 years of age (Frankenburg and Dodds, 1971). The test takes from 15 to 30 minutes to administer and consists of 105 test items selected on the basis of economy and simplicity from developmental and preschool intelligence tests. It provides an overall developmental profile, with items grouped in four sections to cover gross motor development, fine motor/adaptive development, language development, and personal–social skills. The items were administered to a sample of 1036 infants and children between the ages of 2 weeks and 6.4 years, and normative data were computed by calculating the percentage of children in each age group who passed each item. The ages at which 25, 50, 75, and 90% passed each item were then calculated for the entire sample. The test, therefore, is one of the better-standardized screening instruments available. It has also been shown to have adequate reliability (test–retest agreement within 1 week of 97%) and validity (decent correlations with other measures of development), reported in the manual. Unfortunately, predictive studies for the DDST are still lacking. It can, how-

TABLE 6

Neuropsychological screening examinations

Examination	Ages tested	Source
General Developmental Screening Examinations		
Denver Developmental Screening Test	Birth–6 yrs.	Frankenburg & Dodds (1971)
Developmental Profile	Birth–12 yrs.	Alpern & Boll (1972)
Developmental Screening Inventory	1 month–3 yrs.	Knobloch & Pasamanick (1974)
Preschool Screening Examinations		
Florida Kindergarten Screening Battery (FKSB)	Kindgergarten	Satz & Fletcher (1982)
McCarthy Screening Test	4–6 1/2 yrs.	McCarthy (1978)
Neurological Dysfunctions of Children (NDOC)	3–10 yrs.	Kuhns (1979)
Quick Neurological Screening Test (Rev. ed.) (QNST)	Wide range	Mutti, Sterling, & Spalding (1978)
School-Age Screening Examinations		
Bender Visual-Motor Gestalt Test	All ages	Bender (1938)
Children's Neuropsychological Screening Test (CNST)	Approx. 8–13 yrs.	Lowe, Krehbiel, Sweeney, Crumley, Peterson, Watson, & Rhodes (1984)
Clinical Neuropsychological Evaluation Instrument (CNE)	Approx. 12–20 yrs.	Majovski, Tanguay, Russell, Sigman, Crumley, & Goldenberg (1979a, 1979b)
Neurological Dysfunctions of Children (NDOC)	3–10 yrs.	Kuhns (1979)
"Screening for MBD" (Peters' "Special" Neurological Examination for School-Age Children)	6–14 yrs.	Peters, Davis, Goolsby, Clements, & Hicks (1973)
Quick Neurological Screening Test (Rev. ed.) (QNST)	Wide range	Mutti, Sterling, & Spalding (1978)

ever, be a reliable and useful device for the *early* screening of developmental disabilities or general lags in development. It is particularly useful for screening of infants and very young children.

The Developmental Profile (Alpern & Boll, 1972) has a much different format. This test is actually a formalized interview, designed to be given to a parent or any other person who knows the child well. It is designed to assess physical, self-help, personal–social, and communication development, as well as academic achievement (for older children). It can be used to screen children from birth to about age 12 years, and it can take from 20 to 40 minutes to administer. The 218 interview items (questions) were formulated so that the person being interviewed can answer yes or no, and they were placed into age levels at which 75% of the normative population could pass. The Developmental Profile was standardized on 3008 children ranging in age from 1 month to 12 years. There were 16 age groups, with an average of 225 children per group, and boys and girls approximately equally represented. Reliability studies of test–retest reliability and interobserver agreement were conducted with very high reliability noted. Validity studies are almost nonexistent, with the studies only being done on the academic scale, and thus are not considered here. Overall, the Developmental Profile, despite methodological problems, holds potential as a screening test of general development for older children, and the interview format can be useful for screening younger children who are otherwise uncooperative or unavailable.

The last developmental screening test reviewed is the Developmental Screening Inventory (DSI) of Knobloch and Pasamanick (1974). This exam was based directly on the work of Gesell and Amatruda and is not formally standardized. It consists of the systematic application of items selected from the Gesell Developmental Schedules in each of five areas: adaptive, gross motor, fine motor, language, and personal–social skills. A level of function (maturity level) is obtained for each of the five areas. An evaluation is then made of whether the child falls more nearly into the normal, questionable, or abnormal developmental range for each age level. The test is designed for children from about 1 month of age to 3 years. The DSI is administered in about 20 to 30 minutes in an interview format to the parent, and by direct observation of the child. Reliability and validity data are scanty for the test, but it generally does meet clinical acceptability levels. One of the major benefits of the DSI is its use of enjoyable, well-composed items for the children, but this is also a major pitfall, in that the inventory also depends heavily on the examiner developing the necessary rapport with the child. Fairly great sophistication is also required for interpretation and, although there are no restrictions placed on its use, only people experienced in the evaluation of development in young children should use the DSI.

Screening Preschool Children

Screening children in the age range of about 4 to 6 years of age can be considered preschool screening (Lichenstein & Ireton, 1984), with its major purpose, unlike developmental screening, being the identification of children at high risk for disorders that will interfere with academic progress. However, while it may have a more restricted goal, its scope is very large because many neurological and behavioral disorders can lead to academic difficulties in early schooling. Thus, early identification of learning disabilities is a major focus of preschool screening. One of the major difficulties in preschool screening is the establishment of *predictive validity* for the screening instrument; it is especially important in predicting school failure that the test be able to accurately classify children at risk for school difficulties in a predictive manner. Unfortunately, because of the expense involved in such an endeavor, few longitudinal studies have been conducted during this age range.

Only a few preschool screening tests are reviewed here (see Table 6); the reader is referred to the book by Lichenstein and Ireton (1984) for further information. The tests described in detail are the Florida Kindergarten Screening Battery and the McCarthy Screening test; the NDOC and QNST, described in more detail earlier, as measures of soft signs, have also been presented as neuropsychological screening measures in preschool children, and they are discussed, but briefly.

The Florida Kindergarten Screening Battery (FKSB) is designed for the early identification (in kindergarten) of learning disorders. Its manual (Satz & Fletcher, 1982) states that it has the very restricted goal of predicting "the likelihood that an individual kindergarten child will manifest learning problems 3 years later (end of grade 2)" (p. 1). The FKSB was developed from a study, now known as the "Florida Longitudinal Project" (Fletcher et al., 1982; Satz et al., 1978), which was conceived as a large-scale multivariate prediction study designed to investigate the neuropsychological factors associated with reading success and failure in elementary school. With its emphasis on neuropsychological prediction, the study showed that it was possible to predict second-grade reading-achievement levels from their tests (which now form the FKSB) given at the beginning of kindergarten (Satz et al., 1978). The main features of the predictive aspect of the study have been retained, and the tests have now been pulled together and incorporated into a battery for neuropsychological screening.

The FKSB now consists of four individually administered tests, requiring approximately an hour to administer. These include a Recognition–discrimination test, an Alphabet Recitation test, an optional supplementary measure, the Finger Localization test, and two previously published tests, the Peabody Picture Vocabulary Test–Revised (PPVT-R) and the Beery Developmental Test of Visual–Motor Integration (Beery DVMI). The battery can be administered in either the four- or five-test versions.

The standardization of the FKSB was carried out on a complete sample of 497 *boys* who entered kindergarten in 1970 in one county in Florida and the prediction equations were derived from the collapsing of data from this original longitudinal sample with the results of a cross-validation study of 181 very similar boys. As Gates (1984) has pointed out, the nature of this type of restricted standardization sample (white, middle- to upper-class boys) gives cause for concern in limiting generalizability of the results unless further comparative research has been undertaken. One of the most interesting features of the FKSB is that rather than predictions based on the presence–absence of dysfunction, predictive classification is done according to a range of possible predicted and actual outcome categories (severe, mild, average, and superior). This use of graded-outcome categories obviates the typical overemphasis on hit rates in screening tests and provides, on a longitudinally based predictive basis, much more clinically meaningful information. Reliability studies for the tests of the FKSB are reported in the manual as having "generally high reliabilities" (p. 14), although as Gates (1984) points out, several of the tests (the Alphabet Recitation Test in particular) have no reliabilities reported at all.

Overall, the FKSB is a neuropsychological screening instrument with a restricted goal; to predict reading or learning failure in grade two from neuropsychological tests administered in preschool. (Gates, 1984, however, does note ambiguity in the interchangeable use of the terms "reading" and "learning" problems by the authors.) Although Gates (1984) also criticizes the FKSB as not being ready for off-the-shelf use, the battery, with its excellent application of multivariate predictive methodology, stands today as one of the true screening tests in the neuropsychological assessment of children.

The McCarthy Screening Test (MST) (McCarthy, 1978), however, is not such an instrument. Although it has a similar purpose in screening preschool age children for future academic success, it does not incorporate a predictive methodology but instead uses a concurrent validity methodology based on cross-sectional, not longitudinal, data. The MST is designed only to be a general screening instrument that is brief to administer and that identifies a child who appears to be developing at a slower rate than his or her peers, in which case a further evaluation is recommended. Thus, the MST classifies children into a not-at-risk or an at-risk group for school problems, based on the results of the test. The MST is composed of 6 of the 18 subtests that form the original *McCarthy Scales of Children's Abilities*. The 6 subtests were chosen on the basis of content, level of difficulty, time for administration, and ease of scoring (the MST can be given and scored by teachers or other paraprofessionals with sufficient training). They are Right–Left Orientation, Verbal Memory,

Draw-a-Design, Numerical Memory, Conceptual Grouping, and Leg Co-ordination. Unlike the original Scales, the MST takes about 20 minutes to administer and is only given to children ages 4 to $6\frac{1}{2}$ years. Thus, the MST is clearly a preschool screening instrument.

The MST uses the standardization sample of 1032 normal children from the original, well-developed McCarthy Scales. Reliability (test–retest stability) for the MST subtests varies from .32 to .69 and are not high enough to warrant making fine distinctions within a group. Thus, screening decisions are made on the basis of multiple hurdles. Based on some validity studies of the MST, reported in the manual, a variety of criteria can be used to determine classification of the children. Classification is typically determined by grading each subtest as passed or failed at a given percentile; so that a general classification rule would put a child into the at-risk classification if the child failed 3 or more tests at the 30th percentile. Using the accuracy tables provided in the manual, users of the test can decide for themselves the cutoff values used and can thus determine their own hit rates. The MST is a very useful test for screening for general neuropsychological and academic difficulties and, while not predictive, uses a good standardization and adequate methodology for decision making.

As described in the previous section in this chapter, the NDOC and QNST were considered measures of subtle neurobehavioral dysfunction. Both of these tests have also been proposed as useful in the screening of children for neurobehavioral dysfunction. They are considered here as screening tests for preschool- (and later school-) age children because they each cover a rather wide age range. Specific descriptions of the tests have already been provided. As a neurobehavioral screening test, the NDOC is claimed to have both face validity and an acceptable level of screening validity. Screening validity was obtained by calculating the level of agreement between the results of the test (in terms of clusters) and a pediatric neurologist's and other specialists' follow-up evaluations of the child. Acceptable levels of agreement were obtained on these concurrent measures in two independent studies with samples of 28 and 66 children; unfortunately, ages of the children screened are not reported. While these results do not provide overwhelming evidence for the screening utility of the NDOC, it does suggest that it may be a useful clinical measure for children which deserves to be evaluated more fully.

The QNST, on the other hand, does not have as much research evidence to back up its claims as a screening test. It does provide ranges of classification for the total test score of high, suspicious, and normal, and it suggests that suspicious and high scores represent the children at risk for learning disabilities. But except for correlational (between normal and LD overall scores) studies, no hit rates or other predictive or concurrent validity data are provided. The reader of the manual is, unfortunately, left to infer what to do with scores in these ranges (or even how the cutoffs were decided). Nevertheless, as with the NDOC, the QNST has items that appear face valid, and with the fairly comprehensive theoretical explanations of the items in the manual, it can probably be used to provide screening-type decisions if administered by a well-trained individual.

Screening School-Age Children

The neuropsychological screening of school-age children has received a different kind of attention in the past because predictive screening for academic difficulties has not been as much of a focus as has the general (concurrent) detection of subtle neurobehavioral deviations (organicity). Thus, the identification of school-age children who have, up to that point, missed detection of brain damage has been the primary concern. A related implication has been the cost-effectiveness of providing this screening with as few resources as are necessary; hence, the neuropsychological screening of school-age children has had a major emphasis on the use of *single* tests sensitive to brain dysfunction or specific abnormalities. Examples of such tests include the Bender-Gestalt (Koppitz, 1963, 1975), the Purdue Pegboard (Rapin, Tourk, & Costa, 1966), the Reitan Aphasia Screening test (Reitan, 1984; Wolf & Tramontana, 1982), and Schiller et al.'s (1982) screening test for dysnomia. Only in the last several years have composite screening batteries for school-age children been developed (Table 6).

The scope of this chapter (and its orientation) does not allow detailed exploration of the many single tests for the screening of brain dysfunction. The one discussed here is one of the most common, and most widely used: the Bender–Gestalt Test of Visual–Motor Integration (Bender, 1938; Lacks, 1984). Bigler and Ehrfurth (1981) have criticized the singular use of the Bender–Gestalt as an omnibus measure of brain damage, although as Lacks (1984) points out, this criticism tends to ignore the reality of the testing situation and ignores evidence favoring a general-effect view of brain damage. In fact, because the Bender-Gestalt test involves such a wide range of abilities, presumably tapping broad areas of the brain, its use as a screening test is probably enhanced due to its broad sensitivity. The Bender–Gestalt is also firmly entrenched in many clinical and school psychologists' practice, and therefore, deserves at least recognition as a useful tool (based on the assumption that it provides some type of useful information).

A brief description is in order. The Bender–Gestalt test consists of nine geometrical figures presented one at a time to the child and the child is required to copy these figures as accurately as possible onto one or more pieces of paper. There is no time limit. Thus, in terms of administration, the Bender–Gestalt is a very brief, nonverbal, standardized, perceptual–motor test which has been scored and interpreted in a multitude of ways (Lacks, 1984; Koppitz, 1963, 1975).

Koppitz (1975) views the developmental changes seen in Bender–Gestalt performance to be a reflection of brain-based changes in visuomotor and higher-order integrative skills that mature only gradually. Disturbance thus represents global dysfunction. Such is the view also taken by Lacks (1984) and other users of the Bender–Gestalt who feel that it can be useful as a marker for dysfunction per se even though it does not indicate the precise source, diagnosis, or degree of impairment. Readers wanting to acquire further information on interpretation or screening with the Bender–Gestalt are referred to Lacks (1984) or Koppitz (1963, 1975) for details. It is sufficient to say here that interpretations based solely on the results of this one test are questionable and require a great deal of experience on the examiner's part. Until now, scoring and reliability have also remained controversial issues surrounding the Bender–Gestalt (Lacks, 1984).

The NDOC and QNST, as screening tests, have been described earlier and are not discussed further here; the same difficulties with screening validity apply for school-age children as for preschool children. Until a greater research base for these tests has been developed, decisions made on the basis of their use only rest on face validity and clinical interpretation. Similar problems exist for another soft signs measurement instrument that can be used for screening school-age children: Peters et al.'s (1973) Screening for MBD evaluation. Along with their "special" neurological examination, Peters et al. provide in their handbook a variety of office screening procedures (designed primarily for physicians) that can screen for psychological, language, educational, or other preschool difficulties. Most of the items have been taken from other examinations and have been pulled together into this one sourcebook. Unfortunately, the authors omitted providing other useful information about the tests (like norms, reliabilities etc.) that preclude the use of these procedures as standardized instruments. They also omit any description of the validity of the procedures, although they tend to have a great deal of face validity and can probably serve a useful clinical function.

Finally, two further neuropsychological screening instruments for school-age children have been developed and described in the literature. Both of these exams have been developed solely for the purpose of neuropsychological screening of a variety of CNS impairments. The Clinical Neuropsychological Evaluation (CNE) Instrument was developed by Majovski et al. (1979a, 1979b) as a clinical research tool designed to screen for disturbances of higher cortical functions in adolescents. It was based on the work of the Soviet A. R. Luria's clinical neuropsychological evaluation and is basically a foreshortened version of a full clinical neuropsychological evaluation. Thus, its main benefits for screening purposes are that it is brief and covers a wide range of functions.

It consists of 72 items arranged into nine sections: Motor functions, acousticomotor organization, higher visual functions, impressive speech, expressive speech, reading and writing, arithmetical skill, mnestic processes, and intellectual processes. The items have been published in their second publication (Majovski et al., 1979b). Each of the items on the CNE is scored from 0 (no impairment) to 3 (severe impairment), and their papers provide objective scoring criteria. Majovski et al. (1979a) calculated the interrater agreement for the CNE with a limited sample of 5 subjects, but Goehring and Majovski (1984) have now included a sample of 20 subjects and demonstrate that intraclass correlation coefficients (measures of interrater reliability) for the various measures of the CNE range from .79 to .99, thus supporting its potential as a clinical and research assessment tool. The authors (Majovski et al., 1979a) carefully point out that, while the CNE offers some potential advantages as a screening device (such as efficiency, breadth of coverage, and underlying conceptual framework), limitations regarding validity abound. They emphasize, however, that the CNE was not intended as a psychometric instrument but rather, as intended by Luria, to be *descriptive* of possible neural dysfunctions.

Lowe et al. (1984) have recently presented the Children's Neuropsychological Screening Test (CNST) as an adaptation of the CNE more culturally appropriate to the United States and designed for a slightly lower age range (approximately 8–13 years in pilot work). Their only published article (Lowe et al., 1984) describes the results of an initial pilot study using the CNST, which attempted to discriminate normal from at-risk learning-disabled children. The test made a discrimination between normals and special groups at a statistically significant level, but of course this type of research is only suggestive, not demonstrative, of the CNST's potential screening utility. Until further studies appear, the CNST, while attractive as a screening device, retains only its face validity and its conceptual underpinnings (like the CNE) as useful features for the clinician.

Clinical Implementation of Neuropsychological Screening

The use of neuropsychological screening by the clinician requires careful consideration of the purposes of the screening technique and the particular evaluation. On an individual-child level, the screener needs to consider the advantages and disadvantages of the vast array of screening devices available. Some of the considerations that need to be considered were discussed previously: reliability and validity of the procedure, appropriateness, cost-effectiveness, et cetera. Validity of the procedure, especially as a predictive instrument is a critical concern in developing a screening test for children and needs to be considered by the person using the device as well.

There is another level at which neuropsychological screening requires careful consideration; this is at the level of implementing screening programs for many children. Demonstrated validity becomes even more important here as the cost of ineffective techniques can rise astronomically with greater numbers of children. The same practical and methodological considerations by the designer of the program (whether it is the neuropsychologist, the school psychologist, or someone else) need to be taken into account. In addition, further practical considerations are involved, such as acquiring the cooperation of the school system and parents, training the appropriate personnel in use of the screening procedures, et cetera. Therefore, the clinical implementation of neuropsychological screening techniques has to be done on a rational, well-thought-out basis because it involves so many people (children and adults); yet it can serve a tremendously useful function in secondary prevention.

CONCLUSIONS

This chapter has provided an overview of a particularly nonspecific area in child neuropsychology. The current myths and beliefs that abound are based on a great deal of presumptive evidence (see also Fletcher & Taylor, 1984) and work against the drawing of any *specific* conclusions about the status of soft neurological signs and screening tests in the neuropsychological assessment of children. Nevertheless, it should be apparent from the review that some statements can be made about particular aspects of the measurement of subtle CNS manifestations in children and that this measurement can be useful in a clinical setting.

Soft neurological signs, though nonspecific, can be reliably assessed. In general, the screening tests thus far developed also tend to be reliable. Both topics, as sides of our assessment coin, have been shown to demonstrate a fair amount of face validity, but research has not provided a complete understanding of the theoretical basis of these soft signs and neuropsychological screening techniques. As was noted at the beginning of the chapter, the topics of neuropsychological screening and soft signs deal with some of the most complex issues confronting clinicians and researchers in child neuropsychological assessment—issues and questions for which there is no easy solution. Finding the answers to these questions is of paramount importance for the children that are examined.

Are we then left with questionable techniques to use and no understanding of how best to apply them? Certainly not. There is a long history of the use of similar techniques in neuropsychology, and we are now ready to put screening and soft signs into the context of a more full evaluation of the child—a more clinical evaluation. Thus, screening techniques and measurement of soft signs both serve useful functions, but only as *part* of a broader assessment process. If we consider the early identification (screening) and more full description (including soft signs) of neuropsychological impairments as an early goal in assessment, we can understand the necessity for follow-up to gain a more complete clinical picture of any given child. Several models are available for such a process. Yule (1978) proposes a full developmental psychological assessment, incorporating assessment of a wide range of both neurological and behavioral measures, while H. G. Taylor et al.'s (1984) functional model looks at the child's manifest disabilities, basic competencies, biological factors, and the influence of moderator variables. Screening and soft-sign measurement are not substitutes for these more complete assessment processes, only lead-ins. To end with continuance of our metaphor: The screening and soft signs assessment coin is only part of a pocketful of change.

REFERENCES

Abercrombie, M., Lindon, R., & Tyson, M. (1964). Associated movements in normal and physically handicapped children. *Developmental Medicine and Child Neurology, 6,* 573–580.

Adams, R. M., Kocsis, J. J., & Estes, R. E. (1974). Soft neurological signs in learning-disabled children and controls. *American Journal of Disabled Children, 128,* 614–618.

Alpern, G. D., & Boll, T. J. (1972). *Developmental profile manual.* Indianapolis: Psychological Developmental Publications.

American Psychological Association. (1974). *Standards for educational & psychological tests.* Washington, DC: Author.

Barlow, C. F. (1974). "Soft signs" in children with learning disorders. *American Journal of the Disabled Child, 128,* 605–606.

Bax, M., & Whitmore, K. (1973). Neurodevelopmental screening in the school-entrant medical examination. *Lancet,* August 18, 368–370.

Bender, L. (1938). *A visual–motor Gestalt test and its clinical use.* New York: American Ortho psychiatric Association.

Bender, L. (1947). Childhood schizophrenia: Clinical study of one hundred schizophrenic children. *American Journal of Orthopsychiatry, 17,* 40–56.

Benton, A. L. (1973). Minimal brain dysfunction from a neuropsychological point of view. *Annals of the New York Academy of Sciences, 205,* 29–37.

Berger, E., & Berger-Margulies, J. (1978). Frequency of minor nervous dysfunction in school children. *Journal of Neurology, 219,* 205–212.

Bigler, E. D., & Ehrfurth, J. W. (1981). The continued inappropriate singular use of the Bender Visual Motor Gestalt test. *Professional Psychology, 12,* 562–569.

Boll, T. J. (1978). Diagnosing brain impairment. In B. B. Wolman (Ed.), *Clinical diagnosis of mental disorders.* New York: Plenum.

Boll, T. J. (1983). Neuropsychological assessment of the child: Myths, current status, and future prospects. In C. E. Walker & M. C. Roberts (Eds.), *Handbook of clinical child psychology.* New York: Wiley.

Boll, T. J., & Barth, J. T. (1981). Neuropsychology of brain damage in children. In S. B. Filskov & T. J. Boll (Eds.), *Handbook of clinical neuropsychology.* New York: Wiley (Interscience).

Bortner, M., Hertzig, M. E. & Birch, H. G. (1972). Neurological signs and intelligence in brain-damaged children. *Journal of Special Education, 6,* 325–333.

Camp, J. A., Bialer, I., Sverd, J., & Winsberg, B. G. (1978). Clinical usefulness of the NIMH Physical and Neurological Examination for Soft Signs. *American Journal of Psychiatry, 135,* 362–364.

Clements, S. D. (1966). *Minimal brain dysfunction in children—Terminology and identification.* Washington, DC: U. S. Public Health Service.

Cohen, H. J., Taft, L. T., Mahadeviah, M. S., & Birch, H. G. (1967). Developmental changes in overflow in normal and aberrantly functioning children. *Journal of Pediatrics, 71,* 39–47.

Connolly, K., & Stratton, P. (1968). Developmental changes in associated movements. *Developmental Medicine and Child Neurology, 10,* 49–56.

Copple, P. J., & Isom, J. B. (1968). Soft signs and scholastic success. *Neurology, 18,* 304.

Dawson, P., Cohrs, M., Eversole, C., Frankenburg, W. F., & Roth, M. L. (1979). Cost effectiveness of screening children in health centers. *Public Health Reports, 94,* 362–365.

Delaney, R. C. (1982). Screening for organicity: The problem of subtle neuropsychological deficit and diagnosis. *Journal of Clinical Psychology, 38,* 843–846.

Denckla, M. B. (1973). Development of speed in repetitive and successive finger movements in normal children. *Developmental Medicine and Child Neurology, 15,* 635–645.

Denckla, M. B. (1978). Minimal brain dysfunction. In J. S. Chall & A. F. Mirsky (Eds.), *Education and the brain.* Chicago: University of Chicago Press.

Fletcher, J. M., Satz, P., & Morris, R. (1982). The Florida Longitudinal Project: A review. In S. A. Mednick & M. S. Harway (Eds.), *Longitudinal projects in the United States* (pp. 313–348). Boston: Nijhoff.

Fletcher, J. M., & Taylor, H. G. (1984). Neuropsychological approaches to children: Towards a developmental neuropsychology. *Journal of Clinical Neuropsychology, 6,* 39–56.

Fog, E., & Fog, M. (1963). Cerebral inhibition examined by associated movements. In R.

MacKeith & M. Bax (Eds.), *Minimal cerebral dysfunction* (C.D.M. No. 10). London: Heinemann.

Frankenburg, W. K., & Camp, B. W. (Eds.). (1975). *Pediatric screening tests*. Springfield, IL: Charles C. Thomas.

Frankenburg, W. K., & Dodds, J. B. (1971). The Denver Developmental Screening Test. *Journal of Pediatrics, 79*, 988.

Friedlander, S., Pothier, P., Morrison, D., & Herman, L. (1982). The role of neurological–developmental delay in childhood psychopathology. *American Journal of Orthopsychiatry, 52*, 102–108.

Gaddes, W. H. (1981). An examination of the validity of neuropsychological knowledge in educational diagnosis and remediation. In G. W. Hynd & J. E. Obrzut (Eds.), *Neuropsychological assessment and the school-age child*. New York: Grune & Stratton.

Gardner, R. A. (1979). *The objective diagnosis of minimal brain dysfunction*. Cresskill, NJ: Creative Therapeutics.

Garfield, J. C. (1964). Motor impersistence in normal and brain-damaged children. *Neurology, 14*, 623–630.

Gates, R. D. (1984). Florida Kindergarten Screening Battery (Test Review). *Journal of Clinical Neuropsychology, 6*, 459–465.

Goehring, M. M., & Majovski, L. V. (1984). Interrater reliability of a clinical neuropsychological screening instrument for adolescents. *International Journal of Clinical Neuropsychology, 6*, 35–41.

Gomez, M. R. (1967). Minimal cerebral dysfunction (maximal neurologic confusion). *Clinical Pediatrics, 6*, 589–591.

Guy, W. (1976). Physical and Neurological Examination for Soft Signs (PANESS). In W. Guy (Ed.), *ECDEU assessment manual for psychopharmacology* (pp. 383–393). Rockville, MD: National Institute of Mental Health.

Hart, A., Rennick, P. M., Klinge, V., & Schwartz, M. L. (1974). A pediatric neurologist's contribution to evaluations of school underachievers. *American Journal of Diseases of Children, 128*, 319–323.

Helper, M. M. (1980). Follow-up of children with minimal brain dysfunctions: Outcomes and predictions. In H. E. Rie & E. D. Rie (Eds.), *Handbook of minimal brain dysfunctions*. New York: Wiley (Interscience).

Herbert, M. (1964). The concept and testing of brain-damage in children: A review. *Journal of Child Psychology and Psychiatry, 5*, 197–216.

Hertzig, M. E. (1981). Neurological 'soft' signs in low-birthweight children. *Developmental Medicine and Child Neurology, 23*, 778–791.

Hertzig, M. E. (1982). Stability and change in nonfocal neurologic signs. *Journal of the American Academy of Child Psychiatry, 21*, 231–236.

Hertzig, M. E., Bortner, M., & Birch, H. G. (1969). Neurologic findings in children educationally designated as "brain-damaged". *American Journal of Orthopsychiatry, 39*, 437–446.

Hertzig, M. E., & Shapiro, T. (in press). The assessment of non-focal neurologic signs in school-aged children. In D. E. Tupper (Ed.), *Soft neurological signs: Manifestations, measurement, research, and meaning*. Orlando, FL: Grune & Stratton.

Holden, E. W., Tarnowski, K. J., & Prinz, R. J. (1982). Reliability of neurological soft signs in children: Reevaluation of the PANESS. *Journal of Abnormal Child Psychology, 10*, 163–172.

Hynd, G. W., Quackenbush, R., & Obrzut, J. E. (1980). Training school psychologists in neuropsychological assessment: Current practices and trends. *Journal of School Psychology, 18,* 148–153.

Ingram, T. T. S. (1973). Soft signs. *Developmental Medicine and Child Neurology, 15,* 527–530.

Jones, B. P., & Butters, N. (1983). Neuropsychological assessment. In M. Hersen, A. E. Kazdin, & A. S. Bellack (Eds.), *The clinical psychology handbook.* New York: Pergamon Press.

Kennard, M. A. (1960). Value of equivocal signs in neurologic diagnosis. *Neurology, 10,* 753–764.

Kennard, M. A. (1969). EEG abnormality in first grade children with "soft" neurological signs. *Electroencephalography and Clinical Neurophysiology, 27,* 544.

Kenny, T. J., & Clemmens, R. L. (1971). Medical and psychological correlates in children with learning disabilities. *Journal of Pediatrics, 78,* 273–277.

Kenny, T. J., Clemmens, R. L., Cicci, R., Lentz, G. A., Nair, P., & Hudson, B. W. (1972). The medical evaluation of children with reading problems. *Pediatrics, 49,* 438–442.

Kinsbourne, M. (1973). Minimal brain dysfunction as a neurodevelopmental lag. *Annals of the New York Academy of Sciences, 205,* 268–273.

Knobloch, H., & Pasamanick, B. (Eds.). (1974). *Gesell and Amatruda's developmental diagnosis.* New York: Harper & Row. (Esp. chap. 17)

Koppitz, E. M. (1963). *The Bender–Gestalt Test for Young Children.* New York: Grune & Stratton.

Koppitz, E. M. (1975). *The Bender–Gestalt Test for Young Children: Vol. 2. Research and application, 1963–1973.* New York: Grune & Stratton.

Kuhns, J. W. (1979). *Neurological dysfunctions of children.* Monterey, CA: Publishers Test Service.

Lacks, P. (1984). *Bender–Gestalt Screening for Brain Dysfunction.* New York: Wiley (Interscience).

Lerer, R. J., & Lerer, M. P. (1976). The effects of methylphenidate on the soft neurological signs of hyperactive children. *Pediatrics, 57,* 521–525.

Lezak, M. D. (1983). *Neuropsychological assessment* (2nd ed., pp. 147–153). New York: Oxford University Press.

Lichenstein, R., & Ireton, H. (1984). *Preschool screening: Early identification of school problems.* Orlando, FL: Grune & Stratton.

Lowe, J., Krehbiel, R., Sweeney, J., Crumley, K., Peterson, G., Watson, B., & Rhodes, J. M. (1984). A screening battery for identifying children at risk for neuropsychological deficits: A pilot study. *International Journal of Clinical Neuropsychology, 6,* 42–45.

MacKeith, R., & Bax, M. (Eds.). (1963). *Minimal cerebral dysfunction* (C.D.M. No. 10). London: Heinemann.

Majovski, L. V., Tanguay, P., Russell, A., Sigman, M., Crumley, K., & Goldenberg, I. (1979a). Clinical Neuropsychological Screening Instrument for assessment of higher cortical deficits in adolescents. *Clinical Neuropsychology, 1*(3), 3–8.

Majovski, L. V., Tanguay, P., Russell, A., Sigman, M., Crumley, K., & Goldenberg, I. (1979b). Clinical Neuropsychological Screening Instrument: A clinical research tool for assessment of higher cortical deficits in adolescents. *Clinical Neuropsychology, 1*(3), 9–19.

McCarthy, D. (1978). *Manual for the McCarthy Screening Test.* New York: Psychological Corporation.

McMahon, S. A., & Greenberg, L. M. (1977). Serial neurologic examination of hyperactive children. *Pediatrics, 59,* 584–587.

Meehl, P. E., & Rosen, A. (1955). Antecendent probability and the efficiency of psychometric signs, patterns, or cutting scores. *Psychological Bulletin, 52,* 194–216.

Mikkelsen, E. J., Brown, G. L., Minichiello, M. D., Millican, F. K., & Rapoport, J. L. (1982). Neurologic status in hyperactive, enuretic, encopretic, and normal boys. *Journal of the American Academy of Child Psychiatry, 21,* 75–81.

Mutti, M., Sterling, H. M., & Spalding, N. V. (1978). *QNST: Quick Neurological Screening Test* (rev. ed.). Novato, CA: Academic Therapy Publications.

Nichols, P. L., & Chen, T.-C. (1981). *Minimal brain dysfunction: A prospective study.* Hillsdale, NJ: Lawrence Erlbaum Associates.

Owen, F. W., Adams, P. A., Forrest, T., Stolz, L. M., & Fisher, S. (1971). Learning disorders in children: Sibling studies. *Monographs of the Society for Research in Child Development, 36*(4, Serial No. 144).

Page-El, E., & Grossman, H. J. (1973). Neurologic appraisal in learning disorders. *Pediatric Clinics of North America, 20,* 599–605.

Paulsen, K. A., & O'Donnell, J. P. (1980). Relationship between minor physical anomalies and "soft signs" of brain damage. *Perceptual and Motor Skills, 51,* 402.

Peter, N. M., & Spreen, O. (1979). Behavioral and personal adjustment of learning disabled children during adolescence and early adulthood: A follow-up study. *Journal of Clinical Neuropsychology, 1,* 17–37.

Peters, J. E., Davis, J. S., Goolsby, C. M., Clements, S. D., & Hicks, T. J. (1973). *Physician's handbook: Screening for MBD.* Summit, NJ: Ciba Pharmaceuticals.

Peters, J. E., Romine, J. S., & Dykman, R. A. (1975). A special neurological examination of children with learning disabilities. *Developmental Medicine and Child Neurology, 17,* 63–78.

Prechtl, H. F. R., & Stemmer, C. J. (1962). The choreiform syndrome in children. *Developmental Medicine and Child Neurology, 4,* 119–127.

Quitkin, F., Rifkin, A., & Klein, D. F. (1976). Neurologic soft signs in schizophrenia and character disorder. *Archives of General Psychiatry, 33,* 845–853.

Rapin, I. (1982). *Children with brain dysfunction: Neurology, cognition, language, and behavior.* New York: Raven Press. (Esp. Chap. 3)

Rapin, I., Tourk, L. M., & Costa, L. D. (1966). Evaluation of the Purdue Pegboard as a screening test for brain damage. *Developmental Medicine and Child Neurology, 8,* 45–54.

Reitan, R. M. (1984). *Aphasia and sensory–perceptual deficits in children.* Tucson: Reitan Neuropsychology Laboratories.

Rie, E. D., Rie, H. E., Stewart, S., & Rettemnier, S. C. (1978). An analysis of neurological soft signs in children with learning problems. *Brain and Language, 6,* 32–46.

Rie, H. E., & Rie, E. D. (Eds.). (1980). *Handbook of minimal brain dysfunctions.* New York: Wiley (Interscience).

Rimm, D. (1963). Cost efficiency and test prediction. *Journal of Consulting Psychology, 27,* 89–91.

Ross, A. O. (1973). Conceptual issues in the evaluation of brain damage. In J. L. Khanna, (Ed.), *Brain damage and mental retardation: A psychological evaluation* (2nd ed.). Springfield, IL: Charles C. Thomas.

Rourke, B. P. (1981). Neuropsychological assessment of children with learning disabilities. In S. B. Filskov & T. J. Boll (Eds.), *Handbook of clinical neuropsychology.* New York: Wiley (Interscience).

Rourke, B. P., Bakker, D. J., Fisk, J. L., & Strang, J. D. (1983). *Child neuropsychology: An introduction to theory, research, and clinical practice*. New York: Guilford Press.

Rudel, R. G., Healy, J., & Denckla, M. B. (1984). Development of motor coordination by normal left-handed children. *Developmental Medicine and Child Neurology, 26,* 104–111.

Rutter, M. (1981). Psychological sequelae of brain damage in children. *American Journal of Psychiatry, 138,* 1533–1544.

Rutter, M. (1982). Syndromes attributed to "minimal brain dysfunction" in childhood. *American Journal of Psychiatry, 139,* 21–33.

Rutter, M., Chadwick, O., & Schachar, R. (1983). Hyperactivity and minimal brain dysfunction: Epidemiological perspectives on questions of cause and classification. In R. E. Tarter (Ed.), *The child at psychiatric risk*. New York: Oxford University Press.

Rutter, M., Graham, P., & Yule, W. (1970). *A neuropsychiatric study in childhood*. (C.D.M. Nos. 35/36). London: Heinemann.

Satz, P., & Fletcher, J. M. (1979). Early screening tests: Some uses and abuses. *Journal of Learning Disabilities, 12,* 65–69.

Satz, P., & Fletcher, J. M. (1980). Minimal brain dysfunctions: An appraisal of research concepts and methods. In H. E. Rie & E. D. Rie (Eds.), *Handbook of minimal brain dysfunctions*. New York: Wiley (Interscience).

Satz, P., & Fletcher, J. M. (1982). *Manual for the Florida Kindergarten Screening Battery*. Odessa, FL: Psychological Assessment Resources.

Satz, P., Taylor, H. G., Friel, J., & Fletcher, J. M. (1978). Some developmental and predictive precursors of reading disabilities: A six-year follow-up. In A. L. Benton & D. Pearl (Eds.), *Dyslexia: An appraisal of current knowledge* (pp. 313–347). New York: Oxford University Press.

Schiller, J. J., DeSimone, J. R., Gross, R., Hoey, J. A., McGuire, J. P., Smith, E. A., & Torres, P. A. (1982). A screening instrument for the assessment of dysnomia of children. *Clinical Neuropsychology, 4,* 22–25.

Schmitt, B. D. (1975). The minimal brain dysfunction myth. *American Journal of Diseases of Children, 129,* 1313–1318.

Shafer, S. Q., Shaffer, D., O'Connor, P. A., & Stokman, C. J. (1983). Hard thoughts on neurological "soft signs." In M. Rutter (Ed.), *Developmental neuropsychiatry*. New York: Guilford Press.

Shaffer, D. (1978). "Soft" neurological signs and later psychiatric disorder—a review. *Journal of Child Psychology and Psychiatry, 19,* 63–65.

Shaffer, D. (1980). An approach to the validation of clinical syndromes in childhood. In S. Salzinger, J. Antrobus, & J. Glick (Eds.). *The ecosystem of the "sick" child* (pp. 31–45). New York: Academic Press.

Shaffer, D., O'Connor, P. A., Shafer, S. Q., & Prupis, S. (1983). Neurological "soft signs:" Their origins and significance for behavior. In M. Rutter (Ed.), *Developmental neuropsychiatry*. New York: Guilford Press.

Shapiro, T., Burkes, L., Petti, T. A. & Ranz, J. (1978). Consistency of "nonfocal" neurological signs. *Journal of the American Academy of Child Psychiatry, 17,* 70–79.

Silver, A. A. (1978). Prevention. In A. L. Benton & D. Pearl (Eds.), *Dyslexia: An appraisal of current knowledge*. New York: Oxford University Press.

Sloan, W. (1955). The Lincoln–Oseretsky motor development scale. *Genetic Psychology Monographs, 51,* 183–252.

Small, L. (1982). *The minimal brain dysfunctions: Diagnosis and treatment*. New York: Free Press. (Esp. Chap. 5)

Spreen, O. (1981). The relationship between learning disability, neurological impairment, and delinquency: Results of a follow-up study. *Journal of Nervous and Mental Disease, 169*, 791–799.

Spreen, O., & Benton, A. L. (1965). Comparative studies of some psychological tests for cerebral damage. *Journal of Nervous and Mental Disease, 140*, 323–333.

Spreen, O., & Gaddes, W. H. (1969). Developmental norms for 15 neuropsychological tests age 6 to 15. *Cortex, 5*, 170–191.

Spreen, O., Tupper, D., Risser, A., Tuokko, H., & Edgell, D. (1984). *Human developmental neuropsychology*. New York: Oxford University Press.

Stangler, S. R., Huber, G. J., & Routh, D. K. (1980). *Screening growth and development of preschool children: A guide for test selection*. New York: McGraw-Hill.

Sterling, H. M., & Sterling, P. J. (1977a). Experiences with the QNST. *Academic Therapy, 12*, 339–342.

Sterling, H. M., & Sterling, P. J. (1977b). Further experiences with the QNST. *Academic Therapy, 12*, 487–490.

Sterling, P. J., & Sterling, H. M. (1980). Neurological status vs. QNST status in 557 students. *Academic Therapy, 15*, 317–323.

Stine, O. C., Saratsiotis, J. B., & Mosser, R. S. (1975). Relationship between neurological findings and classroom behavior. *American Journal of Diseases of Children, 129*, 1036–1040.

Strauss, A. A., & Kephart, N. C. (1955). *Psychopathology and education of the brain-injured child* (Vol. II). New York: Grune & Stratton.

Strauss, A. A., & Lehtinen, L. E. (1947). *Psychopathology and education of the brain-injured child*. New York: Grune & Stratton.

Taber's cyclopedic medical dictionary. (1973). C. L. Thomas (Ed.), 12th ed. Philadelphia: Davis.

Tarter, R. E. (1983). Vulnerability and risk: Assessment and prediction of outcome. In R. E. Tarter (Ed.), *The child at psychiatric risk*. New York: Oxford University Press.

Taylor, E. (1983). Measurement issues and approaches. In M. Rutter (Ed.), *Developmental neuropsychiatry*. New York: Guilford Press.

Taylor, H. G. (1983). MBD: Meanings and misconceptions. *Journal of Clinical Neuropsychology, 5*, 271–287.

Taylor, H. G., & Fletcher, J. M. (1983). Biological foundations of "specific developmental disorders": methods, findings and future directions. *Journal of Clinical Child Psychology, 12*, 46–65.

Taylor, H. G., Fletcher, J. M., & Satz, P. (1984). Neuropsychological assessment of children. In G. Goldstein & M. Hersen (Eds.), *Handbook of psychological assessment*. New York: Pergamon Press.

Telzrow, C. F. (1983). Making child neuropsychological appraisal appropriate for children: Alternative to downward extension of adult batteries. *Clinical Neuropsychology, 5*, 136–141.

Touwen, B. C. L. (1978). Minimal brain dysfunction and minor neurological dysfunction. In A. F. Kalverboer, H. M. van Praag, & J. Mendlewicz (Eds.), *Minimal brain dysfunction: Fact or fiction?* (Advances in Biological Psychiatry, Vol. 1). Basel: Karger.

Touwen, B. C. L. (1979). *Examination of the child with minor neurological dysfunction* (2nd ed.). London: Heinemann.

Touwen, B. C. L., & Sporrel, T. (1979). Soft signs and MBD. *Developmental Medicine and Child Neurology, 21*, 528–530.

Tucker, G. J. (1979). Sensorimotor disturbances in psychotics. In L. Bellak (Ed.), *Psychiatric aspects of minimal brain dysfunction in adults*. New York: Grune & Stratton.

Voeller, K. (1981). A proposed extended behavioral, cognitive, and sensorimotor pediatric neurological examination. In R. Ochroch (Ed.), *The diagnosis and treatment of minimal brain dysfunction in children.* New York: Human Sciences Press.

Weiss, G. (1980). MBD: Critical diagnostic issues. In H. E. Rie & E. D. Rie (Eds.). *Handbook of minimal brain dysfunctions: A critical view.* New York: Wiley (Interscience).

Werry, J. S., & Aman, M. G. (1976). The reliability and diagnostic validity of the Physical and Neurological Examination for Soft Signs (PANESS). *Journal of Autism and Childhood Schizophrenia, 6,* 253–262.

Werry, J. S., Minde, K., Guzman, D., Weiss, G., Dogan, K., & Hoy, R. (1972). Studies on the hyperactive child. VIII: Neurological status compared with neurotic and normal children. *American Journal of Orthopsychiatry, 42,* 441–450.

Wolf, B. A., & Tramontana, M. G. (1982). Aphasia screening test interrelationships with complete Halstead–Reitan test results for older children. *Clinical Neuropsychology, 4,* 179–186.

Wolff, P. H., & Hurwitz, I. (1973). Functional implications of the minimal brain damage syndrome. In S. Walzer & P. H. Wolff (Eds.), *Minimal cerebral dysfunction in children.* New York: Grune & Stratton.

Yule, W. (1978). Diagnosis: Developmental psychological assessment. In A. F. Kalverboer, H. M. van Praag, & J. Mendlewicz (Eds.), *Minimal brain dysfunction: Fact or fiction?* (Advances in Biological Psychiatry, Vol. 1). Basel: Karger.

Chapter 7

Standard Neuropsychological Batteries for Children

PHYLLIS ANNE TEETER

Department of Educational Psychology
University of Wisconsin at Milwaukee
Milwaukee, Wisconsin 53201

INTRODUCTION

There has been a proliferation of literature in recent years discussing the neuropsychological basis of learning. The ability to perform language and cognitive tasks, such as reading, writing, mathematics calculation, and spelling, is dependent on a complex interaction between intact neural systems, neurochemistry, and other motivational and environmental factors. The central nervous system (CNS), especially those areas of the cerebrum dedicated to higher functions, mediates the learning process (Gaddes, 1980; Tarnopol & Tarnopol, 1977). Clinical studies have demonstrated that when these brain areas are dysfunctional, the learning process is disrupted (Luria, 1966). In order to determine how cortical dysfunction affects human behavior, neuropsychologists have developed test batteries that assess the integrity of the brain. Subsequently, neuropsychological assessment methods have been used with children to better understand the nature of learning failure, and to determine which instructional strategies will be beneficial (Hartlage & Hartlage, 1977).

Recently, there has been considerable interest in neuropsychology as it

187

CHILD NEUROPSYCHOLOGY, VOL. 2
Copyright © 1986 by Academic Press, Inc.

relates to the practice of child clinical psychology. First, early explorations into reading and learning disabilities were intricately tied to the neuropsychological theory of the time (Clements, 1966; Cruickshank & Hallahan, 1975; Myklebust, 1968; Strauss & Lehtinen, 1947). Hynd and Obrzut (1981) have also identified several other factors that have contributed to this renewed interest, including research linking cognitive development and cerebral lateralization, and neuropsychological remediation techniques with learning-disabled children. As the field of child neuropsychology grows, it becomes increasingly important for child clinical psychologists to become familiar with this body of knowledge. Perhaps one of the most compelling statements comes from Rourke (1975). After years of investigating the etiology of learning disorders, he concludes "that at least one crucial factor limiting the satisfactory adaptation of children with learning disabilities is cerebral dysfunction" (p. 918). This viewpoint has received widespread acceptance as evidenced by the (1981) definition by the National Joint Committee for Learning Disabilities, which states that this disorder is "presumed to be due to central nervous system dysfunction" (Hammill, Leigh, McNutt, & Larsen, 1981, p. 336). It seems imperative that psychologists reconceptualize learning disorders in terms of the functional status of the brain by applying neuropsychological assessment and remedial procedures for this population.

In this chapter, two major neuropsychological assessment approaches for children are discussed: (1) the Halstead–Reitan Neuropsychological Test Batteries and Allied Procedures; and (2) the Luria–Nebraska Neuropsychological Battery for Children. The theoretical basis of each procedure is discussed, including general guidelines for interpretation. Research findings supporting the validity of each battery for assessing brain-damaged and learning-disabled populations are also presented. In order to provide a framework for understanding child clinical neuropsychology, it is necessary first to discuss the general aims of neuropsychological assessment and some developmental factors that affect the neuropsychological investigation of children.

Aims of Clinical Neuropsychological Assessment

Regardless of the age of the patient, the aim of clinical neuropsychological assessment is to investigate the functional status of the brain by analyzing behavioral responses on a variety of tests (Rourke, Bakker, Fisk, & Strang, 1983). A broad range of human behaviors are sampled to provide information concerning the functional integrity of specific neural structures and cortical systems of the brain that mediate mental processes. Neuropsychological batteries are designed to assess global brain functioning, as well as to evaluate the presence of deficits in specific, focalized areas of the cortex (Selz, 1981). A comprehensive approach is taken to measure cognitive, language, sensory–perceptual, motor, and reasoning abilities. It is the aim of standardized test batteries to provide reliable data from which valid descriptions can be made concerning the neuropsychological status of the client. Neuropsychologists do not support a single-test approach, but rather stress the necessity of using a battery for a comprehensive and thorough evaluation of brain function. Clinical neuropsychological procedures assess only cortical functions of the brain and have not been designed to measure the status of subcortical brain areas. Often, psychologists work cooperatively with physical and occupational therapists to obtain information concerning the functional status of cerebellar and lower brainstem structures.

It is important to point out that the goal of neuropsychology is not diagnosis, nor is it simply determining the presence or absence of brain damage. While the procedures have shown clinical validity for differentiating behavioral deficiencies resulting from brain dysfunction, the main objective in neuropsychological evaluation is to provide descriptive information about the brain–behavior relationship (Boll, 1981). The focus of neuropsychology then is to obtain valid descriptive information about the behavioral consequences of neuropathology which can be used to design relevant rehabilitation or remedial programs for individuals with brain-related disorders.

Developmental Factors Affecting Child Neuropsychology

While all neuropsychological assessment is complex, there are a number of factors that increase the complexity of evaluating and interpreting neuropsychological data with children. In this regard, child neuropsychologists have focused on two major questions: (1) What effect does the age of onset of brain damage have on the overall development of the child? and (2) To what extent can findings from adult neuropsychology be generalized to children? Although there is a need for continued research in the area of applied child neuropsychology, extensive studies have generated valuable information concerning the structure, organization and function of the developing brain.

Age of Onset of Brain Damage

Implicit in the question, does age of onset of brain damage affect the overall development of the child, is the broader issue of whether children recover from early brain damage. In order to better understand the effects of the age of onset of brain injury to later development, it is necessary to review the behavioral sequelae accompanying damage due to trauma or insult to the brain. (See Berg, Chapter 5 of this volume for a more thorough discussion.) Damage to the brain results in numerous changes involving greater portions or functions of the brain than the specific site where neurons have been destroyed, including changes of both a transient and a permanent nature (Isaacson, 1976). Isaacson (1976) enumerates the following transient reactions that affect brain functioning: (1) destruction of cells at the site of damage; (2) disruption of cellular activity of nearby cells; (3) phagocytic and astrocytic reactions at the border of the lesion; (4) changes in the blood vessels at and around the site of damage; (5) irritative reactions, including edema; (6) pressure build-up that disrupts activities of healthy cells; (7) changes in cerebrospinal fluid; (8) loss of enervation of cells that were at one time controlled or monitored by the destroyed cells; (9) proliferation of newly generated axon collaterals into regions once enervated by damaged cells; and (10) changes in the size and cellular makeup of the brain if damage occurs early. Many of the behaviors affected by these brain activities are restored subsequent to damage and improve with time, so that functions initially lost are naturally regained when these transient reactions stabilize. Isaacson (1976) points out, however, that some of these transient reactions can result in permanent changes both in the structure of the brain and in its function.

Most of the permanent changes that Isaacson (1976) discusses involve new and abnormal patterns that are formed by axon collaterals invading damaged areas, which results in differential control and regulation of the specific brain region. Some of the changes due to the different input, control, and regulation of a region can be helpful in restoring the loss of a function, but occasionally new synaptic contacts can hinder brain activity. In some instances, major neuronal fiber tracts are formed and move into regions in which they would normally not be found. One of the major points of interest here is the fact that the immature or infant brain is more receptive to these new contacts than is the adult brain, which can result in abnormal activity in the brain (Isaacson, 1976). Perhaps even more important, the infant brain often shows a reduction in size following brain damage, and Isaacson (1976, p. 42) concludes that "from a structural point of view early damage must be considered to be *more* disastrous than damage occurring later." Damage to the mature brain of the adolescent or adult usually shows neither formation of abnormal neuronal tracks nor a reduction of the size of the brain. Consequently, loss of function tends to be more highly localized and specific for the adult.

Isaacson's (1976) research has been supported by earlier studies conducted by Reitan (1974), showing that brain damage affects the developmental potential of the child. In a longitudinal, cross-sectional study comparing children 4, 8, 12, and 16 years of age, Reitan (1981a) found that children sustaining damage at the age of 4 years showed a distinctly different learning curve than older children with brain damage. While all brain-injured subjects showed a decrease in learning compared to nonimpaired children, the older groups eventually approached their normal age peers in performance. The younger groups demonstrated a clear reduction of overall potential throughout their development and never reached the performance levels of their normal counterparts. Reitan (1981a) concluded that the longer the brain is normal, healthy, and intact, the greater is its general and overall capacity to acquire higher-level language and cognitive functions.

Although the research of Isaacson (1976) and Reitan (1974) is convincing, competing plasticity theories indicate that young children show a greater restoration of brain functions following brain damage than do adults. Alajouanine and Lhermitte (1965) found that a majority of children between the ages of 6 and 15 years showed substantial improvement in language functions 1 year after injury to the left hemisphere. Other studies (Basser, 1962; Hecaen, 1976) have also reported that children demonstrate milder deficits in language following left-hemisphere lesions than do adults. Lenneberg (1967) theorizes that both hemispheres are equally capable of assuming language functions for young children, but as the brain becomes more lateralized and specialized with age, damage to the left hemisphere late in life results in more severe and long-term language dysfunctions. Lenneberg postulates that after about age 14, the brain is less successful in transferring language functions from the left to the right hemisphere. However, Golden and Wilkening (1986) indicate that the critical period may be more restricted than Lenneberg suggests. For example, when left-hemisphere damage occurs prior to the age of 2 years, the right hemisphere can assume language functions (Golden & Wilkening, 1986). After 2 years, the transfer of function is less complete, and deficits for children are similar to those of adults. Apparently, there are optimal times when lateralized damage can be minimized, and the earlier the damage the better the chance for transfer of functions.

Studies with hemispherectomy patients show that both hemispheres are specialized at birth, but they are both relatively plastic and functionally capable of assuming activities generally performed by the other hemisphere (Kolb & Whishaw, 1980). When unilateral hemidecortications are performed prior to the development of language (first year of life), Kolb and Whishaw (1980) report that transfer of functions is possible. Specifically, if the left hemisphere is removed, simple language tasks can be performed by the right hemisphere without a decrease in simple or complex visuospatial abilities; and, if the right hemisphere is removed, simple visuospatial abilities can be mediated by the left hemisphere without impairment to simple or complex language functions. While simple tasks can be performed by the remaining hemisphere, more complex tasks cannot be. That is, left hemidecortification results in a loss of complex language functions, whereas right hemidecortication is followed by a loss of complex visuospatial abilities. Kolb and Whishaw (1980) conclude that each hemisphere has the ability to mediate functions of the opposite hemisphere, but neither hemisphere is able to assume all the functions of the other. These studies support the idea of plasticity in the young brain but not equipotentiality, as evidenced by the loss of some complex functions (Kolb & Whishaw, 1980). Other research (Milner, 1975) indicates that general intelligence is also lowered when one hemisphere functions in the absence of the other.

Boll and Barth (1981) make an important point concerning the difference between children who have sustained lateralized damage, which results in the surgical removal of one hemisphere, and children who have experienced generalized brain damage where surgery is not possible. By removing a damaged region or area of the brain, the abnormal influence of this system on mental activity may actually be less than the effects of a continued influence from abnormal or dysfunctional brain tissue (Boll & Barth, 1981). Boll and Barth (1981) also cite studies reporting that the intact hemisphere receives interference or competition from the damaged hemisphere when it attempts to assume a particular function for the abnormal region. For these reasons, milder impairment can actually be more detrimental to the overall functioning of the brain than the complete absence of localized or lateralized brain tissue. Boll and Barth's conclusions are consistent and supportive of Isaacson's (1976) comments on the negative influence of abnormal brain tissue to that of healthy tissue.

Obviously the question, does early injury have a more serious affect on overall mental development than does later injury, cannot be easily answered. Boll and Barth (1981) suggest that many factors concerning the type, size, extent, and location of damage must be considered, as well as the specific mental activity involved and its cognitive complexity. Wilkening and Golden (1982) also show that other factors influence the outcome of injury, including the socioeconomic status (SES) of the family; the results of computerized axial tomography (CAT scan); the presence and length of unconsciousness; and, the treatment of injury (i.e., surgery and/or cranial irradiation). Even when recovery of function occurs, it is impossible to determine if there has been a general reduction of higher-level abstraction or cognitive functioning. Consequently, the relationship of brain injury to later development is dependent on numerous factors; and generally, the brain–behavior relationship in children must be viewed as a complex interaction.

Generalization of Neuropsychological Findings

Caution is exercised when generalizing clinical research findings from adults to children. Children differ from adults on a number of dimensions that preclude valid generalizations. Boll and Barth (1981) refer to neuro-anatomical, neuropathological, and psychological differences that affect behavior following brain injury. First, anatomic neural structures are not fully developed in children, but as myelination and dendritic connections develop, psychological and cognitive changes are observed. Second, the type of damage seen in adults is typically focalized and most often results from cerebral vascular accidents, traumatic (penetrating) head injuries, and intracerebral tumors. On the other hand, children suffer more from generalized disorders, such as epilepsy, anoxia, perinatal trauma, postnatal infections, and closed-head (rather than penetrating) injuries. Very different neuropsychological profiles are present when injury is focalized rather than generalized. Finally, the psychological effects of brain damage as measured by the Wechsler Scales are often different for adults and children (See Boll and Barth, 1981, for a more detailed discussion on this topic.)

In children, there tends to be a consistent problem determining whether the lack of a skill is due to brain damage, pathology, or dysfunction, or whether the absence is due to a lack of acquisition of the skill. The importance of this fact cannot be underestimated, as the confounding effects of developmental factors can result in the misdiagnosis and misunderstanding of the range of variability in normal development for many neuropsychological abilities. This problem is further exacerbated because the premorbid status of children is often more difficult to establish than it is for adults. For example, if a 7-year-old child evidences dyslexia following brain trauma, it is difficult to determine whether deficits are a result of damage to the cortex or whether reading levels are similar to those prior to injury. However, for adults, the level of education and occupational status help to establish premorbid states.

Neuroanatomical Structures and Functions of the Brain

The human cortex is composed of two separate hemispheres that are similar in anatomical structure. The right and left hemispheres are joined

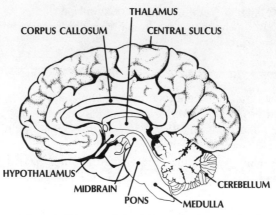

Figure 1. Diagram of the right cerebral cortex showing
the corpus callosum and brainstem structures.

by two major neuronal pathways, the corpus callosum and the anterior
commissure, which allow for interhemispheric communication by transferring information from one hemisphere to the other.

Each hemisphere is organized into four distinct lobes: frontal, parietal,
temporal, and occipital. Kolb and Whishaw (1980) outline the boundaries
separating the four lobes. The frontal lobe is separated from the parietal
area by the central sulcus, and from the temporal lobe by the lateral

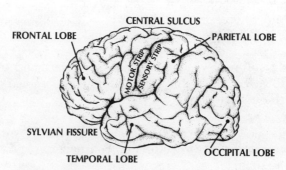

Figure 2. Diagram of the left cerebral cortex showing
major divisions and lobes.

(Sylvian) fissure. The parietal and occipital lobes are separated medially by the parieto-occipital sulcus. Finally, there are no lateral anatomical boundaries between the occipital lobe and the parietal and temporal lobes.

Kolb and Whishaw (1980) point out that the lobes represent anatomical regions of the brain, but because of the functional differences between these areas they can be used in a "descriptive way to indicate functional regions" (p. 16). The relative functional differences between the lobes allow neuropsychologists to identify localized deficits. Localization of cortical function is generally analyzed in quadrants: anterior, posterior, superior, and inferior brain regions. Anterior functions of the cortex (frontal lobe) are assessed by a variety of motor tasks; while posterior functions (posterior to the central sulcus) are measured by tactile–sensory (parietal lobe) and visual (occipital lobe) tasks. The integrity of superior and inferior regions of the cortex are measured by motor and tactile sensory tasks.

Lateralized brain damage or dysfunction is determined by comparing performances of the right and left hemispheres. The two hemispheres are contralaterally organized, so that the right side of the body is primarily controlled by the left hemisphere, and the left side of the body is primarily regulated by the right hemisphere. While the somatosensory, motor, and auditory systems are almost completely crossed, ipsilateral pathways send impulses from the same side of the body to the same hemisphere (e.g., right ear to right hemisphere). However, contralateral pathways are dominant for transmitting signals to and from sense receptors. The visual system is more complex than the other systems because the visual fields (not the eyes) are crossed in the hemispheres. Thus, the left visual field projects to the right visual cortex, and the right visual field projects to the left visual cortex.

Right-left performance differentials on motor and tactile–sensory tasks are analyzed to implicate either the right or the left hemisphere. For example, if a child shows significantly depressed motor speed and consistent sensory imperceptions on the right side of the body, the functional status of the left hemisphere is thought to be impaired. If other higher-level cognitive disabilities, such as significantly low verbal IQ (compared to performance IQ) and reading deficits are also found, then they are most likely a result of left hemisphere dysfunction. Neuropsychologists are cautious when inferring lateralized dysfunction based solely on test data when cognitive deficits are found in the absence of sensory–motor impairments. However other evidence (CAT scans, neurological examination, and medical history) is used to confirm or support signs of lateralized dysfunction.

THE HALSTEAD–REITAN
NEUROPSYCHOLOGICAL TEST BATTERIES
AND ALLIED PROCEDURES

The most well publicized and widely used clinical neuropsychological methods were devised by Ward Halstead, and later expanded and revised by Ralph Reitan (Boll, 1981). According to Boll (1981), Halstead initially focused his investigations on the observations of behavioral characteristics of individuals with brain injury, and subsequently formulated psychological tests to measure these behaviors more systematically. Reitan modified and extended many of Halstead's experimental procedures for clinical use with adults and children. Hartlage and Hartlage (1977) suggest that the tests designed by Halstead and Reitan are the best and most comprehensive neuropsychological batteries available. Periodic revisions by Reitan have strengthened and improved the diagnostic utility of these procedures.

Halstead Neuropsychological Test Battery for
Children (Ages 9 through 14)

Between 1951 and 1953, Reitan modified and extended the Halstead Neuropsychological Test for Adults downward, incorporating test items suitable for children between the ages of 9 through 14 years (Reitan & Davison, 1974). Reitan (1969) and Boll (1981) have described the items as follows:

Category Test. There are a total of 168 items on this test, which are projected onto a screen in front of the child. The child must select the correct stimulus figure, and pull one of four levers on the test apparatus indicating the answer. There is a feedback mechanism, either a bell or a buzzer, informing the child that the answer is right or wrong. The items are divided into sections, and each section has a specific principle consistent throughout. The feedback system allows the child to test certain principles in each section until the correct principle is found. In the instructions, the child is told when a new section is beginning, and that the principle may be the same as the last or it may be different. This test was designed to measure abstract concept formation, mental efficiency, and to some extent, learning skills. The category test is sensitive to general or global brain functioning.

Tactual Performance Test. On this test, there are six figures on a form board, and the child must place the blocks into the correct forms. At no time is the child allowed to see the forms or the board because he or she is blindfolded. The child first uses his or her preferred hand, then the non-

TABLE 1

Subtests of the Halstead–Reitan neuropsychological test batteries for children

Halstead Battery[a] (9–14 years)	Reitan–Indiana Battery (5–9 years)
Category test	Category test
Tactual performance test	Tactual performance test
Finger tapping test	Finger tapping test
Speech-sounds perception test	—
Seashore rhythm test	—
Trail-making test	Marching test
Strength of grip test	Strength of grip test
Sensory perceptual exam	Sensory perception test
Tactile form recognition test	Tactile form recognition test
Tactile finger localization test	Tactile finger localization test
Finger-tip number writing test	Finger symbol writing test
Aphasia screening test	Aphasis screening test
	Color form test
	Progressive figures test
	Matching pictures test
	Target test
	Individual performance tests

[a] Reitan includes the Wechsler Intelligence Scale, the Wide Range Achievement Test (WRAT), and the Lateral Dominance Test.

preferred, and finally both hands to complete the task. Times on each subtrial are analyzed to determine differential performance for each side of the body. After all three trials are finished, the child is instructed to draw as many of the designs from memory as possible. The child's tactile discrimination, manual dexterity, kinesthetic functions, spatial abilities, as well as incidental memory skills are measured by this task. This test measures parietal lobe functioning and can be used to lateralize brain dysfunction. The total time, memory and localization scores can be used to determine general, overall brain integrity.

Finger Tapping Test. On this test, the child is instructed to tap a mounted key (similar to a telegraph key), as quickly as possible. There are five trials with the preferred hand and five trials with the nonpreferred hand, allowing for interpretation of differential tapping speeds for both sides. This task is simply a measure of motor speed.

Speech-Sounds Perception Test. This test is composed of 60 nonsense words on a tape recorder, with different beginning and ending consonant sounds. The child is given a form with three alternatives, and he or she must identify the correct sound. Attentional abilities, auditory discrimination, and crossmodal skills (auditory-input–visual-output) are assessed on this task. This test is used as an indicator of global brain functioning, but depressed scores can accompany specific left-hemisphere dysfunction.

Seashore Rhythm Test. This test was adopted from the Seashore Test of Musical Talent, where pairs of rhythms are presented to the child from a tape recorder. The object of the task is to determine of the rhythms are the same or different. Attention and concentrational skills, as well as auditory perceptual abilities, are assessed on this test.

Allied Procedures

Other subtests in the neuropsychological examination were not originally developed by Halstead or Reitan, but they were included to provide a more comprehensive evaluation. Boll (1981) describes the following subtests.

Trail Making Test. There are two parts on this test, consisting of 15 items. On Trail A, the child is required to connect circles from 1 to 15 as quickly as possible. On Trail B, the child must connect alternating circles from A to G and 1 to 8. These tasks require motor speed, visual perception, sequencing ability, symbol recognition, and simultaneous processing of two series of symbols. Trial B is sensitive to general brain functioning.

Strength of Grip (Hand Dynamometer). Hand strength is measured using an adjustable dynamometer. Alternating trials are administered with the preferred and nonpreferred hand, allowing for analysis of differential hand strength.

Sensory Perceptual Exam. Tactile, auditory, and visual perception are measured both unilaterally (one side of the body) and bilaterally (both sides of the body).

Tactile perception is assessed unilaterally by touching the child's hand or face while the eyes are closed. The child must indicate which side of the body has been touched, and whether double simultaneous (hand–hand or hand–face) stimulation has been presented. One can determine if the child has right- or left-sided tactile–perceptual difficulties on this task.

Auditory perception is assessed by presenting soft stimuli behind the child's back first to one ear, then the other, then simultaneously. Again the child must indicate which ear has been stimulated.

Visual perception is measured by having the child determine whether the examiner is moving one or two hands from a peripheral level. The visual field is tested in quadrants, above and below eye level.

These sensory exams are sensitive to parietal, temporal, and occipital lobe functioning, respectively, and provide methods for lateralizing and localizing brain damage.

Tactile Form Recognition. On this task, the child places one hand through an opening in a board, and the examiner places either a square, a cross, a circle or a triangle into the child's hand. The subject is then asked to point to the object on another board. Both hands are tested for tactile discrimination. Parietal lobe functions are measured by this task, and right–left performance differentials can be used as lateralizing signs.

Tactile Finger Localization. On this test, the examiner touches the child's finger lightly in a prescribed order, and the child indicates which finger is being touched. Tactile localization is assessed for all fingers. Again, lateralizing signs for parietal lobe integrity are measured by this test.

Finger-Tip Number Writing. Using the tip of a pen, the examiner traces a series of numbers in a prescribed order on each of the child's fingers. As a cue, each number is written on the palm of the hand before the trial begins, and the child is informed which numbers will be used. This test is sensitive to parietal lobe functioning.

Aphasia Screening Test. Reitan modified Wepman's Aphasia Screening Test, and it is commonly included in the neuropsychological test battery for children, to assess receptive and expressive aphasia. There are 32 items on the Aphasia Screening Test for older children. The items include naming, copying, spelling, reading, and simple arithmetic calculation tasks.

Reitan–Indiana Neuropsychological Test Battery (Children Ages 5 through 8)

The Reitan–Indiana (Reitan, 1969) battery is a modification of the Halstead Neuropsychological Test Battery, devised for children 5 years through 8 years of age. The following procedural changes were necessary to accommodate for the developmental differences between the older and the younger children (Boll, 1981; Reitan & Davison, 1974).

Category Test. The instrument panel was changed to simplify the response pattern. The test itself was reduced to 80 items arranged in 5 categories. On the first subtest, the child must pull the lever corresponding to the color of the stimulus card, while the other subtests involve principles of size, shape or color. Again, the correct answer is reinforced by a bell.

Tactual Performance Test. The same six-form board was retained from the previous battery, but was turned horizontally to allow the smaller child ample room for exploration.

Strength of Grip and Finger Tapping Test. Modification of the grip strength test was not necessary for younger children, however an electric tapping key is used for the Finger Tapping Test.

Finger Symbol Writing Test. Using the tip of a pen, the examiner writes a series of X's and O's (instead of numbers as for older children) on the child's fingers. The child must indicate which symbol has been traced on his or her finger.

Tactile Finger Localization, Tactile Form Recognition, and Sensory Perceptual Exams. These tests were adopted without modification.

Aphasia Screening Test. Changes were made in the Aphasia Screening Test to simplify the tasks required of the younger children. There were also fewer items included to measure receptive and expressive aphasic disorders. Selected items involved: writing child's own name; copying a square, triangle and cross; identifying pictures of a baby, clock, and fork; reading letters and simple phrases; computing simple arithmetic functions; and, following simple verbal commands.

Rhythm, Speech-Sounds Perception, and Trail Making Test. These tests were not included in the neuropsychological battery for children under 9 years of age.

New Subtests for Young Children

Reitan developed several new procedures for young children. These new procedures were described by Reitan and Davison (1974), and Boll (1981), as follows.

Marching Test. Reitan devised this test to measure gross motor functions and coordination of the upper extremities. The child must follow a sequence of circles connected by lines up a page, by touching each circle as quickly as possible. Both time and accuracy are recorded for each hand. The second part of this test involves using both hands to "march up the page," with the right hand touching the circles on the right side of the page, alternating with the left hand touching the circles on the left side of the page.

Color Form Test. On this task, there are geometric shapes of different colors printed on a tag board. The child is instructed to touch one figure and then another, moving in a sequence of shape–color–shape–color. The child is required to selectively attend to one aspect of the stimulus (e.g., color) and ignore the other (e.g., shape). This test is similar to Part B of the Trail Making Test, where the child moves from numbers to letters, and back to numbers.

Progressive Figures Test. On this test, there are eight large shapes (such as a circle), with smaller shapes (such as a square) inside. The child must move from the small square (inside) to a large figure with the same shape (square). The second large shape may have a smaller triangular shape inside, indicating that the next move will be to a large triangular shape. This task requires visual perception, motor speed, attention, concentration, and flexibility to change sets.

Matching Pictures Test. This test requires the child to match pictures that are initially identical. The task becomes progressively more difficult as generalization is necessary, such that the child must identify pictures that are in the same category but are not identical to the stimulus.

Target Test. This stimulus for this test is an 18 × 18 square-inch card with nine dots printed on it. The child is given a sheet with the same dot configuration. The child is instructed to draw the same design that the examiner has tapped out on the larger sheet. This item requires visual-memory abilities.

Individual Performance Tests (Matching Figures, Matching V's, Concentric Square, and Star). The matching figures subtest requires the child to match a group of figures (printed on a square). The matching V's task involves matching V's that vary in the width of the angle. The concentric square and star tests involve copying complex designs. The individual performance tests measure visual perception and motor abilities.

Reitan systematically includes the Wechsler Intelligence Scale (WISC), the Wide Range Achievement Test (WRAT), and a test of lateral dominance in a comprehensive neuropsychological evaluation with children.

Scoring Procedures

Scoring procedures on the Halstead and the Reitan–Indiana Neuropsychological test batteries vary according to the subtest. For example, sometimes errors are counted (category test), or the number of responses are calculated (finger tapping Test), or the time required to complete the task is recorded (tactual performance test). Reitan completed the standardization procedures after years of developmental research and clinical experimentation, and these are reported in Reitan and Davison (1974). Developmental norms have also been reported by Knights (1966) and Spreen and Gaddes (1969), with similar findings. Spreen and Gaddes (1969) report that intelligence, educational, and motivational factors should be similar to those children described in their normative sample before meaningful comparisons and generalizations can be made with other children.

Neuropsychological Model for Data Interpretation

Scores on the Halstead Neuropsychological Test Battery for Children (9–15 years) and the Reitan–Indiana Test Battery (5–8 years) are interpreted on four dimensions. Selz and Reitan (1979) describe these four levels of inference as (1) analyzing the child's level of performance against a comparison group; (2) analyzing patterns of performance within the battery to determine the child's relative strengths and weaknesses on various tasks; (3) analyzing pathognomonic signs for the presence or absence of abnormalities; and (4) analyzing right–left differences in performance to determine the efficiency of each side of the body.

Level of Performance

The first step in the interpretation of neuropsychological test data involves determining the individual's level of performance, or as Reitan (1981b) succinctly puts it, "How well does the subject do?" This procedure calls for determining whether the child's test scores fall into normal or abnormal ranges that have been determined in previous studies where children with documented brain dysfunction have been compared to groups of learning-disabled and normal children. Rourke (1981) suggests that using a normative approach is absolutely necessary for children in the 5- to 15-year age range because of the developmental nature of many neuropsychological abilities. Because levels of performance can be similar for different brain pathologies, Rourke (1981) further argues that normal or abnormal levels of performance can not unequivocally indicate normal or abnormal brain function. This may be due to the recovery of function phenomenon discussed earlier, where some brain injured children reach normal levels of functioning. In these cases, it is difficult if not impossible to determine if the child's overall capacity was higher prior to brain damage. Rourke (1981) also indicates that interpretation of the level of performance also may result in a great number of false positives, because other factors not related to brain pathology can contribute to low scores, including motivation, emotional disturbance, and language deprivation. Consequently, the clinician must analyze test data for the presence of pathognomonic signs and specific patterns of performance to fully appreciate the adequacy of brain functions.

Despite adequate norms for children 5 to 15 years of age, Reitan (1981b) points out that the developmental variance within normal populations makes the use of level of performance somewhat problematic for children. Further, the age of onset of brain injury, the severity of injury, and the recovery of functions are factors influencing the level of performance.

Consequently, this first approach is complex and cannot be considered in isolation for interpreting how the brain is functioning in young children.

Pathognomonic-Sign Approach

The second approach for analyzing neuropsychological test data involves looking at specific deficit signs that indicate cerebral damage, and these signs often implicate either the right or left hemisphere (Reitan, 1981b). Deficit or pathognomonic signs indicate pathology because they occur almost exclusively in brain-damaged individuals and rarely in "normals"; and, as Rourke (1981) indicates, the sign approach has been one of the most common clinical methods for investigating brain behavior. Wheeler and Reitan (1962) found that a number of specific test items from the Aphasia Screening Test consistently differentiated normal from brain-injured adults; and, these test variables were powerful discriminators for determining right- versus left-hemisphere dysfunction. Wheeler and Reitan (1962) specified that the following aphasia errors frequently occurred in groups with brain damage but not in normals: dyscalculia, central dysarthria, dysnomia, and dysgraphia as indicators of left-hemisphere dysfunction; and, constructional dyspraxia as an indicator of right-hemisphere impairment.

Pathognomonic signs are also difficult to analyze in children because before brain pathology can be inferred, one must be certain that the skill has been developed prior to insult or injury. Reitan (1981b) again points out that it is easier to determine this with adults, as extremely poor performance on certain tasks indicates an impairment or loss of function; whereas, with children poor performance may simply reflect the fact that the skill has never been acquired. However, the lateralizing signs (implicating either the right or the left hemisphere) tend to be similar for adults and children, especially when lesions or damage occur in the child after spatial organization and language abilities have been firmly established (Reitan, 1981b).

Differential Score Approach

The differential score approach has been extensively applied to aid in the identification of special populations, especially brain-damaged and learning-disabled individuals. In a neuropsychological evaluation, patterns between test scores typically include analyzing verbal–performance IQ differences, patterns on the Trail Making Test (Halstead–Reitan Battery), and scores on the Speech-Sounds Perception Test (Reitan, 1981b). Reitan suggests that left hemisphere dysfunction may be present when the verbal IQ is "clearly lower" than the performance IQ, and Wechsler scores are particularly low on the arithmetic and similarities subtests. In contrast, the right hemisphere may be implicated when the performance IQ is clearly lower than the verbal IQ, and Block Design and Picture Arrangement subtests are very low (Reitan, 1981b). The clinician must be cautious when operationally defining what Reitan means by clearly lower and very low. The reader is referred to Kaufman's (1979) research with the Wechsler standardization sample to determine typical verbal–performance discrepancy scores found in normal children before hypotheses concerning lateralized dysfunction can be reasonably made. Again, Reitan uses sensory–motor signs to confirm lateralized brain dysfunction.

Other Wechsler subtest patterns have been consistently found in children with severe reading disabilities, which are reflected by outstandingly poor performance on the arithmetic, coding, information, and digit-span subtests (Rourke, 1981). Rourke suggests that prognosis for normal reading for children with this particular pattern is very poor. In general, Rourke and Reitan both indicate that individuals may have similar or identical levels of performance on the Wechsler that are derived in very different ways; that is, by investigating particular patterns of strengths and weaknesses, clinically relevant neuropsychological differences can be determined from one individual to another.

Patterns of performance can also be compared on the Trail-Making Test found on the Halstead–Reitan Neuropsychological Test batteries. After extensive research, Reitan (1981b) reported that low scores on Part B of the Trails, in comparison to the individual's performance on Part A, was suggestive of left cerebral hemisphere dysfunction. Further, poor performance on the Halstead Speech Sounds Perception test was also indicative of left-hemisphere impairment. Reitan found similar patterns for children and adults for these subtests, again particularly when the child was developmentally capable of performing the task. In instances where longstanding brain pathology was present or damage was incurred early in life, the distinct differential patterns were less obvious (Reitan, 1981b). When reviewing neuropsychological test profiles, Reitan does considerable analysis of the patterns between specific subtests to build a clear case for lateralizing and localizing cerebral dysfunction.

Performance on Two Sides of the Body

Lateralized sensory or motor deficits are among the most valid signs of cerebral dysfunction or damage (Rourke, 1981). Errors on unilateral and bilateral sensory or motor tasks can be analyzed the same for adults and children (Reitan, 1981b). Reitan found that the following motor and sensory signs implicate the left hemisphere for right-dominant individuals: (1) significantly lower (10% slower) finger tapping speed with the right hand as compared to the left hand; (2) lower scores with the right hand on the

Tactual Performance Test; (3) lower grip strength (10% less) for the right hand as compared to the left hand; and, (4) errors on the right side of the body on the sensory–perceptual exams and the tactile perceptual tests (finger localization, finger-tip writing, tactile identification). Indicators for the right hemisphere (for right-dominant individuals) are also present in all of the preceding areas, but individuals with right-hemisphere dysfunction show consistently lower scores on the left side of the body on motor and sensory tasks (Reitan, 1981b).

Validity Studies with Halstead–Reitan Batteries

There have been numerous studies with the Halstead–Reitan neuropsychological test batteries for children. Selz (1981) reports that studies initially focused on comparisons between brain-damaged and normal children, and later included learning-disabled subjects. More recently, studies with the Halstead–Reitan batteries have addressed neurodevelopmental issues and the neuropsychological basis of achievement with normal children.

Differential Diagnosis of Brain-Damaged Children

Reed, Reitan, and Klove (1965) compared the performance of 50 brain-damaged children (aged 10 to 14 years of age) to 50 children with normal brain functioning. The brain-damaged group comprised children with heterogeneous cerebral dysfunctions that were independently diagnosed through neurological examinations and medical history. Subtests of the Wechsler scales and the Halstead–Reitan test battery were analyzed. Of the 27 measures, 24 variables showed statistically significant differences ($p < .005$) between the groups; and, the remaining 3 variables reached significance at the .01 level. In a rank-order comparison, language-related measures appeared most impaired for the brain-damaged children. In a replication study with 27 brain-damaged and 27 normal children, Boll (1974) reported similar findings. Thirty-two of 40 variables reached statistical significance (.05 level), with comparable rank order distributions for the Wechsler and the neuropsychological variables.

In an effort to analyze performance differences on motor and sensory–perceptual measures, Boll and Reitan (1970) compared 35 brain-damaged and 35 control subjects in the 9 - to 14-year age range. Performance on the tactile finger localization, finger tapping, grip strength, and tactual performance tests were significantly different for the two groups. Although specific sensory–motor subtests differentiated normals from brain-damaged groups, Selz (1981) cautions against using an abbreviated battery for a neuropsychological evaluation. A full-battery approach is necessary for an adequate assessment of brain functioning for individuals. In the afore-mentioned studies, level of performance was the only method of inference used for comparison. Although this one approach showed differential validity, Boll (1974), Selz (1981), and Reitan (1974) indicate that all 4 methods of inference are essential for clinical diagnosis.

Validity studies with younger children (5- to 8-year range), have also found functional differences between brain-damaged and normal children. In a matched-group design, with 29 children with cerebral damage and 29 normal children, 40 of 41 variables were statistically significant (Selz, 1981). Although in a rank-order comparison, language abilities were most impaired for the brain-damaged group (Reitan, 1974), deficits on motor and sensory–perceptual measures also differentiated the two groups at a 70–80% accuracy rate (Selz, 1981). In summary, language-related deficits were reported for both older children (Boll, 1974; Boll & Reitan, 1970; Reed et al., 1965) and younger children (Reitan, 1974).

Neuropsychological Classification of Brain-Damaged, Learning-Disabled, and Normal Children: A System of Rules

Selz and Reitan (1979) have developed an actuarial system of rules for the neuropsychological diagnosis and classification of children in the 9- to 14-year range. The system incorporates all 4 methods of inference: level of performance, right–left differences, pathognomonic signs, and patterns of performance. Scores from the Halstead–Reitan test battery, the Trail-Making test, the Reitan–Klove Sensory Perceptual exam, the grip strength test, the Aphasia Screening test, and the Wechsler scales were incorporated into the rules for classifying children as normal, learning disabled, and brain damaged.

The rules were derived from an initial pilot sample of 19 children in each group, and a separate sample of 25 children across each group was used for cross-validational purposes. Children were independently as-signed to each group prior to evaluation. See Selz and Reitan (1979) for criteria of how individuals were assigned to the three groups. Raw scores on each measure were converted to scaled scores as follows: (0) scaled score for normal to superior performance; (1) scaled score for slightly below normal performance; (2) scaled score for below normal perfor-mance; and, (3) scaled score for impaired performance. Cut-off scores were selected based on group means and standard deviations for the total sum of the scaled scores, resulting in the following ranges: 0–19 normal, 20–35 learning disabled, and 36+ brain-damaged. An overall classification accuracy rate of 73.3% was obtained using these cut-off ranges. Misclassi-fications were typically *false negatives,* where signs of pathology or performance appeared less impaired than original group membership might have predicted. This was particularly true for the learning disabled (8 misclassified as normal), and the brain-damaged groups (4 misclassified as normal and 4 misclassified as learning disabled). Based on these results, Selz and Reitan (1979) suggested that some of the learning-disabled children were showing academic problems in the classroom for reasons other than abnormal brain functioning; and a portion of the brain-damaged group may have recovered functions sufficiently to perform in the learning-disabled or normal group.

These results are promising, and provide diagnostic guidelines for identifying brain-related disorders. In fact, the classification rate was the highest for differentiating normals from brain-damaged children (87% accurate). Although the prediction rate was less for the learning-disabled group, 68% of these children fell into categories suggesting moderate to severe impairment, suggesting a neuropsychological basis of this disorder. Selz and Reitan (1979) suggest that this system of rules can be used as a clinical aid for screening purposes to assist in meaningful diagnosis. However, other developmental, medical, and academic history is needed to provide information for the diagnosis and remediation of individual cases.

Reitan (1980a) further analyzed these data to identify the specific kinds of deficiencies the three groups demonstrated. Reitan classified tests into measures of higher-level and lower-level brain functioning. See Table 2 for the specific categorizations. Reitan hypothesized that the control group would score within a normal range on both higher and lower-level measures; children with learning disabilities would score within normal limits on lower-level measures and below normal on higher-level measures; and, brain-injured children would score in the impaired range on both measures. Actual performance showed that the control group did well on both higher- and lower-level measures; the learning-disabled group did poorly on the higher-level tasks and performed better on the lower-level measures; and the brain-damaged group showed the same pattern as the learning-disabled group (Reitan, 1980a). From this perspective, the learning-disabled group was more similar to the brain-damaged group than the control group on neuropsychological measures.

In an earlier study, Reitan and Boll (1973) compared the neuropsychological functioning of normal, brain-damaged, and children with minimal brain dysfunction (MBD) aged 5 to 8 years. The entire set of data from the Reitan–Indiana test battery were analyzed using the four methods of inference. Using blind judgements, Reitan and Boll (1973) had an overall hit rate of 84.4% for predicting group membership. In the control group, 64% were correctly classified and 36% were misclassed as mildly im-

TABLE 2

Categorization of tests form the Halstead–Reitan battery

Measures of higher-level brain function	Measures of lower-level brain function
Category	Tactual performance (memory)
Tactual performance (total time)	Tactual performance (localization)
Trails A	Performance IQ
Trails B	Tapping speed (preferred hand)
Speech-sounds	Tapping speed (nonpreferred hand)
Rhythm	Name writing (preferred hand)
Verbal IQ	Tactile finger recognition (difference)
Name writing (difference score)	Finger-tip number writing (difference)
IQ pattern	Imperception
	Tactile finger recognition (errors)
Aphasia Screening Test	Finger-tip number writing (errors)
	Tactile form recognition
Dysnomia	Grip strength (difference)
Spelling dyspraxia	Tapping (difference)
Dysgraphia	Tactual performance (difference)
Dyslexia	
Central dysarthria	Aphasia Screening Test
Dyscalculia	
Right–left confusion	Constructional dyspraxia
Auditory verbal dysgnosia	
Visual number dysgnosia	
Visual letter dysgnosia	
Body dysgnosia	

paired. In the MBD group, 89% were accurately classified, but 11% were judged to have definite abnormal brain functioning. The prediction rate was the highest with the brain-damaged group, with 96% accuracy and only 4% were thought to be mildly impaired. As might be expected, the control group performed the best, the brain-damaged group did the most poorly, and the MBD group fell between the two extreme groups.

In summary, these studies lend support to the validity of the Halstead–Reitan and the Reitan–Indiana Neuropsychological Test Batteries for the diagnosis of brain dysfunction. It should be noted that less experienced neuropsychologists were not able to obtain the same accuracy of classification, based on clinical judgment, that Reitan showed (1980a). However, Reitan suggests that the more objective system of rules should be of help to the less-experienced clinician. Also, it is important to note that these studies demonstrate differences in group not in individual performances.

Although mean scores for brain-injured and control groups differ, individuals within specific groups may or may not fit these group patterns.

Neuropsychological Basis of Achievement with Normal Children

Although the major research thrust in child neuropsychology has focused on children with documented brain damage (Boll & Barth, 1981) or learning disabilities (Gaddes, 1980; Rourke, 1975; Selz & Reitan, 1979), recently there has been an interest in investigating the relationship between neuropsychological functioning and academic achievement in normal children. Townes, Trupin, Martin, and Goldstein (1980) employed a cross-sectional design to determine the neuropsychological basis of early achievement for kindergarten and second-grade students. Ten subtests of the Reitan–Indiana test battery were selected because of their ease of administration and limited time demands, including aphasia screening test, matching pictures test, finger tapping test, progressive figures test, color form test, target test, matching figures test, matching V's test, imperception test, and star–concentric squares test. Townes et al. (1980) found that this abbreviated battery accurately discriminated among high, average, and low readers (75% correct classification) in kindergarten and second grade. This prediction rate was equal to that of WISC scores for the same population.

Variables measuring expressive language abilities, abstract verbal reasoning, and pattern matching were most highly related to early school achievement; while measures of tactile–sensory and motor functioning were less predictive (Townes et al., 1980). Using Reitan's (1980a) classification system, higher-level measures discriminated reading groups better than lower-level measures. Townes et al. (1980) also found sex differences in performance on these tasks and suggested that females have a neurodevelopmental advantage over males on abilities related to early achievement in the first years of schooling.

In a longitudinal study using the same 10 Reitan subtests and the McCarthy Scale of Children's Abilities, Teeter, Jenks, Van Handel, and Zander (1984) also reported that neuropsychological functioning was related to kindergarten and first-grade achievement. The Aphasia Screening Test was the single best neuropsychological predictor variable for the auditory, language, and comprehensive scales of the Metropolitan Readiness Test for kindergarten achievement (Year 1); while the target test was the top predictor for the visual and quantitative scales. Generally, the 10 Reitan subtests were as strong as the McCarthy scales for predicting readiness skills, with the exception of the language scale, where the McCarthy Scales were slightly better. Similar to the Townes et al. (1980)

findings, language-related and abstract reasoning measures were most highly related to kindergarten achievement.

The Aphasia Screening Test, the color form test and the matching pictures test were better than the McCarthy subtests for predicting spelling, reading, and total reading achievement on the Stanford Early Achievement test at the end of first grade. Again, higher-level language and reasoning abilities predicted early achievement over a 2-year period better than did measures of lower-level, sensory-motor skills. Generally, these results indicate that specific predictor variables are relatively stable over a 2-year period, and that the Reitan and the McCarthy subtests have strong psychometric properties.

Implications for Remediation

Reitan (1980b) has developed a rehabilitation program for training children with brain-related disabilities. REHABIT, Reitan Evaluation of Hemispheric Abilities and Brain Improvement Training, materials incorporate neuropsychological principles of the brain–behavior relationshp. The program is organized into three phases (Reitan, 1980b): (1) the evaluation of brain-related deficits using the Halstead–Reitan batteries; (2) the training of deficits using tests from the neuropsychological batteries; and (3) the training of deficits with special REHABIT materials. The first phase is essential, to obtain a comprehensive analysis of the child's functional status and to identify specific deficit areas. For the second phase, Reitan has developed alternate forms for some of the subtests of the Halstead–Reitan batteries for training purposes. The materials for the third phase have been gathered from a variety of training procedures and vary from simple to complex tasks.

Materials (Phase 3) have been organized into five tracts for training general abstraction abilities, which Reitan (1980b) believes are fundamental to overall brain functioning. These tracts are (1) *Tract A,* materials for expressive–receptive language and verbal skills; (2) *Tract B,* materials for abstraction, reasoning, organization, and logical analysis in the verbal–language domain; (3) *Tract C,* materials for general reasoning, abstraction, and organization skills; (4) *Tract D,* materials for abstraction emphasizing visual–spatial, manipulation, and sequential processing; and, (5) *Tract E,* materials for basic visuospatial and manipulation skills. Based on results from the Halstead–Reitan batteries, materials are selected from each tract depending on the type and severity of deficits identified. Reitan (1980b) suggests that training should begin at a level where the individual can be successful, then rehabilitation should proceed to more-complex materials.

Reitan provides a comprehensive list of materials, describes the ability functions necessary for completing the tasks, and indicates the primary brain areas involved. A list of publishers and distributors of these materials is also provided (Reitan, 1980b).

Although there have been no studies to date that empirically test the REHABIT procedures, Reitan (1980b) reports that this program has been used with success for a number of years at the Reitan Neuropsychological Laboratory at the University of Arizona. The procedures and materials available through this program do provide a preliminary step in the much-needed link between assessment and remediation of brain-related disorders. The program also has a strong theoretical basis and has been clinically tested. However, controlled research studies are needed to validate these procedures.

THE LURIA–NEBRASKA NEUROPSYCHOLOGICAL BATTERY FOR CHILDREN

Neuropsychologists have long recognized A. R. Luria's work in clinical neuropsychology, including his theoretical exposes (Golden, Hammeke, & Purisch, 1978). Luria's unique contributions are best exemplified in his theory of the functional units of the brain. It is imperative to have an understanding of this theory as a framework for investigating Luria's neuropsychological assessment techniques.

Luria's theory incorporates aspects of both localization and equipotential theories of brain functioning, and provides an integrative, developmental approach for analyzing the brain–behavior relationship (Wilkening & Golden, 1982). Localization theory evolved as a result of clinical findings that damage to localized cortical regions produced highly specific cognitive deficits. The cerebral cortex was considered to be composed of distinct anatomic structures responsible for complex human behaviors. For example, damage to Wernicke's area in the temporal cortex produced receptive aphasia, while damage to Broca's area in the frontal lobe produced expressive aphasia. Damage to other cortical regions did not result in these types of highly specific deficits. Conversely, because recovery of function often follows brain damage, the theory of equipotentiality postulates that the brain is composed of undifferentiated neuronal tissue and that brain areas are equipotential in terms of mediating specific behaviors (Golden & Wilkening, 1986). Supporters of this theory suggest that all brain regions contribute equally in the execution of complex tasks. According to equipotential theory, the severity and extent of brain damage is determined by the amount of tissue destroyed and not the specific site injured.

These two competing theories do not sufficiently account for many behaviors observed in some patients with brain damage. For example, the localization theory is unable to explain the fact that damage to specific brain areas do not always result in the types of deficits that might be expected (Golden & Wilkening, 1986). Also, some patients display specific deficits even when the associated cortical region is intact. Golden and Wilkening (1986) also indicate that the equipotential theory has similar problems explaining the behavioral sequelae of some patients following brain injury. For example, sometimes damage to very small areas of the brain produce more serious behavioral deficits than do lesions involving larger portions of the cortex.

Luria's Functional Systems of the Brain

Luria attempted to integrate the localization and equipotential theories and to provide a theory of brain functioning that could account for the inconsistencies of these two theoretical approaches (Golden & Wilkening, 1986). In *Higher Cortical Functions in Man,* Luria (1980) provided an extensive theory of functional systems as an alternative paradigm. Fundamental to Luria's theory is the supposition that the brain comprises highly specialized cortical regions that are connected to other cortical and subcortical areas, producing complex functional systems (Luria, 1980). Luria does not believe that specific areas of the brain are responsible for certain behaviors, such as reading or writing, but rather these specialized areas interact with other specialized areas to mediate complex behaviors. Golden and Wilkening (1986) conclude that brain tissue is physiologically and behaviorally specialized (consistent with localization theory), and these areas interact with large portions of the brain to produce behaviors (consistent with equipotential theory).

Specific behavioral deficits can result from a variety of different lesions. Luria (1980, p. 71) states that "higher mental functions may be disturbed by a lesion of one of the many different links of the functional systems; nevertheless, they will be disturbed differently by lesions of different links." Consequently, damage to a link in a functional system might result in a collapse of that system, or it may become reorganized with another functional system so that the behavior may be performed by a new chain (Luria, 1980). Luria's neuropsychological assessment techniques were designed to evaluate these functional systems and to assess the integrity of separate links. Behaviors are tested in a variety of ways by changing input and output demands, thereby altering the links that are operating at any point in time.

Luria (1973) postulated that the brain was divided into three functional units: (1) the arousal unit; (2) the sensory receptive and integrative unit; and (3) the planning and organizational unit. See Golden (1981) and Golden and Wilkening (1986) for an in-depth discussion of the functional systems.

Development of the Standardized Luria-Nebraska Battery for Children—Revised

Luria developed a variety of tasks that assess the functional units of the brain. Luria's original procedures were not standardized, and varied across patients depending on the type of dysfunction present. Consequently, it was difficult to replicate Luria's assessment methods and to learn his techniques. Anne-Lise Christensen first attempted to compile and organize Luria's methods into a test battery (Christensen, 1975). Golden and his associates further refined Luria's techniques into a standardized test battery for adolescents and adults (Golden, Hammeke, & Purisch, 1980), and later developed a standardized battery for children. Initially, the adult Luria–Nebraska was administered to children with average to above-average intelligence (Wilkening, Golden, MacInnes, Plaisted, & Hermann, 1981). Difficult items were eliminated, instructions were revised, and new items were developed for children between the ages of 8 to 12 years. The child's battery went through four separate revisions prior to its final format (Plaisted, Gustavson, Wilkening, & Golden, 1983).

The Luria–Nebraska Neuropsychological Battery–Children's Revision (Children's LNNB) presently comprises 149 items. The administration time is approximately $2\frac{1}{2}$ hours, which is considerably less than the administration time for the Reitan battery. Test items were selected that identify and localize brain dysfunction, including motor functions; acousticomotor organization; tactile functions; visual functions; receptive and expressive speech abilities; writing, reading, and arithmetic skills; memory functions; and intellectual processes.

Description of the Battery

The 11 scales of the Luria–Nebraska Neuropsychological Battery for Children are described as follows (Golden, 1981; Plaisted et al., 1983).

Motor Skills. There are 34 activities on this scale, requiring the child to carry out simple and complex hand movements; execute oral movements with the tongue and cheeks; reproduce a circle, a square, and a triangle; and perform simple actions that are regulated by the examiners' directions. The child's speed, coordination, imitation, and construction abilities on motor tasks are assessed on this scale.

Acoustico-Motor Organization (Rhythm). The eight items on this scale require the perception of tones, reproduction of melodies, evaluation of auditory stimuli, and motoric reproduction of rhythms. The items on this scale measure the child's auditory perception, discrimination, and reproduction of sounds and rhythmic patterns.

Higher Cutaneous and Kinesthetic Functions (Tactile). This section comprises 16 items where the child is required to identify, discriminate, and localize simple and complex tactile information. Both right- and left-side competencies are assessed.

Visual Functions. On this scale, there are seven items measuring visual perception, where the child is required to identify common pictures and objects; specify similarities and differences between stimuli; and memorize and reproduce stimuli. The stimuli presented range from simple to complex, with varied spatial components and three-dimensional qualities.

Receptive Speech. Receptive speech abilities are assessed on 18 items, evaluating the child's discrimination of phonemes, identification of words, and comprehension of words, sentences, and complex grammatical structures. This scale also measures the child's ability to follow simple commands and verbal instructions with visual cues.

Expressive Speech. On this 21-item scale, the child is asked to repeat and to read letters, sounds, series of words, and sentences. Automatic speech, description of pictures, identifying objects from descriptions, and short speech making are also measured by this scale.

Writing. On the seven items in this scale, the child must copy and write letters, graphemes, words, and phrases from dictation. Performance on these tasks measure the child's ability to write, spell, copy, and analyze letter sequences.

Reading. Seven reading items have been incorporated into this scale. On these tasks, the child is instructed to read letters, words, phrases, sentences, and complete passages.

Arithmetic. There are nine items designed to assess arithmetic skills, including: number recognition, comprehension of number values, and simple computation in addition, subtraction, and multiplication.

Memory. Memory competencies are assessed on a variety of verbal and nonverbal tasks. The child is asked to repeat a series of words that are unrelated, recall pictures exposed on a card, remember three positions that the examiner demonstrates with his or her hand, remember a list of words with and without interference, and recall words with visual cues. There are eight items on the scale.

Intellectual Process. Many of the items on this scale resemble those on the WISC-R, especially the picture arrangement, picture completion, vocabulary, comprehension, arithmetic, and similarities subtests. The 15 items measuring intellectual processes require the child to place cards in a sequence that makes sense, describe what is happening in a picture, identify what is foolish about a picture, analyze a story that has been read, define words, indicate ways in which things are similar and different, find logical relationships between concepts, and figure basic arithmetic problems.

Additional Clinical Summary Scales

Three additional clinical summary scales have been developed for the Children's LNNB which provide further information concerning the functional status of the brain: (1) the Pathognomonic, (2) the Left Sensory–Motor, and (3) the Right Sensory–Motor scales (Sawicki, Leark, Golden, & Karras, 1984). The items that make up these scales were statistically derived and provide for maximum differentiation of brain-injured from normal children. See Table 3 for the specific items of the Children's LNNB that constitute the Pathognomonic, Left Sensory–Motor, and Right Sensory–Motor Scales.

Scoring Procedures

The scoring procedures for the Children's LNNB are based on a three-point scale: (0) representing normal performance; (1) representing performance between 1 and 2 standard deviations below the mean; and, (2) representing performance more than 2 standard deviations below the mean (Gustavson, Golden, Wilkening, Hermann, Plaisted, & MacInnes, 1981). Separate age norms were necessary for some test items. These age norms were derived from a sample of 125 normal children, 25 subjects in each age range from 8 to 12 years. Raw scores were then converted to *t*-scores for each of the 11 scales.

Data Interpretation

Test data from the Children's LNNB-Revised are interpreted from a quantitative–normative and a qualitative perspective. Normative interpretation is accomplished by examining *t*-score distributions across the 11 scales. This allows the examiner to determine the relative strengths and

TABLE 3

Description of scale items from the LNNB-C for the pathognomonic, left sensory–motor, and right sensory–motor scales

Pathognomonic scale		Left sensory–motor scale		Right sensory–motor scale	
Item no.	Description	Item no.	Description	Item no.	Description
2	Touch fingers sequentially (left hand)	1	Touch fingers sequentially (right hand)	2	Touch fingers sequentially (left hand)
3	Touch fingers sequentially (both hands)	4	Repeat finger position (right hand)	5	Repeat finger position (left hand)
17	Tap rhythm	43	Touch localization (errors on right)	43	Touch localization (errors on left)
35	Compare auditory tones	45	Tactile discrimination (errors on right)	46	Tactile discrimination (errors on left)
65	Rotate squares	47	Tactile discrimination (errors on right)	48	Tactile discrimination (errors on left)
79	Spoken directions	49	2-Point discrimination (right hand)	50	2-Point discrimination (left hand)
118	Paragraph reading	51	Directional sensation (errors on right)	52	Directional sensation (errors on left)
127	Count backwards	53	Graphesthetic sensation (right)	54	Graphesthetic sensation (left)
128	Learn 7 words (5 trials)	57	Stereognostic sensation (errors on right)	57	Stereognostic sensation (errors on left)
131	Memorize words				
146	Part–whole comprehension				
149	Math problem				

weaknesses on individual profiles for the different ability areas measured. Although the quantitative method of interpretation is helpful for identifying deficit areas, a qualitative method of interpretation is necessary to develop a clinical picture of the functional systems involved. Also, the 11 scales are not homogeneous in composition, so while the motor scale contains items tapping primary and secondary frontal regions, they are not all pure motor measures. For example, some items involve tasks measuring frontal–temporal regions (e.g., "If I say 'red' squeeze my hand, if I say 'green,' do nothing"), or tasks measuring frontal–parietal regions (e.g., "With your eyes closed, put your other hand the same way I put this one"—left thumb and middle finger pressed together). Therefore an elevated t-score on the motor scale can be a result of a number of different types of deficits in the frontal cortex and/or associated brain regions. Qualitative item analysis is used to isolate damaged links in each of the functional systems.

There are also some instances when t-scores may not be significantly elevated on a scale, but neuropathology may still be present. That is, a patient may answer most of the questions correctly but may have difficulty on a few select items (Golden et al., 1980). Item analysis becomes particularly important in these cases for identifying specific disabilities that are relevant for accurate diagnosis and treatment.

The qualitative method of interpretation for diagnosing brain pathology requires a highly skilled clinician. Anne-Lise Christensen (1975) and Golden et al. (1980) provide extensive descriptions of the brain regions operating in each task for adults and adolescents. However, there is a lack of specific information for children for item-by-item interpretation.

Validity Studies with the Children's LNNB: Differentiating Brain-Damaged from Normal Children

There are a number of studies available supporting the validity of the Children's LNNB for determining normal and abnormal brain functioning. Wilkening et al. (1981) reported the first validity study with this instrument, where the performance of 76 brain-damaged children was compared to the original normative group ($N = 125$). All subjects in the brain-damaged group were independently diagnosed from neurological evaluations, neurosurgical reports, abnormal EEG findings, or abnormal CT scans (Wilkening et al., 1981). Children with minimal brain dysfunction or learning disabilities were excluded from this study. The normative sample comprised 125 children, with 25 children across the five age ranges from 8 to 12 years. Children in this group were free from developmental anomalies, academic problems, and neurological signs. Also, children with a history of head trauma resulting in a loss of consciousness were not included. Results from multivariate analysis of variance (MANOVAs) and univariate t-tests revealed that the brain-damaged and normal children differed significantly on all 11 scales of the LNNB (Wilkening et al., 1981).

Further discriminant function analysis resulted in a 91.3% classification accuracy for the normal group, and a 65.3% rate for the brain-damaged group, with an 81.6% overall hit rate. In an effort to provide quantifiable criteria for differentiating brain-damaged from normal subjects, Wilkening et al. (1981) established a method for deriving critical cut-off scores. Age and education were entered into a multiple regression formula to predict average t-scores for the 11 scales in the normal group. Age in months was significantly related to performance and weighed heavily in the formula for predicting average t-scores. In order to reduce the number of false positives, 17 points (1.7 standard deviation) were added to the baseline in the critical level formula (Wilkening et al., 1981). The critical cut-off formula was derived as: $82.02 - (.14 \times$ age in months$) =$ average t-score.

When classification as brain-damaged was defined as more than one scale above the critical level, 80% of the normal group and 69.7% of the brain-damaged children were accurately classified, with an overall accuracy rate of 76.2% (Wilkening et al., 1981). Although these percentages are similar to the classification rates for differentiating normals from brain-damaged with the system of rules presented by Selz and Reitan (1979), a direct comparison of these percentages would be misleading because Selz and Reitan employed three different groups (brain-damaged, learning disabled, and normals). It would be difficult to determine the hit rate of the Selz and Reitan study if only two groups had been used. That is, if subjects could only be classified as either brain-damaged or normal, the accuracy rates may have changed when the middle group (learning disabled) was eliminated as an alternative. Further research comparing the LNNB and the Halstead–Reitan tests is needed to determine which battery best differentiates these three groups.

Gustavson et al. (1981) performed a cross-validation of the Wilkening et al. (1981) findings. Gustavson et al. (1981) evaluated a new sample with 91 normals and 58 brain-damaged children. The same criteria for selecting children in each group was used. Again, the brain-damaged and normal groups differed significantly on all 11 scales when MANOVAs and t-tests were conducted. Discriminant function analyses resulted in slightly higher prediction rates than the Wilkening et al. (1981) study. Critical cut-off scores were also employed and yielded a 90% accuracy rate for normals, an 80% rate for the brain-damaged group, with an 85% overall prediction accuracy (Gustavson et al., 1981). Again, these prediction rates were better than those reported by Wilkening et al. (1981). These two studies show that brain-damaged children do perform more poorly on the LNNB than do normals; and, that critical cut-off scores can be helpful for determining abnormal brain functioning. However, both studies caution that individual diagnosis can not be accurately made without a qualitative analysis of performance on the LNNB.

Sawicki et al. (1984) used a discriminant function analysis, including the three additional clinical summary scales, and they found that the pathognomonic scale was the most sensitive measure for predicting membership for two separate clinical groups. Group 1 comprised 125 normals and 76 brain-impaired, and Group 2 comprised 91 normals and 58 brain-impaired children. The overall classification rates were higher than those reported by Wilkening et al. (1981) and by Gustavson et al. (1981). When the 3 clinical summary scales were added to the original 11 scales, the following hit rates were reported: Group 1, 96.7% for normals and 80.9%

for brain-injured; and, Group 2, 95.6% for normals and 79.3% for brain-injured (Sawicki et al., 1984). Sawicki et al. (1984) conclude that diagnostic decisions can be made on the basis of (1) the number of scales above the critical level; (2) an elevated pathognomonic scale (greater than the critical level); (3) qualitative analysis of error patterns; and (4) developmental history with information about medical, social and emotional factors affecting the child.

Gustavson, Golden, Leark, Wilkening, Hermann, and Plaisted (1982) combined data from two validity studies, with 201 children from the Wilkening et al. (1981) investigation and 149 subjects from the Gustavson et al. (1981) project. In the third study, LNNB data were correlated with the WISC-R and the WRAT. High positive correlations were reported for the LNNB and the full scale intelligence quotient (FSIQ) at .86, the verbal intelligence quotient (VIQ) at .83, and the performance intelligence quotient (PIQ) at .83. Correlations with the WRAT and the LNNB were also high: WRAT reading and LNNB .87; WRAT spelling and LNNB .81; and, WRAT arithmetic and LNNB .73.

When the FS IQ was used as a covariate, univariate F tests showed that the brain-damaged and normal children still differed in performance on the rhythm, visual, receptive language, arithmetic, and memory scales of the LNNB. When all three IQ measures were used as covariates, the two groups showed performance differences on the motor, expressive language, and writing scales, in addition to the 5 scales reported with the FSIQ. When the effects of IQ scores were eliminated, the intelligence, tactile and reading scales of the LNNB no longer discriminated between the two groups. While performance on some scales of the LNNB is affected by intelligence abilities, 8 of the 11 scales were not.

When WRAT standard scores were used as covariates, performance on the rhythm, tactile, visual, receptive language, expressive language, arithmetic, memory, and intelligence scales significantly discriminated the brain-damaged and the normal groups. It is reasonable to conclude from these data that while the LNNB is measuring abilities related to IQ and achievement, it is also assessing neuropsychological skills that are distinct from intelligence and achievement (Plaisted et al., 1983).

Carr, Sweet, Rossini, and Angara (1983) tested the ability of the LNNB to discriminate among a group of normals ($N = 32$), psychiatrics ($N = 32$), and neurologically impaired children ($N = 32$). Main effects were reported for diagnostic groups, intelligence, and sex using MANOVA methods. In this study, the neurologically impaired children had the worst performance on the LNNB and the normal children had the best performance. However, when IQ was covaried, the effects of diagnostic groups dropped out. Although the LNNB scales were derived from age norms, the effect of age was still present as the younger children scored lower than the older children. While differences in sex were present using MANOVA, univariate analysis did not show significant differences for males and females on the 11 scales.

Carr et al. (1983) also used a discriminant function analysis to determine which scales best predicted diagnostic group membership. Six scales were identified: motor, rhythm, visual, expressive language, reading, and arithmetic. Classification accuracy was reported to be 84% for the psychiatric group and 78% for the neurologic group, with an overall prediction of 81%.

Clearly, these studies indicate that the LNNB is a valid instrument for differentiating brain-damaged from normal and psychiatric children. Although Plaisted et al. (1983) indicate that the LNNB is a useful neuropsychological battery for children, further research is needed. This is particularly relevant for better understanding the neuropsychological status of children with focalized cortical lesions, and for determining the effects of brain damage at different developmental stages (Plaisted et al., 1983).

Research with Learning-Disabled Children

There have been a number of studies to date investigating the diagnostic utility of the LNNB with learning-disabled (LD) children. Geary, Jennings, and Schultz (1984) tested 15 LD and 15 normal children between the ages of 9 and 12 years. The LD children demonstrated at least average intelligence (above 80 on the WISC-R), and had a 2-year discrepancy between grade placement and academic achievement. All of the LD children were selected from special classes for learning disabilities. Overall classification accuracy for the LNNB was 86.7% for the two groups. The LD and normal groups differed in performance on 10 of the 11 LNNB scales. Correlations ranged from a .30 for the motor scale and WISC-R, to a .70 for the writing scale and WISC-R. While all 15 subjects in the LD group were accurately classified, 3 subjects in the normal group were misclassified as LD based on LNNB scores. While the authors concluded that the LNNB can be useful for identifying LD children, the percentages of false positives indicates that other criteria must be considered for the most accurate diagnosis of children without brain-related disabilities. Plaisted et al. (1983) also suggested that these results be viewed as tentative because the sample size was small.

Nolan, Hammeke, and Barkley (1983) investigated children with specific types of learning disabilities. Three groups were compared: (1) a control group, (2) a reading-spelling LD group, and (3) an arithmetic LD group. The expressive speech, writing, and reading scales of the LNNB were significantly elevated for the reading–spelling LD group when compared to those scores for the other groups. However, scales on the LNNB did not discriminate the arithmetic LD group from the control and the reading–spelling LD group. Nolan et al. (1983) indicate that further research with the arithmetic LD group would be helpful for identifying the neuropsychological correlates of this disability.

In an effort to determine the effectiveness of the LNNB for differentiating mildly and severely learning disabled children, Snow, Hynd, and Hartlage (1984) selected 20 subjects from a resource LD program (mild LD) and 20 subjects from a self-contained LD program (severe LD). The severe LD group showed poorer performance than the mild LD group on the receptive language, writing, reading, and arithmetic scales. Performance differences between the two groups were most pronounced on the achievement-oriented scales. Snow et al. (1984) also used the critical cutoff formula for determining abnormal brain functioning on the LNNB. In this sample, 39 of the 40 LD subjects had 2 or more t-scores above the critical level suggesting abnormal brain functioning. Snow et al. (1984) concluded that the critical cut-off criteria indicating brain pathology may result in too many false positives, and that the formula criteria may not be appropriate for LD students. Snow and Hynd (in press) also conducted a multivariate study to determine the factor structure of the LNNB with LD students. Three factors emerged and were labeled: language–general intelligence factor; academic-achievement factor; and, sensory–motor integration factor.

Teeter, Uphoff, Obrzut, and Malsch (1984) conducted a study with 15 LD and 15 normal children. Federal and state guidelines were used for classifying children as learning disabled. The results of this study showed that the LD children performed more poorly than the normal children on all scales of the LNNB except the visual scale. T-scores for the LD group were particularly elevated (above 70) on the following scales: receptive, language, expressive language, writing, reading, and arithmetic. Apparently deficits in the verbal–language domain severely impaired the acquisition of normal achievement for this group. The critical level approach was used to determine the effectiveness of this method for differentiating LD children from children with normal academic functioning. When 2 or more scales above the critical level were used as criteria for determining abnormal, a 95% overall accuracy rate was obtained. Twenty-eight out of 30 children were accurately classified. While these results are impressive, one must consider how the critical level approach can be used for differentiating LD from brain-impaired children. The criteria of 2 scales above the critical level, suggested by Gustavson et al. (1981), discriminates normal from brain damaged children and normal from LD children. However, this criteria will not differentiate the performance of LD from brain-impaired children. These results confirm those reported by Geary et al. (1984) and Snow et al. (1984).

Finally, the addition of the three clinical summary scales provided further information for differentiating LD from normals. The pathognomonic scale was significantly elevated for 78% of the LD group, while none of the normal children showed elevated scores. Also, 39% of the LD group showed elevated scores on the left sensory–motor scales, indicative of lower-level neuropsychological deficits in the left hemisphere. Other left-hemisphere signs were also found on scales measuring higher-level abilities (i.e., receptive and expressive language, writing, reading and arithmetic). The right sensory–motor scale was elevated for 22% of the LD group and 13% of the normal group. Again, the number of false positives may be a problem with the clinical summary scales, and their addition may not help to differentiate the performance of LD and brain-injured children.

Initial research indicates that the LNNB is useful for discriminating brain-damaged from normal groups, and LD from normal children. However, these results must be considered as preliminary. Further research is necessary to determine the diagnostic validity of this instrument for differentiating brain-damaged from LD children. Information is also needed to determine how children with highly localized or lateralized brain damage differ on the 11 scales.

Implications for Remediation

At the present time, Luria's theory of brain functioning has not been incorporated into a structured rehabilitation program for children. However, Luria's system of functional units and the developmental nature of these systems provide a strong theoretical basis on which predictions can be made concerning the outcome of an injury and the potential for rehabilitation (Golden & Wilkening, 1986). However, Golden and Wilkening (1986) are conservative in their claims about specific outcome predictions. They further indicate that hypotheses must be tested prior to developing a clear understanding of brain functioning. More empirical data is needed to either confirm or refute Luria's principles of brain functioning in the areas of diagnosis and remediation.

Luria (1963) has provided an extensive theory supported by clinical findings in his book, entitled *Restoration of Function after Brain Injury*. In this treatise, Luria describes conditions of brain injury that result in either reversible or irreversible loss of functions. Luria's (1963) treatment of spontaneous restoration of temporally inhibited functions, provides clinical evidence supporting Isaacson's (1976) discussion on transitory reactions in the cortex following brain injury. Luria indicates that, initially reversible and irreversible deficits appear outwardly identical. In the case of reversible loss of function, where cortical tissue is intact, changes in behavior due to metabolic disturbances have been reversed with appropriate drug treatment. In reversible cases where drugs were not effective, Luria (1963) describes another method of restoring functions by altering a patient's mental orientation to reduce the psychological reactions that impede recovery following injury.

In situations where loss of function is due to destruction of specific cells or pathways, recovery of function is quite different than situations where loss of function is a result of psychogenic or metabolic disturbances (Luria, 1963). Recovery of function is also different depending on the site of injury (at primary, secondary, or association areas of the cortex). When injury is sustained to primary areas of the parietal, temporal, occipital, or frontal regions, the reorganization of functional systems typically takes place automatically and quickly, and the patient is often not aware of the recovery of function (Luria, 1963). For example, loss of part of the visual field can be compensated for by using the remaining intact field. However deficits resulting from lesions to secondary areas can be overcome "either by internal reorganization of its preserved elements or by the replacement of the lost cerebral link by another which is still intact" (Luria, 1963, p. 55). Special training aimed at conceptual reorganization is necessary when damage occurs at secondary cortical regions. This is usually accomplished by pairing an intact functional system with the impaired system to achieve reorganization.

Luria (1963) presented a case study of a patient with damage to the secondary left temporal cortex, affecting the auditory analyzer. The subject was unable to differentiate simple sounds, such as /s/ and /z/. Although the patient was unable to distinguish sounds in isolation, with training he was able to learn to classify sounds into groups (/t/ is the same for "tone" and "tots"). Finally, the patient learned to recognize the sound /s/ was the same as in "seal," and /z/ was the same as in "zeal" (Luria, 1963). In this patient, the intact visual system was paired with the dysfunctional auditory system to achieve some restoration of function.

At this time, Luria's work can only be used as a theoretical basis for designing remedial programs. However, by using a viable theory of brain functioning, the clinician can avoid trial-and-error or hit-or-miss approaches to the remediation of brain-related deficits. There is no doubt that controlled research of the diagnosis–remediation link is needed before treatment based on neuropsychological theories can be fully accepted and their clinical usefulness can be ascertained.

CONCLUSIONS

In this chapter, two major standardized neuropsychological test batteries for children were reviewed. Current studies with these batteries were also presented to provide initial support of these instruments as clinical and research tools. However, there are a number of issues that are relevant to clinical child neuropsychology which should be mentioned. First, pediatric neuropsychology is a relatively new field (Wilkening & Golden, 1982). There is still much to learn about brain development in normal children, and the effects of damage to the developing nervous system. Second, more research is needed with highly controlled and adequately described populations. Typically, children identified as brain-damaged show a variety of disorders and pathologies. When groups are heterogeneous, important behavioral differences may be masked. More homogeneous samples need to be studied where children are matched on relevant variables such as type, severity, and age of onset of injury. Third, research comparing the Reitan batteries and the Children's LNNB is needed to determine how these assessment procedures are related. And fourth, research in the remediation area is needed to determine the validity of present theories of brain functioning in children.

Although these issues suggest that some conclusions are tentative, this does not detract from the knowledge generated from the growing body of literature in child neuropsychology. The neurosciences as a whole have made enormous advances since the early 1980s, and much of what was once believed about the human brain has either been abandoned or modified. Recent improvements in medical technology have also expanded the methods available for measuring brain functions. Research linking these more direct measures of cortical activity with neuropsychological assessment findings will undoubtedly have a significant impact on our understanding of child neuropsychology.

REFERENCES

Alajouanine, T., & Lhermitte, F. (1965). Acquired aphasia in children. *Brain, 88,* 653–662.
Basser, L. (1962). Hemiplegia of early onset and the faculty of speech with reference to the effects of hemispherectomy. *Brain, 85,* 427–460.
Boll, T. J. (1974). Behavioral correlates of cerebral damage in children aged 9–14. In R. M. Reitan & L. Davison (Eds.), *Clinical neuropsychology: Current status and application.* Washington, DC: Hemisphere.
Boll, T. J. (1981). The Halstead–Reitan neuropsychological battery. In S. Filskov & T. Boll (Eds.), *Handbook of clinical neuropsychology.* New York: Wiley (Interscience).
Boll, T. J., & Barth, J. T. (1981). Neuropsychology of brain damage in children. In S. Filskov & T. J. Boll (Eds.), *Handbook of clinical neuropsychology.* New York: Wiley (Interscience).
Boll, T. J., & Reitan, R. M. (1970, May). *Motor and sensory-perceptual deficits in brain-*

damaged children. Paper presented at the meeting of the Midwestern Psychological Association.

Carr, M. A., Sweet, J. J., Rossini, E., & Angara, V. K. (1983, August). *Diagnostic accuracy of the Luria–Nebraska Neuropsychological Battery—Children's Revision.* Paper presented at the meeting of the American Psychological Association, Anaheim, CA.

Christensen, A. L. (1975). *Luria's neuropsychological investigation.* New York: Spectrum.

Clements, S. D. (1966). *Minimal brain dysfunction in children* (NINDS Monograph No. 3, U.S. Public Health Service Publication No. 1415). Washington, DC: U.S. Government Printing Office.

Cruickshank, N. M., & Hallahan, D. P. (Eds.). (1975). *Perceptual and learning disabilities in children* (Vol. 1). Syracuse, NY: Syracuse University Press.

Gaddes, W. H. (1980). *Learning disabilities and brain function: A neuropsychological approach.* New York: Springer-Verlag.

Geary, D. C., Jennings, S. M., & Schultz, D. D. (1984). *The diagnostic accuracy of the Luria–Nebraska Children's Battery for 9–12 year-old learning disabled children. School Psychology Review, 13*(3), 375–380.

Golden, C. J. (1981). The Luria–Nebraska children's battery: Theory and formulation. In G. W. Hynd & J. E. Obrzut (Eds.), *Neuropsychological assessment and the school-age child: Issues and procedures.* New York: Grune & Stratton.

Golden, C. J., Hammeke, T. A., & Purisch, A. D. (1978). Diagnostic validity of a standardized neuropsychological battery derived from Luria's neuropsychological tests. *Journal of Consulting and Clinical Psychology, 46,* 1258–1265.

Golden, C. J., Hammeke, T. A., & Purisch, A. D. (1980). *The Luria–Nebraska neuropsychological battery: Manual.* Los Angeles: Western Psychological Services.

Golden, C. J., & Wilkening, G. N. (1986). Neuropsychological basis of exceptionality. In R. Brown & C. Reynolds (Eds.), *Psychological perspectives on childhood exceptionality.* New York: Wiley (Interscience).

Gustavson, J. L., Golden, C. J., Leark, R. A., Wilkening, G. N., Hermann, B. D., & Plaisted, L. R. (1982). *The Luria–Nebraska Neuropsychological Battery—Children's Revision: Current research findings.* Paper presented at the meeting of American Psychological Association, Washington, DC.

Gustavson, J. L., Golden, C. J., Wilkening, G. N., Hermann, B. P., Plaisted, J. R., & MacInnes, W. D. (1981, August). *The Luria–Nebraska Neuropsychological Battery—Children's Revision: Validation with brain-damaged and normal children.* Paper presented at the meeting of the American Psychological Association, Los Angeles.

Hammill, D. D., Leigh, J. E., McNutt, G., & Larsen, S. C. (1981). A new definition of learning disabilities. *Learning Disability Quarterly, 4,* 336–342.

Hartlage, L. C., & Hartlage, P. L. (1977). Application of neuropsychological principles in the diagnosis of learning disabilities. In L. Tarnopol & M. Tarnopol (Eds.), *Brain function and reading disabilities.* Baltimore: University Park Press.

Hecaen, H. (1976). Acquired aphasia in children and the ontogenesis of hemisperic functional specialization. *Brain and Language, 3,* 114–134.

Hynd, G. W., & Obrzut, J. E. (1981). School neuropsychology. *Journal of School Psychology, 19,* 45–50.

Isaacson, R. L. (1976). Recovery "?" from early brain damage. In T. D. Tjossem (Ed.), *Intervention strategies for high risk infants and young children.* Baltimore: University Park Press.

Kaufman, A. S. (1979). *Intelligent testing with the WISC–R*. New York: Wiley (Interscience).

Knights, R. M. (1966). *Normative data on tests for evaluating brain damage in children from 5 to 14 years of age* (Research Bulletin No. 20). London: University of Western Ontario.

Kolb, B., & Whishaw, I. Q. (1980). *Fundamentals of human neuropsychology*. San Francisco: Freeman.

Lenneberg, E. H. (1967). A biological perspective of language. In E. H. Lenneberg (Ed.), *New directions in the study of language*. Cambridge, MA: MIT Press.

Luria, A. R. (1963). *Restoration of function after brain injury*. New York: Macmillan.

Luria, A. R. (1966). *Higher cortical functions in man*. New York: Basic Books.

Luria, A. R. (1973). *The working brain*. New York: Basic Books.

Luria, A. R. (1980). *Higher cortical functions in man* (2nd ed.). New York: Basic Books.

Milner, B. (1975). Psychological aspects of focal epilepsy and its neurological management. *Advances in Neurology, 8,* 299–321.

Myklebust, H. (1968). Learning disabilities: Definition and overview. *Progress in learning disabilities* (Vol. 1). New York: Grune & Stratton.

Nolan, D. R., Hammeke, T. A., & Barkley, R. A. (1983). A comparison of the neuropsychological performance in two groups of learning disabled children. *Journal of Clinical Child Psychology 12*(1), 13–21.

Plaisted, J. R., Gustavson, J. L., Wilkening, G. N., & Golden, C. J. (1983). The Luria–Nebraska Neuropsychological Battery—Children's Revision: Theory and current research findings. *Journal of Clinical Child Psychology, 12,* 13–21.

Reed, H. B., Reitan, R. M., & Klove, H. (1965). Influence of cerebral lesions on psychological test performances of older children. *Journal of Consulting Psychology, 29,* 247–251.

Reitan, R. M. (1969). *Manual for administration of neuropsychological test batteries for adults and children*. Indianapolis, IN: Author.

Reitan, R. M. (1974). Psychological effects of cerebral lesions in children of early school age. In R. M. Reitan & G. A. Davison (Eds.), *Clinical neuropsychology: Current status and application*. Washington, DC: Hemisphere.

Reitan, R. M. (1980a). *Manual for studying the neuropsychological bases of learning disability*. Tucson: Reitan Neuropsychology Laboratory and the University of Arizona.

Reitan, R. M. (1980b). *REHABIT—Reitan evaluation of hemispheric abilities and brain improvement training*. Tucson: Reitan Neuropsychology Laboratory and University of Arizona.

Reitan, R. M. (1981a, July). *Effects of age-of-onset of brain damage on later development*. Presented at the Reitan Neuropsychological Workshop, Chicago.

Reitan, R. M. (1981b). *Neuropsychological methods of inferring brain damage in adults and children*. Unpublished manuscript, University of Washington, Seattle.

Reitan, R. M., & Boll, T. J. (1973). Neuropsychological correlates of minimal brain dysfunction. *Annals of the New York Academy of Sciences, 203,* 65–88.

Reitan, R. M., & Davison, L. A. (Eds.). (1974). *Clinical neuropsychology: Current status and applications*. Washington, DC: V. H. Winston & Sons.

Rourke, B. P. (1975). Brain–behavior relationships in children with learning disabilities: A research program. *American Psychologist, 30,* 911–920.

Rourke, B. P. (1981). Neuropsychological assessment of children with learning disabilities. In S. B. Filskov & T. J. Boll (Eds.), *Handbook of clinical neuropsychology*. New York: Wiley (Interscience).

Rourke, B. P., Bakker, D. J., Fisk, J. L., & Strang, J. D. (1983). *Child neuropsychology: An introduction to theory, research, and clinical practice*. New York: Guilford Press.

Sawicki, R. F., Leark, R., Golden, C. J., & Karras, D. (1984). The development of the pathognomonic, left sensori-motor and right sensori-motor scales of the Luria Nebraska Neuropsychological Battery—Children's Revision. *Journal of Clinical Child Psychology, 13,* 165–196.

Selz, M. (1981). Halstead–Reitan neuropsychological test batteries for children. In G. W. Hynd & J. E. Obrzut (Eds.), *Neuropsychological assessment and the school-age child: Issues and procedures*. New York: Grune & Stratton.

Selz, M., & Reitan, R. M. (1979). Rules for neuropsychological diagnosis: Classification of brain function in older children. *Journal of Consulting and Clinical Psychology, 47,* 258–264.

Snow, J. H., & Hynd, G. W. (in press). Factor structure of the Luria–Nebraska Neuropsychology Battery—Children's Revision with learning disabled children. *Journal of School Psychology*.

Snow, J. H., Hynd, G. W., & Hartlage, L. C. (1984). Differences between mildly and more severely learning disabled children on the Luria–Nebraska Neuropsychological Battery—Children's Revision. *Journal of Psychoeducational Assessment, 2,* 23–28.

Spreen, O., & Gaddes, W. H. (1969). Developmental norms for 15 neuropsychological tests age 6 to 15. *Cortex, 5,* 171–191.

Strauss, A., & Lehtinen, L. (1947). *Psychopathology and education of the brain injured child*. New York: Grune & Stratton.

Tarnopol, L., & Tarnopol, M. (1977). *Brain function and reading disabilities*. Baltimore: University Park Press.

Teeter, P. A., Jenks, G., Van Handel, K., & Zander, E. (1984, April). *The neuropsychological basis of academic achievement: Years 1 and 2 of a longitudinal study*. Paper presented at the meeting of the National Association of School Psychologists, Philadelphia.

Teeter, P. A., Uphoff, C., Obrzut, J., & Malsch, K. (1984). *Diagnostic utility of the critical level formula and clinical summary scales of the Luria–Nebraska Neuropsychological Battery—Children's Revision with learning disabled children*. Unpublished manuscript.

Townes, B. D., Turpin, E. W., Martin, D. C., & Goldstein, D. (1980). Neuropsychological correlates of academic success among elementary school children. *Journal of Consulting and Clinical Psychology, 6,* 675–684.

Wheeler, L., & Reitan, R. M. (1962). The presence and laterality of brain damage predicted from responses to a short aphasia screening test. *Perceptual and Motor Skills, 15,* 783–799.

Wilkening, G. N., & Golden, C. J. (1982). Pediatric neuropsychology: Status, research and theory. In P. Karoly, J. J. Steffen, & D. J. O'Grady (Eds.), *Child health psychology: Concepts and issues*. Elmsford, NY: Pergamon Press.

Wilkening, G. N., Golden, C. J., MacInnes, W. D., Plaisted, J. R., & Hermann, B. P. (1981, August). *The Luria–Nebraska Neuropsychological Battery—Children's Revision: A preliminary report*. Paper presented at the meeting of the American Psychological Association, Los Angeles.

Chapter 8

Neuropsychological Assessment of Children: Alternative Approaches

CLARE STODDART
ROBERT M. KNIGHTS

Department of Psychology
Carleton University
Ottawa, Ontario, Canada K1S 5B6

INTRODUCTION

There has been a rapid growth in the use and application of neuropsychological assessment procedures with children. While much of our knowledge of brain–behavior relationships is based on adult studies, there has been an increasing trend to use neuropsychological approaches to investigate a wide variety of developmental disorders. Currently, the two most frequently used standardized neuropsychological test batteries are adaptations for children of adult assessment procedures: the Halstead–Reitan Battery (Reitan, 1974) and the Luria–Nebraska Battery (Golden, 1981).

DEVELOPMENTAL NEUROPSYCHOLOGY

There are a number of issues that should be considered in the interpretation of brain–behavior relationships in children as compared to adults

229

CHILD NEUROPSYCHOLOGY, VOL. 2

(Knights & Stoddart, 1984). First, a major difference between adults and children is that many childhood disorders are prenatal or perinatal in origin, and thus the child has never experienced the functioning of a normal brain. The child grows up having to adapt to his or her cognitive limitations without being aware of a specific loss of function. For example, a large number of children referred for neuropsychological assessment suffer from disorders such as epilepsy, anoxia, hydrocephalus, and the syndrome of minimal brain dysfunction (MBD). This is in contrast to many adult disorders that result in a loss of a previously established normal skill or ability. Adults referred for neuropsychological assessment have frequently suffered recent cerebral vascular accidents, tumors, or degenerative diseases such as Parkinson's or Alzheimer's disease, which result in a loss of cognitive ability.

Second, related to the etiological differences resulting in cerebral dysfunction in children and adults, is the fact that very few childhood disorders result in localized lesions. It is, therefore, very difficult to determine the differential effects of the diffuse nature of the brain dysfunction and the postulated plasticity of the young brain. For example, discrete lesions in the left hemisphere associated with cerebral vascular accidents in adults may result in specific types of aphasia, whereas in children, not only are cerebral vascular accidents rare, but also those that do occur are generally associated with a global aphasia of a brief duration.

Third, it cannot be assumed that tests that have validated brain–behavior relationships in adults with known lesions will show similar results with children. The number of published studies of children with documented localized lesions is very limited, and one cannot assume that a simpler version of an adult test may necessarily be a measure of the same brain–behavior patterns as in adults (Golden, 1981). For an excellent discussion of the problems in the underlying assumptions made when generalizing from adult to developmental neuropsychology, the reader is referred to an article by J. M. Fletcher and Taylor (1984).

Another issue that should be considered in developmental neuropsychology concerns the purpose of the assessment procedure. The recent technical developments of specialized neurological diagnostic procedures such as the electroencephalogram (EEG), computerized tomography (CT) scan and positron emission tomography (PET) have led to a change in emphasis in neuropsychology from assisting in the diagnosis of lesion type and location to one of assessing the functional capacities of the child in order to make recommendations for management and rehabilitation.

Standardized Batteries

In neuropsychological assessment, the value of using a standardized battery versus selection of tests on an individual basis remains somewhat controversial at the present time (Rourke, Bakker, Fisk, & Strang, 1983; Lezak, 1983). Each method has a number of advantages and disadvantages associated with it, and the choice may reflect the individual clinician's training and orientation to the role of neuropsychological assessment. Another pragmatic factor that often has a strong influence on the choice of approach is whether the cost of assessment must be paid directly by the patient or is covered by state or provincial health plans. For example, Canadian neuropsychologists and their technicians are usually salaried from general hospital funds received from provincial health plans, in contrast to the United States, where direct patient billing is more frequently the case. For this reason, Canadian neuropsychologists tend to favor standardized batteries (see Teeter, this volume, for a review of standardized batteries).

One of the advantages of the standardized battery is that it is typically administered by a highly trained psychometric technician, which ensures a very standardized procedure with high reliability. The disadvantages, however, include the loss of clinical information that could be gained in direct personal contact on the part of the psychologist. In addition, the patient may be required to spend an unnecessarily long period of time in the testing situation.

Other practical issues to be considered in choosing which method of assessment is preferable relate to the purpose of the neuropsychological assessment. As mentioned previously, there has been a change in emphasis away from diagnosis toward the use of neuropsychological assessment for counseling and rehabilitation. Either the battery or the individual approach may provide relevant information for these purposes. A determining factor in deciding between the two approaches may depend on whether the clinician is engaged in ongoing research. For purposes of reasearch, the use of a standardized battery may be preferable because it results in the collection of the same information on each child, thereby allowing statistical comparisons among children with different conditions (Knights & Stoddart, 1981). In addition, this approach allows the determination of patterns of abilities and deficits associated with specific syndromes.

An interesting example of current research that is dependent on the administration of standardized batteries is the classification of learning disabled children into subtypes through the use of multivariate statistical techniques such as Q factor analysis and cluster analysis. This area of research has the potential for establishing reliable classification of subtypes of learning disabled children. It allows the evaluation of differential treatment strategies for the different subtypes. A comprehensive and insightful review of the subtype literature is presented by McKinney (1984), and a book on this topic has been published (Rourke, 1986).

A number of modifications have been made to the Halstead–Reitan Neuropsychological Test Battery for Children 9 to 14 years old and the Reitan–Indiana Neuropsychological Test Battery for Children 5 to 8 years old. Most of these batteries include additional tests to assess language functioning and psychoeducational skills (Knights & Norwood, 1980; Trites, 1977; Matthews & Klove, 1964). These additions are particularly relevant in situations where the neuropsychologist assesses a large number of children with learning disabilities. The use of a neuropsychological approach in school systems has increased dramatically in recent years and reflects the current interest in brain–behavior relationships (Hynd & Obrzut, 1981). The possibility of misinterpretation of neuropsychological test information by nontrained individuals in the school system has been extensively discussed by Gaddes (1980). Moreover, there is a general tendency to presume that any learning disability or behavioral abnormality is directly related to brain dysfunction. The ramifications of this fallacious assumption has been presented by J. M. Fletcher and Taylor (1984) and Satz and Fletcher (1981). Nevertheless, the standardized Halstead–Reitan battery has been shown to be sensitive to brain dysfunction in a variety of developmental disorders, such as asthma (Dunleavy & Baade, 1980), autism (Dawson, 1983), Gilles de la Tourette's syndrome (Bornstein, King, & Carroll, 1983), juvenile delinquency (Yeudall, Fromm-Auch, & Davies, 1982), muscular dystrophy (Knights, Hinton, & Drader, 1973) and epilepsy (Herman, 1982). Studies using the Luria-Nebraska Neuropsychological Battery for Children have been published, reporting the sensitivity of the battery for discriminating between learning disabled and normal children (Geary & Gilger, 1984; Nolan, Hammeke, & Barkley, 1983). As indicated, the use of a standardized battery does allow the neuropsychologist to make meaningful comparisons across a wide spectrum of developmental disorders.

Individual or Deficit Approach

A number of neuropsychologists working with both adults and children have rejected the use of standardized assessment procedures such as the Halstead–Reitan and Luria–Nebraska batteries and recommend an individual approach to assessment following the methods of Luria (1973).

Tests are selected on an individual basis to test toward the specific deficit of each patient. This approach has the advantage of reducing the lengthy testing time required, particularly for the Halstead–Reitan battery. This deficit method of assessment, therefore, may frequently be chosen in situations where the neuropsychologist administers the tests rather than a trained technician. The neuropsychologist is, therefore, in a position to use his or her own clinical judgement to select tests to determine the specific nature of the problems presented by the patient. This approach has the advantage of providing more information of specific deficits but may not provide detailed assessment of the child's cognitive strengths and is highly dependent on the level of clinical expertise of the individual neuropsychologist.

Selected Batteries

Some neuropsychologists have selected a series of tests on an eclectic basis rather than follow a specific approach such as the Halstead–Reitan or Luria–Nebraska batteries (see Obrzut, 1981, for such an approach). Provided that tests are selected to measure a wide range of abilities, including intelligence, abstract reasoning, achievement, memory, language, auditory and visual processing, motor–spatial, and sensory skills, the possibility of overlooking impairments that may not be evaluated in the deficit approach is avoided. One of the difficulties, however, with this approach is that it may assume a more precise knowledge of brain–behavior relationships in children than currently exists, and the tests selected may not be comprehensive enough.

For example, Harness, Epstein, and Gordon (1984) advocate the use of a "Cognitive Laterality Battery" in which tests were selected on an a priori basis to sample right and left hemisphere functioning in children. One of the tests included in a study of children with reading difficulties was the presentation of sequences of well-known sounds such as a baby crying or a rooster crowing. This test was assumed to sample left-hemisphere functioning. One could argue that the perception and recall of such sounds are primarily mediated by the right hemisphere and that their conclusion of left-hemisphere dysfunction in the poor readers is an artifact of the test classification.

A further example of a selected neuropsychological test battery is that used by Obrzut, Hynd, and Obrzut (1983) in a comparison of learning disabled (LD) and normal children. Two of the Halstead–Reitan tests were included (Category and Tactual Performance Test) as well as a laterality measure, dichotic listening, and the Wechsler Intelligence Scale for Children—Revised (WISC-R). Interestingly, the authors report the dichotic listening tasks as the most important variables in differentiating group membership. The results of the dichotic listening tasks are considered as providing support for a language-dominant left hemisphere, with the LD group showing less efficient interhemispheric transfer. As the authors themselves point out, the significance of these results in terms of brain–behavior relationships should be interpreted with caution in view of methodological problems and the influence of strategy effects on dichotic listening measures (Bryden, 1982).

Another example of the problems that may occur in a preselected neuropsychological test battery is demonstrated in a study of the neuropsychological performance and CT scans of obsessive–compulsive adolescents (Behar, Rapoport, Berg, Denckla, Mann, Cox, Fedio, Zahn, & Wolfman, 1984). The patients were compared with matched controls on 8 tests, only one of which is usually assumed to sample left-hemisphere functioning (Key Word List Learning). The only significant group differences occurred on two of the spatial tasks (Money's Road Map Test and Stylus Maze Learning). In view of the greater number of spatial tests, it is not surprising that the authors interpret the results to suggest greater right-hemisphere involvement in adolescents with obsessive–compulsive disorders. Here again, the conclusion regarding specific brain–behavior relationships may be an artifact of the test selection used.

Combined Approaches

Many neuropsychologists in clinical practice use a combined approach. That is, they typically have a selected battery of standard tests covering motor, sensory, spatial, language and memory skills, and then they select further tests on the basis of the pattern of abilities and deficits. This approach is best illustrated in adult neuropsychological assessment by Lezak (1983). An interesting example of this approach in children is presented by Gardner (1979), a child psychiatrist. In his assessment procedures for the diagnosis of MBD, Gardner includes both neuropsychological tests and neurological procedures.

This combined approach may also be followed by neuropsychologists who do use a standardized battery but who supplement this information with further assessment procedures selected on the basis of the pattern of neuropsychological test results. Although this is time consuming, it allows retrospective research on specific subgroups of children and at the same time provides clinical information on an individual basis for diagnosis, management, and rehabilitation.

RECENT DEVELOPMENTS

Assessment of Very Young Children

The original Reitan–Indiana Test Battery for Children was designed for children from 5 to 8 years old. The increasing use and acceptance of pediatric neuropsychology has led to an interest in the assessment of children under 5 years of age. A number of intelligence tests such as the Stanford–Binet and the Wechsler Preschool and Primary Scale of Intelligence (WPPSI) have been available for some time. More recent intelligence tests designed for this age group have included a wider range of abilities such as those frequently included in neuropsychological assessments (McCarthy, 1972; Kaufman & Kaufman, 1983). The Kaufman Assessment Battery for Children represents one of the first attempts to incorporate a neuropsychological model in the assessment of intelligence. Specific neuropsychological tests are also being used for younger children. For example, Wilson, Iacoviello, Wilson, and Risucci (1982) have published normative data on a modification of the Purdue Pegboard for use with preschoolers.

It seems likely that the neuropsychologist will be called on more frequently to contribute in the assessment of developmental disorders in the very young child. Due to the lack of differentiation of abilities at this age, the clinician must rely primarily on level of arousal, motor skills, and sensory functioning. These abilities are extensively examined in the young infant by means of behavioral assessments (Brazelton, 1973) and neurological tests (Prechtl & Beintema, 1964).

Screening Batteries

Another use of neuropsychological assessments is the attempt to predict children who will suffer from learning disabilities on the basis of performance on a test battery administered at kindergarten level. These studies are necessarily longitudinal in nature and can only be conducted using a standardized battery approach. The most extensive study of this type is that of Satz and his colleagues (Satz, Taylor, Friel, & Fletcher, 1978). The battery used by Satz et al. includes a variety of tests sampling a wide range of cerebral functions selected on the basis of a theoretical framework of a maturational lag model. His studies have reported surprisingly accurate predictions of children who later experienced various degrees of reading disabilities. The overall hit rate was as high as 88%, and the best predictors included socioeconomic status, alphabet recitation, and finger localization. Similar longitudinal studies of predictor variables have been conducted by Spreen (1978) and Rourke and Orr (1977) with comparable results.

An interesting use of a standardized neuropsychological test battery as a screening procedure is that of Trites (1983). This research on early French immersion programs in Ottawa, Canada investigated the predictive variables that would differentiate between children who experienced difficulties in second-language acquisition versus those who succeeded. The assessment procedures used in this research included an extension of the Halstead–Reitan (Trites, 1977) with other preschool tests. It is reported that children who experience failure in an immersion program differ from those who would normally be classified as LD in a regular classroom situation specifically in their performance on the Tactual Performance Test. Unfortunately, the data presented and analyzed are only for the extreme groups: the high achievers, low achievers, and drop-outs for the French immersion program. There is no indication of the rate of false positives or false negatives for any group in the sample tested.

COMPUTER USE IN NEUROPSYCHOLOGY

There are three main applications of the computer to the area of neuropsychology. First is the automated scoring of standardized tests. Second is the administration of tests via the video display terminal (VDT). Third is the classification and interpretation of test scores based on preprogrammed mathematical formulae.

The increasing application of computer use in clinical practice is illustrated by recent journals entitled "Computers in Psychiatry and Psychology" (Schwartz, 1984a) and "Cognitive Rehabilitation" (Bracy, 1984b), and a book "Using Computers in Clinical Practice" (Schwartz, 1984b).

Scoring

The computer has been efficiently used for a number of years in the scoring of multiple-item adult personality and vocational interest tests such as the Minnesota Multiphasic Personality Inventory (MMPI) and Strong–Campbell Vocational Interest Blank. With the advent of microcomputers, there has been an increase in the use of the computer as an instrument for scoring not only adult but also children's tests. For example, there are several programs now available for scoring the WISC-R. Information on this type of software currently available is published by Mercadal (1984) in a monthly bulletin entitled "Psychologists' Software Club." The WISC-R programs typically require the input of raw scores and provide scale scores, scale score deviations, significance levels, percentiles, and verbal–performance discrepancies. In addition, Bannatyne's (1974) categorizations and Kaufman's (1981) measures of subtest scatter are computed in some of the programs. With respect to neuropsychology, a similar program is now available to score the Halstead-Reitan Battery for adults (Mercadal, 1984). It seems probable that a comparable program will soon be available for the children's battery. One of the issues that should be considered in this use of the computer is the relative trade-off between the amount of time required to input the raw score data and the amount of information generated by the computer beyond that which is normally part of the clinician's everyday expertise.

Administration

The computer has been used for a number of years in the administration of psychological tests often included in neuropsychological batteries. These tests are typically modifications of standardized tests. For example, one of the earliest studies of automated test administration was that of Elwood (1972) with the Wechsler Adult Intelligence Scale (WAIS). Since that time other investigators have automated the Peabody Picture Vocabulary Test (PPVT) (Overton & Scott, 1972; Knights, Richardson, & McNarry, 1973) and the Category Test (Ball, 1979).

In general, these investigations have shown good reliability between the automated and the manually administered versions. In addition, computer administration of tests may be more effective than personal administration for certain subgroups of disadvantaged children (Johnson & Mihal, 1973; Feldman & Sears, 1970; J. D. Fletcher & Atkinson, 1972). It is obvious, however, that some types of tests used in neuropsychological assessment, such as paper and pencil tests, or some sensory tests such as fingertip writing or tactile imperception, could not readily be adapted for computer administration (Knights & Stoddart, 1983).

An alternative approach to the adaptation of previously existing standardized tests is the development of new tests designed to take advantage of the unique capabilities of the computer. These features include speed of stimulus presentation and recording of response, the display of objects in three-dimensional space and the display of moving objects. The computer also has the capability of recording and storing information accurately. This capability is essential in the use of adaptive or tailored testing (Weiss, 1977). In this procedure, test items are administered to an individual based on his or her previous performance on the test. This type of testing requires the availability of a large pool of items, whose item statistics are known, from which appropriate items can be drawn. For example, if an examinee received an initial test item of average difficulty, the correct answer would cause the selection of an item of greater difficulty, whereas an incorrect answer would cause an easier item to appear. This procedure results in better discrimination at any level of ability and avoids administering many easy items to bright individuals or many hard items to the less able person. The advantages of adaptive testing include the use of 50 to 80% fewer items and higher reliability and validity.

A number of programs have been designed for adult rehabilitation by Bracy (1984a) and Gianutsos and Klitzner (1981). Although developed primarily as training programs for rehabilitation, they can also be used as assessment procedures in a variety of areas. For example, these programs include measures of visual and auditory reaction time; visual-motor and visuospatial skills; verbal and spatial memory; and auditory pitch discrimination. The present authors modified the administration procedures of the visual and auditory reaction time tests so that the stimuli are presented to either the left or the right hemisphere. Normative data were collected on a sample of normal children and the efficacy of the tests is now being evaluated for discriminating among children with lateralized brain lesions. Other computerized tests for neuropsychological assessment under development in the authors' laboratory include measures of tapping speed, verbal memory, attention, and abstract reasoning skills.

Classification and Interpretation

Programming the computer to provide diagnostic classifications on the basis of raw score data is a complex task. An example of the complexity involved in this type of program is illustrated in the use of a computerized actuarial strategy for the diagnosis of children with mental retardation or learning disabilities using only measures of intelligence, achievement, and social behavior (Hale & McDermott, 1984). There have been a number of attempts to develop taxonomic rules to allow diagnostic classification based on test results from the Halstead-Reitan battery (Aaron, 1981; Russell, Neuringer, & Goldstein, 1970; Selz & Reitan, 1979). These approaches are particularly suited for automation because the elaborate sequences of decision-making rules are readily programmable for the computer. Whether this type of approach leads to greater accuracy in diagnostic classification than that of a trained clinician remains controversial at the present time (Heaton, Grant, Anthony, & Lehman, 1981).

Automated interpretations are currently available for the Revised Wechsler Intelligence Scales both for adults and for children (Mercadal, 1984). The only interpretive program in neuropsychology known to the authors is for the Halstead–Reitan Battery for adults (Mercadal, 1984).

The listing states that the program evaluates hypotheses for approximately 100 different combinations of tests, but it has yet to be evaluated in clinical practice.

Ethical Issues

The proliferation of software disks for microcomputers for the scoring, administration, classification, and interpretation of psychological and neuropsychological test data raises a number of serious ethical issues. Although most responsible companies that market these disks attempt to restrict their sale to qualified professionals, it is very probable that nontrained individuals will gain access to this type of software. In the case of neuropsychology, it is not sufficient to restrict the sale of such tests to a registered or licensed psychologist because neuropsychology is a specialty requiring several years of specific training. If a psychologist is not familiar with a particular test, he or she may not detect incorrect output based on scoring errors. Of particular concern in the case of interpretive programs is that despite varying degrees of complexity and sophistication, all characteristics related to an individual child's performance can never be taken into account in a computer program. The neuropsychologist, therefore, must be responsible for integrating the computer output with other information, including family and medical history, which may significantly modify the interpretation of certain test scores. In addition, the nature of the test score interpretation by the neuropsychologist in his or her report will vary according to whether the report is being sent to the parent, teacher, family physician, neurologist or neurosurgeon. A detailed discussion of the ethical and legal issues related to the use of computers in psychology is presented by Zachary and Pope (1984).

CONCLUSIONS

This chapter has included a discussion of some of the issues in pediatric neuropsychology. A number of alternative assessment approaches, ranging from a standardized battery to individual assessment procedures, were reviewed. Although each method has specific advantages and disadvantages, some authors tend to present a polarized view of the relative merits of their own assessment approach. In clinical practice, however, even clinicians who use a standardized battery may modify it as a function of patient characteristics, while those who use a deficit approach usually administer a core battery of standardized tests.

The use of neuropsychological assessments in the screening of kindergarten children to predict those who will subsequently have difficulties in school requires a careful and detailed selection of tests and long-term longitudinal follow-up studies. The investigators conducting this type of classification study must take into account the essential subjectiveness of the application of multivariate techniques. In addition, the researcher must be familiar with the problems of differential base rates and report both valid positive and false positive rates rather than one overall correct classification rate (Satz & Fletcher, 1979).

The use of the computer in neuropsychological assessment of children is rapidly expanding and will continue to do so. The computer provides obvious benefits in the accurate recording and storing of information and is inherently appealing to the computer-age child. It also provides the opportunity to develop tests of human abilities not measurable by traditional psychometric methods. However, automated interpretation of neuropsychological test scores raises serious ethical concerns, and it should only be used as an adjunct tool in the practice of child clinical neuropsychology. Ethical guidelines need to be drawn up to monitor the development, availability, and use of psychological software.

The increasing use of neuropsychological assessment procedures for children under 5 years of age is a welcome development and presents a challenge to the professional in this field. This area constitutes a subspecialty of neuropsychology requiring extensive clinical training and an awareness of the difficulties in drawing inferences regarding brain–behavior relationships in this age group. The application of pediatric neuropsychology in applied settings ranging from medical to educational assessments will continue to provide information regarding the nature of brain–behavior relationships in children and to establish developmental neuropsychology as a distinct discipline.

REFERENCES

Aaron, P. G. (1981). Diagnosis and remediation of learning disabilities in children—A neuropsychological key approach. In G. W. Hynd & J. E. Obrzut (Eds.), *Neuropsychological assessment and the school-age child*. New York: Grune & Stratton.

Ball, C. (1979). *Differential effects of feedback on learning in hyperactive children.* Unpublished master's thesis, Carleton University, Ottawa.

Bannatyne, A. (1974). Diagnosis: A note on the recategorization of the WISC–R scaled scores. *Journal of Learning Disabilities, 7,* 272–273.

Behar, D., Rapoport, J. L., Berg, C. J., Denckla, M. B., Mann, L., Cox, C., Fedio, P., Zahn, T., & Wolfman, M. G. (1984). Computerized tomography and neuropsychological test measures in adolescents with obsessive–compulsive disorders. *American Journal of Psychiatry, 1984, 141,* 363–368.

Bornstein, R. A., King, G., & Carroll, A. (1983). Neuropsychological abnormalities in Gilles de la Tourette's Syndrome. *Journal of Nervous and Mental Disease, 171,* 497–502.

Bracy, O. L. (1984a). Psychological Software Services. P.O. Box 29205, Indianapolis, IN, 46229.

Bracy, O. L. (Ed.). (1984b). *Cognitive Rehabilitation.* P.O. Box 29344, Indianapolis, IN, 46220.

Brazelton, T. B. (1973). Neonatal Behavioural Assessment Scale. *Clinics in Developmental Medicine, 50.*

Bryden, M. P. (1982). The behavioral assessment of lateral asymmetry: Problems, pitfalls and partial solutions. In R. N. Malatesha & L. C. Hartlage (Eds.), *Neuropsychology and cognition* (Vol. 2). The Hague: Nijhoff.

Dawson, G. (1983). Lateralized brain dysfunction in autism: Evidence from the Halstead–Reitan neuropsychological battery. *Journal of Autism and Developmental Disorders, 13,* 269–286.

Dunleavy, R. A., & Baade, L. E. (1980). Neuropsychological correlates of severe asthma in children 9–14 years old. *Journal of Consulting and Clinical Psychology, 48,* 564–577.

Elwood, D. L. (1972). Test retest reliability and cost analysis of automated and face to face intelligence testing. *International Journal of Man–Machine Studies, 4,* 1–23.

Feldman, D. H., & Sears, P. S. (1970). Effects of computer-assisted instruction on children's behaviour. *Educational Technology, 10,* 11–14.

Fletcher, J. D., & Atkinson, R. C. (1972). Evaluation of the Stanford CAI program in initial reading. *Journal of Educational Psychology, 63,* 597–602.

Fletcher, J. M., & Taylor, H. G. (1984). Neuropsychological approaches to children: Towards a developmental neuropsychology. *Journal of Clinical Neuropsychology, 6,* 39–56.

Gaddes, W. H. (1980). *Learning disabilities and brain function.* New York: Springer-Verlag.

Gardner, R. A. (1979). *The objective diagnosis of minimal brain dysfunction.* Creskill, NJ: Creative Therapeutics.

Geary, D. C., & Gilger, J. W. (1984). The Luria–Nebraska Neuropsychological Battery—Children's Revision: Comparison of learning disabled and normal children matched on full scale I.Q. *Perceptual and Motor Skills, 58,* 115–118.

Gianutsos, R., & Klitzner, C. (1981). *Computer programs for cognitive rehabilitation.* Bayport, NY: Life Science Associates.

Golden, C. J. (1981). The Luria–Nebraska Children's Battery: Theory and formulation. In G. W. Hynd & J. E. Obrzut (Eds.), *Neuropsychological assessment and the school-age child.* New York: Grune & Stratton.

Hale, R. L., & McDermott, P. A. (1984). Pattern analysis of an acturial strategy for computerized diagnosis of childhood exceptionality. *Journal of Learning Disabilities, 17,* 30–37.

Harness, B. Z., Epstein, R., & Gordon, H. W. (1984). Cognitive profile of children referred to a clinic for reading disabilities. *Journal of Learning Disabilities, 17,* 346–352.

Heaton, R. K., Grant, I., Anthony, W. Z., & Lehman, R. A. W. (1981). A comparison of clinical and automated interpretation of the Halstead–Reitan battery. *Journal of Clinical Neuropsychology, 3,* 121–141.

Herman, B. P. (1982). Neuropsychological function and psychopathology in children with epilepsy. *Epilepsia, 23,* 545–554.

Hynd, G. W., & Obrzut, J. E. (1981). School neuropsychology. *Journal of School Psychology, 19,* 45–50.

Johnson, D. F., & Mihal, W. L. (1973). Performance of blacks and whites in computerized versus manual testing environments. *American Psychologist, 28,* 694–699.

Kaufman, A. S. (1981). Scatter analysis of WISC–R profiles for learning disabled children with superior intelligence. *Journal of Learning Disabilities, 14,* 400–404.

Kaufman, A. S., & Kaufman, N. L. (1983). *Assessment Battery for Children.* Circle Pines, MN: American Guidance Service.

Knights, R. M., Hinton, G. G., & Drader, D. L. (1973). *Changes in intellectual ability with Duchenne muscular dystrophy* (Research Bulletin No. 8). Ottawa: Carleton University, Psychology Department.

Knights, R. M., & Norwood, J. A. (1980). *A neuropsychological test battery for children: Examiner's manual.* Ottawa: Carleton University, Department of Psychology.

Knights, R. M., Richardson, D. H., & McNarry, L. R. (1973). Automated vs. clinical administration of the Peabody Picture Vocabulary Test and the Colored Progressive Matrices. *American Journal of Mental Deficiency, 12,* 696–697.

Knights, R. M., & Stoddart, C. (1981). Profile approaches to neuropsychological diagnosis in children. In G. W. Hynd & J. E. Obrzut (Eds.), *Neuropsychological assessment and the school-age child.* New York: Grune & Stratton.

Knights, R. M., & Stoddart, C. (1983). *Automated assessment of vocational aptitudes: A feasibility study* (NATCON Vol. 4, pp. 69–114). Ottawa: Government of Canada, Employment and Immigration, Occupational and Career Analyses and Developmental Branch.

Knights, R. M., & Stoddart, C. (1986). Pediatric clinical neuropsychology. In L. P. Ivan (Ed.), *Pediatric neurosurgery.* St. Louis: Warren H. Green.

Lezak, M. D. (1983). *Neuropsychological assessment* (2nd ed.). New York: Oxford University Press.

Luria, A. R. (1973). *The working brain.* New York: Basic Books.

Matthews, C. G., & Klove, H. (1964). *Instructional manual for the Adult Neuropsychological Test Battery.* Madison: University of Wisconsin Medical School.

McCarthy, D. A. (1972). *Manual for the McCarthy Scales of Children's Abilities.* New York: Psychological Corporation.

McKinney, J. D. (1984). The search for subtypes of specific learning disability. *Journal of Learning Disabilities, 17,* 43–50.

Mercadel, D. (1984). *Psychologists' Software Club.* 1151 Cheshire, Casper, WY, 82609: Clinician's Digest.

Noland, D. R., Hammeke, T. A., & Barkley, R. A. (1983). A comparison of the patterns of the neuropsychological performance in two groups of learning disabled children. *Journal of Clinical Psychology, 12,* 22–27.

Obrzut, J. E. (1981). Neuropsychological procedures with school age children. In G. W. Hynd & J. E. Obrzut (Eds.), *Neuropsychological assessment and the school age child.* New York: Grune & Stratton.

Obrzut, J. E., Hynd, G. W., & Obrzut, A. (1983). Neuropsychological assessment of learning disabilities. *Journal of Experimental Child Psychology, 35,* 46–55.

Overton, G. W., & Scott, H. G. (1972). Automated and manual intelligence testing: Data on parallel forms of the Peabody Picture Vocabulary Test. *American Journal of Mental Deficiency, 76,* 639–643.

Prechtl, H. F. R., & Beintema, D. (1964). The neurological examination of the full-term newborn infant. *Clinics in Developmental Medicine, 12,* 1–101.

Reitan, R. M. (1974). Psychological effects of cerebral lesions in children of early school age. In R. M. Reitan & L. A. Dawson (Eds.), *Clinical neuropsychology: Current status and applications.* New York: Wiley.

Rourke, B. P. (1986). *Neuropsychology of learning disabilities: Essentials of subtype analysis.* New York: Guilford Press.

Rourke, B. P., Bakker, D. J., Fisk, J. L., & Strang, J. D. (1983). *Child neuropsychology.* New York: Guilford Press.

Rourke, B. P., & Orr, R. R. (1977). Prediction of the reading and spelling performances of normal and retarded readers: A four-year follow-up. *Journal of Abnormal Child Psychology, 5,* 9–20.

Russell, E. W., Neuringer, C., & Goldstein, G. (1970). *Assessment of brain damage—A neuropsychological approach.* New York: Wiley (Interscience).

Satz, P., & Fletcher, J. M. (1979). Early screening tests: some uses and abuses. *Journal of Learning Disabilities, 12,* 56–60.

Satz, P., & Fletcher, J. M. (1981). Emergent trends in neuropsychology: An overview. *Journal of Consulting and Clinical Psychology, 49,* 851–865.

Satz, P., Taylor, H. G., Friel, J., & Fletcher, J. M. (1978). Some developmental and predictive precursors of reading disabilities: A six year follow-up. In A. L. Benton & D. Pearl (Eds.), *Dyslexia: An appraisal of current knowledge.* New York: Oxford University Press.

Schwartz, M. D. (Ed.). (1984a). *Computers in Psychiatry and Psychology,* 26 Trumbull St., New Haven, CT 06511.

Schwartz, M. D. (1984b). *Using computers in clinical practice.* New York: Haworth Press.

Selz, M., & Reitan, R. M. (1979). Rules for neuropsychological diagnosis: Classification of brain function in older children. *Journal of Consulting and Clinical Psychology, 47,* 258–264.

Spreen, O. (1978). *Prediction of school achievement from kindergarten to grade five: Review and report of a follow-up study* (Research Monograph No. 33). Victoria, BC: University of Victoria, Department of Psychology.

Trites, R. L. (1977). *Neuropsychological test manual.* Montreal: Ronalds Federated.

Trites, R. L. (1983). Early immersion in French at school for anglophone children: Learning disabilities and prediction of success. In Y. Lebrun & M. Paradis (Eds.), *Early bilingualism and child development.* Amsterdam: Swets & Zeitlinger.

Weiss, D. J. (1977). *Applications of computerized adaptive testing* (Research Rep. No. 77-1). Minneapolis: University of Minnesota, Department of Psychology.

Wilson, B. C., Iacoviello, J. M., Wilson, J. J., & Risucci, D. (1982). Purdue pegboard performance of normal preschool children. *Journal of Clinical Neuropsychology, 4,* 19–26.

Yacoviello, J. M., Wilson, J. J., & Risucci, D. (1982). Purdue Pegboard Performance of Normal Preschool Children. *Journal of Clinical Neuropsychology, 4,* 19–26.

Yeudall, L. T., Fromm-Auch, D., & Davies, P. (1982). Neuropsychological impairment of persistent delinquency. *Journal of Nervous and Mental Disease, 170,* 257–265.

Zachary, R. A., & Pope, K. S. (1984). Legal and ethical issues in the clinical use of computerized testing. In M. D. Schwartz (Ed.), *Using computers in clinical practice.* New York: Haworth Press.

Chapter 9

Actuarial and Clinical Approaches to Neuropsychological Diagnosis: Applied Considerations

W. GRANT WILLIS

School of Education
University of Colorado at Denver
Denver, Colorado 80202

INTRODUCTION

Approaches to neuropsychological diagnosis and, less specifically, nearly all psychodiagnostic techniques generally may be classified as either actuarial or clinical. Psychologists have engaged in debates for over three decades now regarding the relative assets and liabilities of these approaches (Meehl, 1954), and the dispute remains unresolved. The purpose of this chapter is not to enter into that long-standing controversy. Rather, the necessity for both approaches is recognized in current pediatric neuropsychological practice.

Here, these two approaches are contrasted. Three multivariate procedures used to derive actuarial rules are noted. Univariate procedures have also (but less frequently) been used to differentiate among neuropsychodiagnostic classifications (e.g., Goldstein & Shelly, 1973). Nevertheless,

245

CHILD NEUROPSYCHOLOGY, VOL. 2
Copyright © 1986 by Academic Press, Inc.

it is generally assumed that optimal predictions of membership to diagnostic groups are usually multivariate processes—that is, processes involving more than a single datum (Sawyer, 1966). Moreover, an advantage of multivariate procedures is that assessment data are considered collectively rather than singly, and their relative contributions to diagnostic predictions may be evaluated. Because clinicians are more likely to be involved in applications rather than derivations of actuarial rules, the major emphasis is directed toward evaluations of those rules rather than explanations of their statistical constructions.

Finally, in clinical practice, actuarial data are often unavailable or inappropriate, and pediatric neuropsychologists frequently must rely on professional clinical judgment in contrast to statistically derived rules in order to predict a diagnosis. Although the relative inaccuracy of this approach is well documented (Goldberg & Werts, 1966; Meehl, 1973; Phelan, 1964; Wallach & Schoof, 1965), in the absence of adequate actuarial data and rules, there is a paucity of literature presenting alternative strategies. Thus, the issue of clinical judgment is addressed as well.

ACTUARIAL AND CLINICAL APPROACHES CONTRASTED

The primary distinction between actuarial and clinical approaches to neuropsychological diagnosis is that in the former approach, assessment data collected from a patient are integrated in a statistical fashion, and in the latter approach, data are integrated in more subjective ways. Methods in which assessment data are collected are of little relevance in this dichotomous classification scheme.

The diagnostic tasks of neuropsychologists differ for these two approaches. Actuarial approaches require the clinician to exercise professional expertise in the collection of assessment data; clinical approaches require the clinician to engage in these activities as well but, further, to also exercise professional expertise for the integration of differential assessment data in order to predict a diagnosis. Neuropsychologists who use standardized measures for assessment purposes, where those measures are interpreted in either nomothetic or idiographic fashions (discussed subsequently), are not necessarily actuarial in their approaches to diagnosis. Similarly, neuropsychologists who use informal tasks and interviews for assessment purposes, where the assessment process is analogous to an individualized experiment, are not necessarily employing clinical approaches. For example, Reitan's blind method of interpreting standardized neuropsychological test scores is distinctly clinical in nature

(Selz, 1981), whereas neuropsychological assessment information collected through methods advocated by Luria (1980) could conceivably be coded and subjected to actuarial interpretation.

This primary difference between the two approaches to neuropsychological diagnosis is manifested in at least three contradistinctions (see also McDermott, 1982, pp. 248–249). Issues involved in these contradistinctions are noted in Table 1. First, the probabilities concerning the relationships between assessment data and particular neuropsychological diagnoses are (1) statistically derived for actuarial approaches and (2) experientially derived for clinical approaches. Thus, for clinical approaches, these probabilities might be influenced by such variables as a clinician's memory of previous cases, an understanding of research relevant to the case, and any number of other subjective factors specific to the case of interest (McDermott, 1982). Second, with reference to their relationships to potential diagnoses, various sources of assessment data are considered in a simultaneous fashion for actuarial approaches and in an independent fashion for clinical approaches.

Finally, a specific assessment datum is weighted consistently in terms of its contribution to the diagnosis for actuarial approaches and differentially for clinical approaches. For example, a pediatric neuropsychologist employing a clinical approach to diagnosis might attribute a higher degree of importance to an assessed constructional apraxia for a child with meaningful psychoeducational experiences than for a child who lacks those kinds of experiences. In contrast, for an actuarial approach, unless psychoeducational experiences were coded and entered into an actuarial rule as a separate variable, the assessed constructional apraxia would be weighted equally in terms of its contribution to the diagnosis for both of these children.

EVALUATIONS OF ACTUARIAL RULES

Three of the most common methods for deriving actuarial rules for neuropsychological diagnosis are multiple regression, discriminant analysis, and cluster analysis. All of these methods are multivariate and lead to rules (or equations) by which assessment data may be combined in order to predict a diagnosis. A thorough discussion of the statistical procedures involved in these methods is beyond the scope of this chapter (Huberty, 1975, 1984; Pedhazur, 1982; Tryon & Bailey, 1970). Instead, the major emphasis is directed toward an evaluation of three primary methodological issues involved in the application of the actuarial rules to neuropsychological diagnosis.

TABLE 1

Approaches to integrating assessment data

	Approach	
Issue	Actuarial	Clinical
Probability of relationship between data and diagnosis	Statistically derived	Experientially derived
Consideration of data	Simultaneous	Independent
Contribution of data to diagnosis	Consistently weighted	Differentially weighted

Methods for Deriving Rules

Multiple regression, discriminant analysis, and cluster analysis, besides being multivariate methods, all represent analyses of the variability in diagnoses (or prognoses) through available sources of assessment information. In these situations, a diagnosis (i.e., criterion variable) is predicted from an optimally weighted composite of assessment information (i.e., predictor variables). The resulting equation is an actuarial rule whereby similar kinds of assessment data subsequently can be integrated in a linear fashion in order to predict the most likely diagnosis. Through the use of these equations, clinical judgment is minimized, at least during the data-integration phase of neuropsychodiagnostic activity.

Multiple regression and discriminant analysis are perhaps more closely aligned conceptually with each other than with cluster analysis. In both of the former two methods, particular diagnostic outcomes must be specified prior to the analysis. Subsequently, the relationship between a composite sum of assessment information and a particular outcome is determined. Discriminant analysis can be considered, at least at an elementary level, as a special case of multiple regression where diagnostic outcomes are scaled in nominal as opposed to metric units. Thus, because of the scales used to measure outcomes, multiple regression tends to lend itself more toward the prediction of degrees of some criterion, a process important for prognosis. Discriminant analysis, however, tends to lend itself more toward prediction of group membership, a process important for diagnosis.

In contrast to multiple regression and discriminant analysis, in the method of cluster analysis, diagnostic outcomes are not specified prior to the analysis; instead, relatively homogeneous groups are determined with reference to particular patterns and combinations of assessment information. This method, consequently, does not rely on the assumption that conceptually derived neuropsychodiagnostic groups comprise homogeneous samples that are distinct from each other, at least with respect to assessment data. Cluster analysis, however, is similar to discriminant analysis, in that outcomes may be considered in terms of nominal units. Thus, cluster analysis also readily lends itself to the process of diagnostic classification.

Of these three methods for deriving actuarial rules for neuropsychological diagnosis, discriminant analysis has perhaps received the most use. This is because, prior to the analysis, nominally scaled outcome variables are designated as criterion groups (e.g., right vs. left vs. diffuse cerebral hemispheric impairments), and linear combinations of predictor variables (i.e., assessment data) are formulated to maximally separate the groups. Descriptive aspects of the discriminant analysis are related to an explanation and interpretation of differences among the diagnostic groups; predictive aspects are related to (1) the derivation of an actuarial rule to predict membership to a particular neuropsychodiagnostic classification, and (2) the evaluation of the accuracy of that rule in terms of the proportion of correct classifications—that is, hit rate (Huberty, 1984). It is the predictive aspects of discriminant analysis that have been most directly applied to actuarial neuropsychological diagnosis.

Regardless of the method used to derive an actuarial rule, it is important for clinical neuropsychologists to understand inherent methodological issues so that appropriate discretion may be used in the application of that rule for individual patients. In this respect, three salient issues concern (1) the stability and generalizability of the actuarial rule when applied to assessment data from patients other than those from which that rule was derived, (2) the validity and generalizability of the neuropsychodiagnostic classifications used as criterion measures in the derivation of the actuarial rule, and (3) the prior probabilities that a patient from a given neuropsychological clinic or department belongs to particular neuropsychodiagnostic groups—that is, base rates in the population of interest.

Stability

Actuarial rules for neuropsychological diagnosis often lack stability in the absence of proper cross-validation. Multivariate classification methods (such as those previously described) capitalize on all variability present among assessment data, even variability due to random factors. Consequently, resultant actuarial rules can potentially classify patients into neuropsychodiagnostic categories largely on the basis of chance variation in assessment information.

Such a possibility is a potential problem in nearly all classification procedures; it represents an even greater hazard, however, in neuropsychological diagnosis because of the unique circumstances surrounding this specialty. Pediatric neuropsychological evaluations typically include a large number of background, psychometric, clinical-neurologic, informal, and interview measures (Hynd & Obrzut, 1981). Moreover, the number of patients afflicted with particular neuropsychological impairments who are available for the research necessary to develop actuarial rules is frequently limited. Such a large number of assessment measures, coupled with a small number of patients given particular diagnoses, leads to a high probability that resultant actuarial rules will be largely determined on the basis of chance variation. Actuarial rules determined in this fashion may lack stability and generalizability in their application to assessment information collected from other patients. A critical index in this regard is the ratio of the number of patients to the number of assessment measures. Low values of this ratio (i.e., ratios approaching 1) lead to potentially greater errors in neuropsychological diagnosis than higher values when the actuarial rule is applied to new patients (Fletcher, Rice, & Ray, 1978). In order to determine the influence of these factors on the accuracy of the actuarial rule, that rule must be cross-validated.

Cross-validation is a method whereby an actuarial rule is applied to assessment data collected from a different group of patients. The application of the actuarial rule for this different group yields predicted diagnostic (or prognostic) outcomes for each patient. Subsequently, the relationship between the predicted outcomes and the actual outcomes for this group of patients is determined. The resulting index of relationship is almost always lower than the comparable relationship calculated for the original group involved in the derivation of the actuarial rule. This is because, as previously noted, the original analysis takes advantage of chance fluctuations in assessment data. The lowering of the relationship between the composite sum of assessment data and diagnostic outcome is referred to as *shrinkage*.

Unless actuarial rules are properly cross-validated, clinical neuropsychologists should exercise caution in applying those rules to individual patients; more appropriately, actuarial rules that have not been cross-validated should not be used for clinical purposes at all. In order to illustrate this caveat, Willson and Reynolds (1982) conducted a secondary analysis of nine studies that derived actuarial rules for neuropsychological diagnosis. Although the results of these studies reported 12 significant indexes of relationship between composite sums of assessment data and diagnostic outcomes, after estimates of shrinkage were made, only about half of those indexes remained significant. Thus, many of the results reported were due to chance variation in assessment data. It was recommended that studies reporting actuarial rules that have not been cross-validated should not be published because of the potential dangers to patients associated with the premature applications of those rules. It is also important for clinical neuropsychologists to gain an understanding of the limited stability and generalizability of actuarial rules that have not been cross-validated, as well as a familiarity with appropriate methods for conducting such replications and estimations thereof (Cattin, 1980; Herzberg, 1969; Lachenbruch, 1967; Mosier, 1951).

Validity and Generalizability

The validity and generalizability of the neuropsychodiagnostic classifications used as criterion measures in derivations of actuarial rules is another salient methodological issue. The accuracy of diagnostic predictions based on actuarial rules must be evaluated in terms of external criteria. Thus, the validity of an actuarial rule is limited by the validity of its criterion. Moreover, similar to any other measure, the validity of the criterion is limited by its own reliability.

The criteria selected against which the accuracies of actuarial rules are evaluated should be independent of the assessment data used in the derivation of those rules. Given the highly inferential nature of neuropsychological evaluations, particularly with pediatric populations, the selection of reliable, valid, and independent criteria for establishing distinct neuropsychological diagnoses is a difficult task. For example, reliance on neurological histories and physical examinations as criteria may be inappropriate because clinical neurological examinations are typically only grossly standardized and may be less sensitive to cerebral impairment that other procedures (including neuropsychological tests). Further, some procedures included in typical pediatric neurological examinations are common to neuropsychological tests, hence, the two evaluations lack independence (Anthony, Heaton, & Lehman, 1980).

In addition to case histories and clinical neurological examinations, however, there are a number of other procedures available to assess the presence, process, and localization of neuropsychological impairment. Such procedures include psychiatric examinations, electroencephalograms, various radiological and laboratory procedures, and autopsies. Thus, there is a hierarchy of procedures that may be used to assess these three aspects of impairment (Russell, Neuringer, & Goldstein, 1970), but although these procedures become increasingly definitive in progressing through this hierarchy, they also become increasingly invasive, hence are often unacceptable.

Because of problems associated with the selection and application of criteria for establishing definitive neuropsychological diagnoses, typically only assessment data collected from patients with clearly localized neuro-psychological impairments are used to derive actuarial rules for neuropsy-chological diagnosis. This common practice frequently results in the ex-clusion of significantly large proportions of patients from research. Thus, actuarial rules are often based on a minority of patients. For example, in one investigation 90% of the total pool of 1500 patients were eliminated in order to ensure certainty with respect to lesion presence and location (Anthony et al., 1980). The remaining 10% (or 150 nonrandom patients) were used to cross-validate actuarial rules for neuropsychological diagno-sis. Basing neuropsychodiagnostic decisions on actuarial rules derived for such highly selected samples may be inappropriate even if those rules have been cross-validated. At least, clinical neuropsychologists should develop a skepticism toward the generalizability of such rules for the particular group of patients with whom they are involved. Thus, in one respect, it is important to establish reliable, valid, and independent crite-ria for diagnostic classification, and in another (perhaps opposing) re-spect, a minority of patients are afflicted with such distinct neuropsycho-logical impairments. In order to apply actuarial rules with appropriate discretion, clinical neuropsychologists need to carefully evaluate the in-verse relationship between precision–accuracy versus generalizability of those rules.

Base Rates

The final methodological issue discussed concerns the prior probabili-ties that a patient belongs to particular neuropsychodiagnostic groups. These probabilities are influenced by the specific neuropsychological clinic or department in which the patient is evaluated and are typically expressed as base rates.

As previously noted, the accuracies of actuarial rules for neuropsycho-logical diagnosis are commonly evaluated in terms of the proportions of patients correctly classified into particular neuropsychodiagnostic groups. These important criteria for actuarial interpretations are called hit rates. Evaluations of hit rates, however, are largely dependent on base rates. In order to be of pragmatic value, actuarial rules must predict a higher number of correct diagnoses than could be predicted given base rates alone. In some instances, using an actuarial rule to predict a neuro-psychological diagnosis can actually decrease the likelihood of a correct classification (Willis, 1984). In order for a positive diagnosis to be more likely accurate than inaccurate, the ratio of positive to negative base rates in the examined population must be greater than the ratio of the false positive rate to the valid positive rate identified by the actuarial rule

(Meehl & Rosen, 1955). Hence, it is important to evaluate the accuracies of actuarial rules developed for neuropsychological diagnoses in terms of base rates in the population sampled. Further, the population sampled must be clearly specified because base rates may vary accordingly. For example, the base rates for diffuse neuropsychological impairments differ widely for children referred to a neuropsychologist in a hospital setting versus children referred to a school psychologist in an educational setting.

Two criteria proposed by Huberty (1984) are useful for assessing the accuracies of actuarial rules for neuropsychological diagnosis in terms of base rates (Willis, 1984). In one such assessment, a comparison is made between the overall hit rate and the proportion of patients in the largest diagnostic group. Huberty labeled this proportion the *maximum-chance criterion;* it is calculated by dividing the number of patients in the largest diagnostic group by the total number of patients in all groups. The maximum-chance criterion represents the probability of diagnosing the patients in the sample correctly by chance. In the other assessment, a comparison is made between the hit rate for a given diagnostic group and the proportion of patients in that particular group. This proportion is calculated by dividing the number of patients in the diagnostic group of interest by the total number of patients in all groups. It is useful in those instances where a neuropsychologist is interested in the probability of a particular diagnosis being correct by chance. In order for actuarial rules to be of any pragmatic diagnostic value, overall and separate-group hit rates must at least exceed chance criteria. In order to determine if potential differences between these hit rates and base rates are statistically reliable, the frequencies on which they are based may be compared using standardized normal statistics (Huberty, 1984).

In addition, Huberty (1984) proposed a statistic that is useful to neuropsychologists who are interested in determining the degree of improvement in diagnostic accuracy that may be attained by using an actuarial rule over chance assignment of patients to groups. This statistic (I) is calculated by dividing the difference between the hit rate and the base rate by the difference between 1 and the base rate. I represents the proportion of error in diagnostic accuracy that is reduced by using the actuarial rule rather than assigning diagnoses to patients on the basis of chance.

When actuarial rules for neuropsychological diagnoses are published, hit rates are usually reported in order to demonstrate diagnostic accuracies. Unless hit rates are compared with population base rates, however, those diagnostic accuracies cannot be properly evaluated. A secondary analysis of five investigations that derived actuarial rules for neuropsychological diagnosis found that, of 26 hit rates presented, only 17 reliably exceeded base rates; in five instances, base rates and hit rates did not

TABLE 2

Information for sample sizes, base rates, and hit rates for criterion groups in each investigation[a,b]

Information	Criterion group					
	L	R	D	NBD	All	BD
Anthony, Heaton, & Lehman (1980)						
n	37	47	29	NA	NA	113
Base rate	.33	.42	.26	NA	NA	.42
Hit rate	.54**	.72**	.34	NA	NA	.57**
Goldstein & Shelly (1982)						
n	41	49	300	NA	NA	390
Base rate	.11	.13	.77	NA	NA	.77
Hit rate	.51**	.67**	.45**	NA	NA	.48**
Russell, Neuringer, & Goldstein (1970)						
n	21	16	43	24	104	80
Base rate	.20	.15	.41	.23	.41	.54
Hit rate	.62**	.56**	.44	.71**	.56**	.51
Swiercinsky & Warnock (1977)						
n	22	17	143	78	260	182
Base rate	.08	.07	.10	.30	.55	.79
Hit rate	.27**	.35**	.43**	.49**	.43**	.40**
Wedding (1983)						
n	6	6	6	12	30	18
Base rate	.20	.20	.20	.40	.40	.33
Hit rate	.67**	.33	.50*	.75**	.60*	.50

[a] From Willis (1984, p. 568). Copyright 1984 by the American Psychological Association. Reprinted by permission.

[b] L = left-hemisphere lesions; R = right-hemisphere lesions; D = diffuse lesions; NBD = no brain damage; All = all four criterion groups; BD = all three brain-damaged criterion groups; NA = not applicable; *$p < .05$; **$p < .001$.

differ significantly and, in four instances, base rates reliably exceeded hit rates (Willis, 1984). Tables 2 and 3 are presented to illustrate the calculations of base rates and I values, respectively, for each of the five investigations analyzed. Such indexes should be calculated and evaluated routinely by clinical neuropsychologists before actuarial rules are applied to individual patients.[1] Even when these calculations demonstrate that using

[1] Formulas for determining the statistical significance of differences between base rates and hit rates are presented by Huberty (1984).

TABLE 3

I **Values for criterion groups** [a,b]

	Criterion group					
Study	L	R	D[c]	NBD	All[c]	BD[c]
Anthony et al. (1980)	.31	.52	ns	NA	NA	.26
Goldstein & Shelly (1982)	.45	.62		NA	NA	
Russell et al. (1970)	.53	.48	ns	.62	.25	ns
Swiercinsky & Warnock (1977)	.21	.30	.37	.27		
Wedding (1983)	.59	ns	.38	.58	.33	ns

[a] From Willis (1984, p. 569). Copyright 1984 by the American Psychological Association. Reprinted by permission.

[b] L = left-hemisphere lesions; R = right-hemisphere lesions; D = diffuse lesions; NBD = no brain damage; All = all four criterion groups; BD = all three brain damaged criterion groups; NA = not applicable; ns = not significant.

[c] Lack of an entry indicates that the base rate exceeded the hit rate.

an actuarial rule significantly improves diagnostic accuracy over chance, however, clinical neuropsychologists must assess the degree of similarity between the setting of their practice versus the setting in which that rule was derived. This is because, as previously noted, population base rates differ markedly in different settings.

CLINICAL JUDGMENT

Research supporting the relatively greater predictive accuracy of actuarial over clinical approaches to diagnosis generally assumes that actuarial rules are readily available to clinicians and, further, that those rules are free from the methodological issues discussed. Moreover, the costs associated with making different kinds of diagnostic errors are assumed to be constant. For example, costs associated with diagnosing a normal child as afflicted with a neuropsychological impairment would be assumed to be comparable to costs associated with diagnosing an afflicted child as normal. In clinical practice, of course, these three assumptions are often violated; however, neuropsychodiagnostic decisions are not robust to such violations. Thus, the clinical judgment of the neuropsychologist frequently becomes a source of data to be considered concomitantly with other assessment information. Consequently, good diagnostic decisions are based on a combination of actuarial and clinical factors. Three of those clinical factors concern (1) adopting a consistent and appropriate orientation to the nomothetic or idiographic interpretation of standardized neuropsychological measures, (2) understanding cognitive heuristics associated with diagnostic errors, and (3) reducing confounding influences in assessments through aggregating information across sources, methods, and settings.

Nomothetic and Idiographic Interpretations

Pediatric neuropsychologists who use clinical judgment to combine assessment information can approach the interpretation of standardized neuropsychological measures in either nomothetic (i.e., normative) or idiographic (i.e., ipsative) fashions. In the former approach, the child's performances on differential components of the evaluation are considered with reference to the normative group for which various tests were standardized; in the latter approach, the child's performances are considered with reference to that child's own mean level of performance (Kaufman, 1979; Kaufman & Kaufman, 1983; Reynolds, 1982; Reynolds & Clark, 1983; Reynolds & Gutkin, 1981). Pediatric neuropsychologists who interpret standardized measures in either nomothetic or idiographic fashions, however, should be aware of at least two cautions.

First, a common source of error in diagnostic decision making is associated with inconsistencies due to applying principles derived from antithetical orientations (McDermott, 1981). Thus, neuropsychologists should approach interpretations in consistent fashions. Clinicians who interpret one source of assessment information in a nomothetic fashion and another source of assessment information in an idiographic fashion are far more likely to misdiagnose a child than clinicians who are more consistent in their interpretive orientations.

Second, in order to be interpreted appropriately (regardless of orientation), differential components of evaluations must possess an adequate amount of specificity (Kaufman, 1979; Kaufman & Kaufman, 1983; Snow & Hynd, 1984). The specificity of a component (or task) refers to the unique abilities that are reliably measured by that component. For example, nomothetic or idiographic interpretations of unique skills measured by most subtests of the Kaufman Assessment Battery for Children (Kaufman & Kaufman, 1983) are possible (although not ordinarily recommended) because those subtests possess an adequate amount of specificity. In contrast, similar interpretations for the Luria–Nebraska Neuropsychological Battery (Golden, Hammeke, & Purisch, 1980) may be inappropriate because subscale specificities for that instrument have not yet been substantiated (Shelly & Goldstein, 1982; Snow & Hynd, 1984).

Cognitive Heuristics

Research conducted regarding errors in clinical judgment has revealed common, cognitive heuristics that frequently result in inaccurate decisions, especially in situations concerning the likelihood of uncertain events such as neuropsychological diagnosis. A discernment of these heuristics and associated errors is important because such understanding can often lead to more accurate diagnoses (Arkes, 1981; Tversky & Kahneman, 1974; Willis & Gelardo, 1984). Many diagnostic errors are related to heuristics associated with the three contradistinctions previously noted between actuarial and clinical approaches to neuropsychological diagnosis (see Table 1).

First, when probabilities of relationships between assessment data and diagnoses are derived on the basis of prior experience, clinicians often rely on heuristics involving the degree to which a particular case is representative of a neuropsychological diagnostic category. The use of such heuristics, however, is frequently associated with dangerous stereotypes of particular diagnostic groups and an insensitivity to the actual prevalence of the neuropsychological impairment in the population of interest (Kahneman & Tversky, 1973). Moreover, experientially derived probabilities are also likely to be influenced by biases due to the clinician's selective retrievability of prior cases. This selective retrievability may be affected by factors such as familiarity and salience (Tversky & Kahneman, 1973) in contrast to more appropriate factors (in terms of neuropsychodiagnostic accuracy) such as frequency and probability.

Second, when various sources of assessment data are considered in an independent fashion, the interdependent nature of those data are not recognized. Consequently, two highly correlated sources of assessment information may be weighted doubly in terms of their contributions to a diagnostic prediction. Further, there may be a tendency to express more confidence in such a prediction when the assessment data to be combined are highly congruent. Such congruence is rarely interpreted as redundancy, although if it were, clinicians would probably realize that a diagnostic prediction based on independent assessment data is more likely to be accurate than a prediction based on correlated measures (Kahneman & Tversky, 1973). Diagnostic errors arising from considering assessment data in an independent fashion are thus related to heuristics associated with overconfidence in diagnoses based on congruent assessment information. Here, the predictive accuracy of a diagnosis cannot be determined by summing the squared simple correlation coefficients between that diagnosis and particular sources of assessment data. This is because the intercorrelations among the assessment data are likely to be greater than 0. Although difficult to accomplish in the absence of actuarial aides, simultaneous consideration of assessment data appropriately reduces such a spuriously inflated sum by the degree to which those data are congruent.

Finally, when a particular source of assessment data is weighted differentially for each case, neuropsychological diagnoses are influenced by potential biases. The implicit assumption underlying the subjective manipulation of weights (i.e., degrees of importance attributed to particular data) is that the data are differentially predictive of neuropsychological diagnoses depending on unique circumstances surrounding individual cases. When the perceived correlation between assessment data and diagnosis is derived by the clinician in the absence of empirical techniques, however, that correlation is likely to be illusory (Chapman, 1967; Chapman & Chapman, 1967, 1969; Golding & Rorer, 1972; Kurtz & Garfield, 1978; Lueger & Petzel, 1979; Starr & Katkin, 1969) or at least subject to the influences of selective retrievability of prior cases. Errors inherent within this kind of logic are well illustrated by misguided attempts to adjust psychometric measures for particular minority groups (Mercer & Lewis, 1978) even though the predictive accuracy of those measures is often comparable across those groups (e.g., Jensen, 1973; Mitchell, 1967; Scarr-Salapatek, 1971).

Arkes (1981) suggested three strategies to minimize the impact of cognitive heuristics such as these on clinical judgment: (1) actively considering alternative diagnostic outcomes, (2) decreasing reliance on memory, and (3) focusing attention on data that are often ignored, such as population base rates. The latter suggestion has received recent empirical support (Willis & Gelardo, 1984), at least in a psychodiagnostic analogue situation. Preservice psychologists improved psychodiagnostic accuracy subsequent to training in Bayesian statistics that required active consideration of base-rate information. All three of these suggestions have the potential to improve diagnostic accuracy, primarily by reducing errors associated with cognitive heuristics that often bias clinical judgment. Continued empirical studies will be useful in testing this assumption.

Confounding Influences

Finally, wise clinical judgment demands that assessment information be aggregated over different sources, methods, and settings. Such aggregation reduces confounding influences that may be present in the neuropsychological evaluation and therefore minimizes the probability of misrepresenting a child's impairment through an inaccurate diagnosis. Three important environments in which children interact are the clinic, home, and school. Although most pediatric neuropsychologists are cognizant of the potentially limited generalizability of particular clinic behaviors to these other two settings, such cognizance often does not enter into diagnostic decisions. Even when the home and school environments are assessed, the source and method of assessment are frequently confounded with the setting in which it occurs. For example, pediatric neuropsychologists may use clinical judgment to integrate standardized assessment measures collected by themselves or their technicians in the clinic, interview information from parents pertaining to the home, and observational or rating scales from teachers pertaining to the school.

Given this kind of procedure, potential neurobehavioral differences may be associated with source, method, setting, or some combination of these factors. Unless efforts are made to reduce the inherent confounding influence, such as using multiple sources and methods for assessment in each setting, it is inappropriate to attribute such potential differences to a single factor. As the amount of assessment data increases, however, neuropsychologists who rely on clinical judgment should exercise greater caution in integrating those data so that duplicative information is not overly weighted in terms of its contribution to the diagnostic prediction. Appropriately collecting and integrating assessment information from multiple sources, methods, and settings is an expensive and time-consuming procedure but is probably cost-effective in most cases because of its potential for more accurate neuropsychological diagnoses than less comprehensive evaluations.

SUMMARY

Both actuarial and clinical approaches to diagnosis are necessary in current pediatric neuropsychological practice. These two approaches are distinguished primarily in terms of the fashions in which assessment information collected from a patient is integrated. For actuarial approaches, data integration is statistical; for clinical approaches, data integration is subjective.

The relative superiority of actuarial over clinical approaches has been well documented in terms of diagnostic accuracy. Supporting research, however, generally assumes that actuarial rules are free from methodological flaws. This assumption is frequently violated in clinical practice, and pediatric neuropsychologists must evaluate actuarial rules developed through various multivariate methods in terms of (1) their stability when applied to new patients, (2) the validity and generalizability of measures used to establish criterion groups, and (3) base rates of neuropsychological impairments in populations of interest.

Typically, good diagnostic decisions are based on both actuarial and clinical factors. Clinical judgment, however, can often lead to misdiagnoses unless clinicians are cognizant of and endeavor to minimize factors that frequently contribute to diagnostic errors. Those factors include inconsistent or inappropriate nomothetic and idiograthic interpretations of standardized neuropsychological measures, common cognitive heuristics associated with the clinical approach to diagnosis, and failure to eliminate the confounding influences of sources, methods, and settings in neuropsychological assessments. Proper evaluations of actuarial rules combined with appropriate clinical judgment may lead to a greater degree of neuropsychodiagnostic accuracy than either approach in isolation.

REFERENCES

Anthony, W. Z., Heaton, R. K., & Lehman, R. A. W. (1980). An attempt to cross-validate two actuarial systems for neuropsychological test interpretation. *Journal of Consulting and Clinical Psychology, 48,* 317–326.

Arkes, H. R. (1981). Impediments to accurate clinical judgment and possible ways to minimize their impact. *Journal of Consulting and Clinical Psychology, 3,* 323–330.

Cattin, P. (1980). Note on the estimation of the squared cross-validated multiple correlation of a regression model. *Psychological Bulletin, 87,* 63–65.

Chapman, L. (1967). Illusory correlation in observational report. *Journal of Verbal Learning and Verbal Behavior, 6,* 151–155.

Chapman, L., & Chapman, J. (1967). Genesis of popular but erroneous psychodiagnostic observations. *Journal of Abnormal Psychology, 72,* 193–204.

Chapman, L., & Chapman, J. (1969). Illusory correlation as an obstacle to the use of valid psychodiagnostic signs. *Journal of Abnormal Psychology, 74,* 271–280.

Fletcher, J. M., Rice, W. J., & Ray, R. M. (1978). Linear discriminant function analysis in neuropsychological research: Some uses and abuses. *Cortex, 14,* 564–577.

Goldberg, L. R., & Wertz, C. E. (1966). The reliability of clinical judgments: A multitrait–multimethod approach. *Journal of Consulting Psychology, 30,* 199–206.

Golden, C. J., Hammeke, T., & Purisch, T. (1980). *Luria–Nebraska Neuropsychological Battery.* Los Angeles: Western Psychological Services.

Golding, S. G., & Rorer, L. (1972). Illusory correlation and subjective judgment. *Journal of Abnormal Psychology, 80,* 249–260.

Goldstein, G., & Shelly, C. H. (1973). Univariate vs. multivariate analysis in neuropsychological test assessment of lateralized brain damage. *Cortex, 9,* 204–216.

Goldstein, G., & Shelly, C. H. (1982). A further attempt to cross-validate the Russell, Neuringer, and Goldstein neuropsychological keys. *Journal of Consulting and Clinical Psychology, 50,* 721–726.

Herzberg, P. A. (1969). The parameters of cross-validation. *Psychometrika, Monograph Supplement* (No. 16).

Huberty, C. J. (1975). Discriminant analysis. *Review of Educational Research, 45,* 543–598.

Huberty, C. J. (1984). Issues in the use and interpretation of discriminant analysis. *Psychological Bulletin, 95,* 156–171.

Hynd, G. W., & Obrzut, J. E. (Eds.). (1981). *Neuropsychological assessment and the school-age child.* New York: Grune & Stratton.

Jensen, A. (1973). *Education and group differences.* New York: Harper & Row.

Kahneman, D., & Tversky, A. (1973). On the psychology of prediction. *Psychological Review, 80,* 237–251.

Kaufman, A. S. (1979). WISC-R research: Implications for interpretation. *School Psychology Digest, 8,* 5–27.

Kaufman, A. S., & Kaufman, N. L. (1983). *Kaufman Assessment Battery for Children.* Circle Pines, MN: American Guidance Service.

Kurtz, R. M., & Garfield, S. L. (1978). Illusory correlation: A further exploration of Chapman's paradigm. *Journal of Consulting and Clinical Psychology, 46,* 1009–1015.

Lachenbruch, P. A. (1967). An almost unbiased method of obtaining confidence intervals for the probability of misclassification in discriminant analysis. *Biometrics, 23,* 639–645.

Lueger, R. J., & Petzel, T. P. (1979). Illusory correlation in clinical judgment: Effects of amount of information to be processed. *Journal of Consulting and Clinical Psychology, 47,* 1120–1121.

Luria, A. R. (1980). *Higher cortical functions in man.* New York: Basic Books.

McDermott, P. A. (1981). Sources of error in the psychoeducational diagnosis of children. *Journal of School Psychology, 19,* 31–44.

McDermott, P. A. (1982). Actuarial assessment for the grouping and classification of school children. In C. R. Reynolds & T. B. Gutkin (Eds.), *The handbook for school psychology* (pp. 243–272). New York: Wiley.

Meehl, P. E. (1954). *Clinical versus statistical prediction: A theoretical analysis and a review of the evidence.* Minneapolis: University of Minnesota Press.

Meehl, P. E. (1973). *Psychodiagnosis: Selected papers.* Minneapolis: University of Minnesota Press.

Meehl, P. E., & Rosen, A. (1955). Antecedent probability and the efficiency of psychometric signs, patterns, or cutting scores. *Psychological Bulletin, 52,* 194–216.

Mercer, J. R., & Lewis, J. F. (1978). *System of Mulicultural Pluralistic Assessment.* New York: Psychological Corporation.

Mitchell, B. (1967). Predictive validity of the Metropolitan Readiness Test and the Murphy–Durrell Reading Readiness Analysis for white and Negro pupils. *Educational and Psychological Measurement, 27,* 1047–1054.

Mosier, C. I. (1951). Problems and designs of cross-validation. *Educational and Psychological Measurement, 11,* 5–11.

Pedhazur, E. J. (1982). *Multiple regression in behavioral research* (2nd ed.). New York: Holt, Rinehart & Winston.

Phelan, J. G. (1964). Rationale employed by clinical psychologists in diagnostic judgment. *Journal of Clinical Psychology, 20,* 454–458.

Reynolds, C. R. (1982). Determining statistically reliable strengths and weaknesses in the performance of single individuals on the Luria–Nebraska Neuropsychological Battery. *Journal of Consulting and Clinical Psychology, 50,* 525–529.

Reynolds, C. R., & Clark, J. H. (1983). Assessment of cognitive abilities. In K. D. Paget & B. A. Bracken (Eds.), *The psychoeducational assessment of preschool children* (pp. 163–189). New York: Grune & Stratton.

Reynolds, C. R., & Gutkin, T. B. (1981). Statistics for the interpretation of Bannatyne reorganizations of WPPSI subtests. *Journal of Learning Disabilities, 14,* 446–467.

Russell, E. W., Neuringer, C., & Goldstein, G. (1970). *Assessment of brain damage: A neuropsychological approach.* New York: Wiley.

Sawyer, J. (1966). Measurement and prediction, clinical and statistical. *Psychological Bulletin, 66*, 178–200.

Scarr-Salapatek, S. (1971). Race, social class, and IQ. *Science, 174*, 1285–1295.

Selz, M. (1981). Halstead–Reitan neuropsychological test batteries for children. In G. W. Hynd & J. E. Obrzut (Eds.), *Neuropsychological assessment and the school-age child: Issues and procedures* (pp. 195–235). New York: Grune & Stratton.

Shelly, C., & Goldstein, G. (1982). Psychometric relations between the Luria–Nebraska and Halstead–Reitan in a neuropsychiatric setting. *Clinical Neuropsychology, 7*, 128–133.

Snow, J., & Hynd, G. W. (1984). Determining neuropsychological "strengths" and "weaknesses" on the Luria–Nebraska: Good practice or wishful thinking? *Journal of Consulting and Clinical Psychology, 52*, 695–696.

Starr, J. G., & Katkin, E. (1969). The clinician as an aberrant actuary: Illusory correlation and the Incomplete Sentence Blank. *Journal of Abnormal Psychology, 74*, 670–675.

Swiercinsky, D. P., & Warnock, J. K. (1977). Comparison of the neuropsychological key and discriminant analysis approaches in predicting cerebral damage and localization. *Journal of Consulting and Clinical Psychology, 45*, 808–814.

Tryon, R. C., & Bailey, D. E. (1970). *Cluster analysis*. New York: McGraw-Hill.

Tversky, A., & Kahneman, D. (1973). Availability: A heuristic for judging frequency and probability. *Cognitive Psychology, 5*, 207–232.

Tversky, A., & Kahneman, D. (1974). Judgment under uncertainty: Heuristics and biases. *Science, 185*, 1124–1131.

Wallach, M. S., & Schoof, K. (1965). Reliability of degree of disturbance rating. *Journal of Clinical Psychology, 21*, 273–275.

Wedding, D. (1983). Comparison of statistical and actuarial models for predicting lateralization of brain damage. *Clinical Neuropsychology, 5*, 15–20.

Willis, W. G. (1984). Reanalysis of an actuarial approach to neuropsychological diagnosis in consideration of base rates. *Journal of Consulting and Clinical Psychology, 52*, 567–569.

Willis, W. G., & Gelardo, M. S. (1984). Clinical judgment and school psychology: A technique for improving accuracy [Summary]. *Proceedings of the 16th Annual Convention of the National Association of School Psychologists*, 310–311.

Willson, V. L., & Reynolds, C. R. (1982). Methodological and statistical problems in determining membership in clinical populations. *Clinical Neuropsychology, 4*, 134–138.

Part III

Intervention and Treatment

Chapter 10

Educational Intervention in Children with Developmental Learning Disorders

CYNTHIA R. HYND

Division of Developmental Studies
Georgia State University
Atlanta, Georgia 30303

INTRODUCTION

Neuropsychologists often find themselves in the position of having to make pertinent recommendations for treatment of subjects that have been diagnosed as having neurologically based learning problems. Instructors of students with learning disabilities often complain that, although theoretical discussions by neuropsychologists are provocative in terms of adding to their understanding of the underlying problem, they often have little to do with the practical apsects involved in working with these children on a day-to-day basis. The translation of theory into practice is slow and often hampered by the fact that many neuropsychologists are not trained in instructional methodology. Another problem is that the variability of human behavior is so great that research aimed at testing the efficacy of instructional methodology has been equivocal. It is true that neuropsy-

265

CHILD NEUROPSYCHOLOGY, VOL. 2
Copyright © 1986 by Academic Press, Inc.
All rights of reproduction in any form reserved.

chological research has not yet provided us with definitive answers to theoretical issues in a detailed enough manner to provide us with clearcut treatment programs that have been proven successful. However, treatment must take place. It would seem infinitely more reasonable to pursue a course of treatment grounded in theory than to pursue a course of treatment based on the promises of materials-publishers that their programs will work.

This chapter, then, attempts briefly to discuss the current research and theory regarding neuroanatomical correlates of learning and then to demonstrate how this knowledge can be used to provide a basis for instructional decision making. It is not claimed that the instructional decisions made for purposes of illustration in this chapter have been proven by research to be effective. Rather, the teaching techniques and strategies offered in illustration are discussed in terms of what appears to make sense when an instructor tries to match materials and techniques to a particular style of learner. While the chapter deals with developmental reading disorders, the methods discussed could be applied just as easily to instruction of children with acquired disorders, because the neuroanatomical correlates of acquired and developmental dyslexia are, in many cases similar.

The areas of theoretical importance that are discussed include the research relating to (1) neuroanatomical functioning, (2) subtyping, and (3) aptitude–treatment interactions. As much of this research has been mentioned in other chapters in this volume, these discussions are necessarily brief.

The section dealing with practical applications to theory include a discussion of (1) the rationale for using particular approaches with certain populations, (2) the process involved in decision making; and (3) a number of strategies that can be used with these populations.

Because reading is of such critical importance and is so very often the major problem in children with learning disabilities, this chapter focuses on the research in the neuroanatomical basis of reading and its practical implications. It is believed, however, that the same type of decision-making process can be used in any instructional endeavor if it is based on a solid knowledge of neuropsychological theory.

THE RESEARCH RELATING TO
BRAIN–BEHAVIOR RELATIONS

Recent neuropsychological research has contributed to our theoretical understanding of brain–behavior relations as they relate to learning, particularly reading. However, in the past our understanding of brain-behavior relations has been confusing at best. Morgan (1896), Bastian (1898), and Hinshelwood (1900, 1902, 1909) provided evidence for the idea that neurodevelopmental deficits in the region of the angular gyrus were responsible for congenital word blindness. Their evidence was used to advance a strict localizationist perspective. Lashley (1938), on the other hand, provided evidence that brain function was not so neatly localized. His work suggested that the brain acted as a whole, and he advanced the notion of mass action. The idea of a reading center in the brain (i.e., the angular gyrus) appeared to be discounted by mass-actionist theory. Orton (1937) further complicated matters by suggesting that reading problems resulted from incomplete establishment of cerebral dominance for language function, allowing the two cerebral hemispheres to compete in the interpretation of visual stimuli.

Current work regarding neuroanatomical correlates of reading, however, suggests that neither a strict localizationist perspective nor a mass-actionist perspective is quite correct. And research has not supported the notion of incomplete cerebral dominance (Berlin, Hughes, Lowe-Bell, & Berlin, 1973; Hynd & Obrzut, 1977). Electrical mapping research with disabled readers (Duffy, Denkla, Bartels, & Sandini, 1980) and autopsy studies of dyslexic brains (Galaburda & Kemper, 1979; Galaburda, Sherman, & Geschwind, in press) have, rather, supported the notion that some basic functions, such as vision, sensation, and coordination, are fairly well localized, but that higher-level processes are not. Rather, higher mental processing such as reading takes place through the interaction of several localized cortical zones. The interaction of these zones forms a functional cognitive system. The functional system for reading, for instance, includes localized areas in both the right and the left hemispheres because reading requires the integration of visual perception, imagery, auditory perception, linguistic awareness, memory, and expression, to name but a few. If there is a weak point in this functional system, then the reading process begins to break down (Hynd & Hynd, 1984).

The question is what causes the weak point in this system. Evidence from autopsy studies suggests that structural abnormalities in brain tissue are present in the brains of dyslexic subjects (Galaburda & Kemper, 1979). These abnormalities could, hypothetically, be genetic, be brought about through lack of stimulation, be caused by some type of viral infection, et cetera. In other words, learning problems may be the result of brain damage, but they may also be the result of brain *difference*. In fact, the genetic nature of a fairly large percentage of reading disabilities is fairly well documented (Sladen, 1970; Decker & Defries, 1981).

If learning disabled children suffer some developmental deficit caused by any number of etiologies, then there should also be any number of possibilities as to the location and type of deficit in terms of central nervous system (CNS) functioning, especially if one assumes that these deficits manifest themselves in a somewhat random fashion (Hynd & Hynd, 1984). Therefore, it would seem unwise to say that all dyslexics, for instance, have the same disorder. There probably exists a number of different types of disorders that manifest themselves in an extreme difficulty with reading. Therefore, research that has been done to identify subtypes of reading disabilities is of interest.

SUBTYPES OF READING DISABILITY

Many researchers, because of the extension of knowledge concerning neuropsychological correlates of reading, have modified their views concerning the nature of neurologically based reading disabilities. Reading disability is no longer regarded as a heterogeneous disorder. In fact, numerous subtypes have been identified. The number of subtypes identified by any one study ranges from two (Pirozzolo, 1979) to six (Lyon & Watson, 1981), depending on the theoretical construct used in determining them.

At times, subtypes have been determined on the basis of a number of psychological variables (Petrauskas & Rourke, 1979). In these studies, there has generally been a failure to evaluate the reading dysfunction in detail. Other studies have determined subtypes on the basis of some measure of reading. In these studies, there has generally been a failure to integrate the results with the neuropsychological variables. In nearly all studies, subtypes have been determined without examining the full extent of phonological, graphological, motor, semantic, syntactic, and schematic aspects to successful reading and comprehension of text. With the amount of variability evident in the methods of determining subtypes, it is surprising to find a great deal of agreement in their results. Most subtype researchers would agree that there are basically three types of dyslexia: one involving difficulty with sound–symbol relations, which may include other language difficulties; one involving difficulty with the visuospatial aspects of reading; and a mixed type.

These results would be encouraging if they lent themselves to practical implications. However, the researchers have, as mentioned, based their findings on a rather distorted view of reading, in that they make their subtyping decisions on the basis of performance on measures of oral reading or spelling of single words (i.e., the Wide Range Achievement Test [WRAT] [Jastak & Jastak, 1978] or the Boder [Boder & Jerrico, 1982]) or on the basis of underlying psychological variables. Because of this distorted view, they are tied to beginning-reading instruction aimed at teaching successful word calling, using either a phonological or sight-word approach. They do not deal at all with the variable of comprehension or the role of context.

It seems much more logical to first analyze reading subskills or variables, find students who are deficient in these variables, and then study these students in depth using neuropsychological measures. It makes more sense to do this because we know from reading research that (1) comprehension of text can take place even when a child may have difficulty reading orally (Furniss & Graves, 1980); (2) a child who can read orally does not necessarily have good comprehension; (3) what a child comprehends when reading orally may be different from what he or she comprehends when reading silently (Harris & Sipay, 1975; Spache, 1973); (4) based on how much prior knowledge a child has concerning a topic, a child's reading and understanding of two otherwise equivalent passages may be vastly different (Pearson & Spiro, 1982); (5) the reading of connected discourse is much different from the reading of single words (Graesser, 1981); and (6) reading is a recursive rather than a sequential process in which confirmation or revision of predictions takes place constantly (Goodman, 1968).

Knowing these things about reading, it seems that researchers could construct more meaningful subtypes of reading-disabled populations. If students are found deficient in specific aspects of the reading act, then these findings could possibly be used to construct some well-defined neuropsychological models of reading.

Actually researchers who focus on the acquired alexias in adults have already enjoyed some success using just such an approach (Kertesz, 1979, 1983; Marshall & Newcombe, 1973). They base their breakdown of reading variables on a psycholinguistic–information-processing model introduced by Marshall and Newcomb (1973, 1980) and elaborated by cognitive psychologists and neuropsychologists. They have defined disorders in terms of symptom complexes and then related them to anatomically based models by correlating a subject's symptom complexes with the site of his or her lesion (Kertesz, 1983). These symptom complexes still do not adequately describe all the variability observed in many children. There are developmental issues in trying to compare the symptoms of adult readers to those of children who are still in the process of learning to read. Bakker (1973), for instance has found a shifting of attention from one cerebral hemisphere to another in the course of learning to rely on different reading strategies. The researchers using this model, too, are still too concerned with individual words rather than with connected discourse. But they do take into account semantic and syntactic variables—hence, the role of comprehension of text. With an approach such as this, one can move beyond the typical recommendations for a phonetic or a sight-word approach when discussing implications for rehabilitation based on research.

Marshall (1984) holds this same view. He states that the subtyping literature heretofore has been based on

> groups of children with reading disorder, where the grouping is determined by the associated symptomatology. Such taxonomies typically fail to specify in any detail the precise *nature* of the reading disorder that the children mainfest; they also fail to establish whether the associated deficits constitute necessary and/or sufficient conditions for the emergence of reading impairment. Such group studies are severely limited in terms of both the theoretical insight that they generate and the practical value of whatever therapeutic measures they may suggest. (p. 46)

It is believed that the understanding of neuropsychologically based reading disorders must be based on an approach that takes into account the type of reading symptomatology first. This can be accomplished by observations of disabled and good readers at several developmental levels, using measures of not only word recognition but also of vocabulary knowledge, comprehension of connected text read both orally and silently, and some assessment of prior knowledge. If subtypes were statistically derived using such measures, the students exhibiting these subtypes could be studied in depth for commonalities in deficiencies of cerebral processing. This has not been done. Still, as said before, instruction must take place. Those in charge of treatment are left in the difficult position of having to make theoretically based instructional decisions before the theory is well-enough articulated.

It makes sense, however, that the neurolinguists appear to be on the right track in their work with adults. Although it cannot be assumed that children have the same anatomically based disorders as adults, it seems reasonable that, when children and adults have similar difficulties, we could profit by having similar classification schemes. Marshall (1984), having done considerable research into psycholinguistic subtyping to the acquired alexias, has attempted to relate the categories of acquired alexia to those that have been studied in terms of developmental dyslexia. He suggests several classifications that are pertinent to developmental dyslexia, in that cases have been reported in the literature suggesting these syndromes. The subtypes are (1) developmental surface dyslexia; (2) developmental direct dyslexia; (3) developmental phonological dyslexia; and (4) developmental deep dyslexia. These subtypes, because of their amenability to practical applications of instructional techniques, are discussed in some detail.

Developmental Surface Dyslexia

The reading of someone with surface dyslexia is characterized by an ability to read phonologically regular words, and even nonwords, but an inability or difficulty reading irregular words. These dyslexics find whole-word recognition difficult. In fact, the route from visual analysis of the word to whole-word recognition is essentially unavailable. Holmes (1973) notes that some children with developmental reading disorders found the context-sensitive nature of English text to be a main stumbling block. Researchers concerned with the adult alexias have also found that the surface dyslexic has difficulty using context clues to aid in word recognition. Comprehension presents a difficulty for these readers. Understanding necessarily only occurs after each word has been phonologically decoded. These readers can often read phonetically regular text better orally than silently.

Developmental Direct Dyslexia

In the acquired version of direct dyslexia, it appears that the central linguistic core is disconnected from whole-word recognition. In other words, patients with direct dyslexia can access print through phonological methods or by whole-word recognition systems. However, linguistic analysis of words and comprehension are deficient. The person evidencing this syndrome would be an accomplished oral reader with poor comprehension. Children with this symptom have often been reported in the literature (McClure & Hynd, 1983; Silberberg & Silberburg, 1967) although the syndrome is sometimes called "hyperlexia." Children evidencing this syndrome are able to read aloud much better than they are able to comprehend what they are reading, and they often call words better than they are able to use language in general. They read nonwords and complex irregular—exception words well. However, the lexicosemantic system appears to be bypassed.

Developmental Phonological Dyslexia

This syndrome in adults is characterized by the ability to read familiar words well (especially nouns) but difficulty with phoneme–grapheme correspondence—the application of a phonetic system. Some of these patients also have difficulty with multimorphemic words, in that prefixes and suffixes are often added, dropped, or substituted. However, other cases have been reported where this function was intact (Funnell, 1983). Function words, too, are sources of difficulty. Semantic errors are not a problem, however, and the phonological dyslexic has an average oral vocabulary. Reports of phonological dyslexia in children indicate that oral reading errors are either on words with close visual similarity to the target word or are derivational forms of the target word (Temple & Marshall, in press).

Developmental Deep Dyslexia

The reading of those with acquired deep dyslexia is characterized by difficulty with phoneme–grapheme correspondence, as is the case in phonological dyslexia. It is different from phonological dyslexia, however, in that derivational errors are common, and semantic substitutions do take place. It is often found that concrete nouns are read better than adjectives, verbs, or abstract nouns. Visual confusion errors are also common (e.g., mitten–mutton–sheep), and there is a reliance, according to some researchers, on imageability, concreteness, and word frequency. Finally, there is a context effect, in that subjects with this syndrome can use context clues as an aid to word recognition.

The two main differences in symptoms between phonological and deep dyslexia concern (1) the occurrence of semantic paralexias (e.g., mutton–sheep); and (2) the concrete/abstract dimension. It has been postulated that deep dyslexics, however, are reading by a completely different system, in particular one located in the right cerebral hemisphere (Coltheart, 1980, Saffran, Bogyo, Schwartz, & Martin, 1980). Indeed, deep dyslexics may read exclusively via the semantic–conceptual system.

Functional System of Reading

How does this classification system fit into neuropsychological knowledge concerning brain function and into educational knowledge concerning program placement and remediation? Concerning neuropsychological knowledge, it must be explained that, from electrophysiological data, autopsies, and isotope studies of alexic and dyslexic patients, a rudimentary functional system of reading has been postulated. This system presupposes that incoming visual stimuli (print) is registered in the occipital lobes, where associations are made between visual stimuli and letter strings which form words. The left and right occipital lobes both have this function, but it is believed that the right occipital lobe processes imageable or concrete words while the left may have more-abstract processing abilities. At that point, information is shared with input from other sensory modalities in the angular gyrus, where the temporal, occipital, and parietal lobes juncture. This area might be the region where phoneme–grapheme correspondence takes place. Linguistic–semantic comprehen-

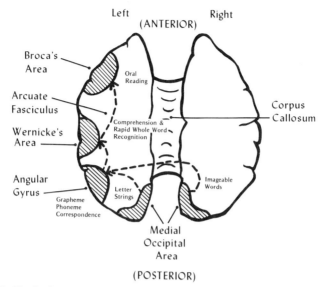

Figure 1. The brain as viewed in horizontal section. The major pathways and cortical regions thought to be involved in reading are depicted. Neurolinguistic processes important in reading are also noted. (From Hynd & Hynd, 1984; reprinted with permission).

sion is thought to be most affected by the region of the planum temporale, and the temporal lobe (Wernicke's area). Information concerning the location of syntactic grammatical disturbances (Kertesz, 1979) indicates that this type of disturbance may be more anterior, whereas semantic disturbances may be more posterior in this general region.

After semantic–syntactic information is shared with phoneme–grapheme information, it (in the case of oral reading) travels via the arcuate fasciculus to Broca's area (the area for speech), where oral reading takes place and the functional system is completed. It must be remembered that this model, while appearing sequential, is probably recursive, in that there may exist many feedback loops. Figure 1 illustrates this proposed functional system of reading.

While it is postulated that most brains are at least grossly organized in a similar fashion, it is likely that the efficiency of certain neural pathways varies considerably from one brain to the next, especially considering the brains of the severely reading disabled, and there are probably weak links to the functional reading chain that result in impaired reading processes. It is important to reiterate at this time that these weak links may be the result of several different factors, including megalovirus or genetic predisposition.

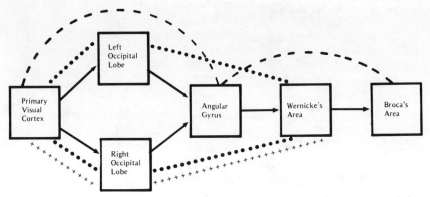

Figure 2. A neurolinguistic model of reading for the surface, phonological, and deep dyslexic (adapted and modified from Sevush, 1983). It should be emphasized that the phonological–nonphonological or visual–nonvisual components of these pattern types are only aspects of the pattern which also includes semantic, syntactic, and imageability components. However, the surface dyslexic could be said to access print through phonological or nonvisual modes. The phonological and deep dyslexic may access print through nonphonological or visual modes. (————), normal reading; (+ + +), deep dyslexia; (●●●), phonological dyslexia; (— — —), surface dyslexia. (From Hynd & Hynd, 1984; reprinted with permission).

Figure 2 offers a hypothetical anatomical view of how reading would seem to take place in subjects with the several aforementioned classifications of dyslexia. Note that the neural pathways are organized the same as in normal brains. It is only that the pathway(s) may be deficient in dyslexic brains, so that the systems depicted by this figure represent only how the reading process would appear to be taking place to an observer.

As to how this model and the neurolinguistic subtypes relate to treatment, there are two issues that must be considered. First, the issue of remediation versus compensation must be discussed, in that these two types of instruction could be characterized as opposites. Secondly, the issue of whether aptitude treatment interactions are positive enough to warrant certain types of treatment programs should be discussed. After these issues are considered, a model for planning treatment programs is offered.

ISSUES RELATING TO TREATMENT

Remediation versus Compensation

If subjects are assumed to have deficiency in learning due to a problem of neurologic origin, then it must also be assumed that, as stated previously, certain neural pathways are operating at depressed or nonfunctioning deficiency levels. It would make little sense, then, to try to teach the skill(s) subsumed by this pathway. Instructors are well aware of the child who has received literally years of instruction in phonics, but still is unable to correctly hear phonetic differences in sound. It is the contention of this author that those in charge of instruction have been involved in a useless activity. If the grapheme–phoneme correspondence system is deficient, then some other pathway to word recognition will need to take its place. Inherent in this argument is the idea of plasticity of function and the notion of neurodevelopmental deficits versus neurodevelopmental delays (Hynd & Hynd, 1984).

It has been documented that there is some plasticity of function when the brains of children are traumatized. In fact, it has been documented that there is often no loss of language function following left hemispherectomy of children suffering from severe cases of epilepsy (Annett, 1973). While this finding argues for the idea that surrounding tissue can take over the functions of diseased tissue, recent evidence suggests that severe trauma must be present for this condition to exist (St. James-Roberts, 1981). Even so, there will probably be slight to moderate deficiencies in the system that has been transferred to other tissue (Dennis, 1977; Levine, Hier, & Calvanio, 1981; Wilson & Wilson, 1980). It is likely, then, based upon the preceding findings, that, without some sort of severe trauma, the brain does not reorganize itself. Therefore, genetic or mild neurological deficiencies are likely to remain.

Indeed, Rapin (1982) says that the new techniques of studying cognitive function of the CNS allow us to tie behavior with brain function, and that these approaches have already "dealt a mortal blow to the idea of equipotentiality of the so-called association areas of the neocortex" (p. 181).

Annett (1973) found that even in infants suffering brain damage of the left hemisphere, plasticity of function is not complete. While the infant can learn to speak, linguistic tasks such as reading and spelling and the perception of complex visual patterns may remain difficult. He says, "it is safe to assume, nevertheless, that genetically determined broad programs for brain development are resistant to change. Therefore, common behavioral deficits in different individuals are more likely than not to reflect dysfunction in analogous systems" (p. 181).

The other issue deals with developmental lag versus developmental deficiency. It has been argued that there is a development of unilateral specialization for language in the left hemisphere as a child develops (Berlin et al., 1973; Lenneberg, 1967; Porter & Berlin, 1975; Satz, Bakker, Teunissen, Goebel, & Van der light, 1975). Others argue that left-hemisphere specialization does not develop slowly, but is present at birth

(Gilbert & Climan, 1974; Hynd & Obrzut, 1977; Kinsbourne & Hiscock, 1977, 1978; Molfese, Freeman, & Palermo, 1975; Schulman-Galambos, 1977). Supporters of developmental lag theories have based their notions on dichotic listening and clinical literature (Hécaen, 1976), and supporters of deficient processing theories have based their notions on dichotic listening, time sharing, and electrophysiological measurement.

Some poor readers do seem to improve dramatically in reading ability around the age of 9 or 10, and this improvement could seem to be indicative that these students had previously been victims of developmental lag and had finally caught up. While this may be true in some cases, it is the contention of this author that this surprising jump in reading ability may really be merely a reflection of the change in reading instruction that takes place around the fourth or fifth grade. At this point, the learning-to-read period, with its emphasis on phonetic word recognition strategies is essentially over, and the reading-to-learn stage is implemented. Silent reading largely replaces oral reading, so that pronunciation problems become less evident. Comprehension of the message is, in many cases, the main tested outcome of the reading lesson.

It will be recalled, both the phonologic and deep dyslexic reader has adequate comprehension for meaningful material and has the ability to use context clues to provide word meaning. Indeed, the deep dyslexic is often able to put words in the right categories or demonstrates knowing the concepts of words he is not able to pronounce. (He can point to a picture depicting the word but will call it something else in the same category.) Therefore, as long as this type of reader has sufficient prior knowledge of subject matter and has adequate vocabulary knowledge, he should be able to demonstrate adequate comprehension of silently read material. It is believed that it is in the case of these types of readers that reading disability appears to be overcome at a certain stage in the course of development.

Therefore, if we consider these two contentions—that (1) dyslexics suffer from deficient processing rather than delayed development of processing; and (2) dyslexics have very little hope of recovering function from neural pathways that are damaged or deficient, then one must conclude that remediation, in the sense of reteaching missed skills, will not be profitable. Trying to teach someone to break a word down into component phonetic units and then blend these components into words seems unprofitable when that process has been impaired because of neurologic abnormalities.

If the student is able to rapidly recognize whole words and morphemic units, then it may be possible to teach this student word recognition without relying on phonics. Putting the stress on meaningful word units seems infinitely more reasonable and profitable. The child who has experienced frustration at not being able to read can now read rudimentary material. Frustration decreases, the child reads more, automaticity develops, et cetera. This child may always experience problems. Experienced normal readers generally rely on phonics to attack unknown words rather than context, and this method of word attack will not be at this child's disposal. But, even though his reading may be somewhat more laborious, this student will be able to derive meaning from text. In other words, instruction, to be productive for learning disabled subjects, should be tailored for them on the basis of their known strengths in processing. These students should be taught to compensate for their impaired processes by using strategies based on strengths.

It may be that some remediation can be of benefit if taught using unique methods, however. For instance, a program such as Auditory Discrimination in Depth (A.D.D.) teaches a student auditory discrimination skills involving letters, but the process is uniquely different from the way phonics is taught in the public classroom, in that the child is taught to pay attention to visual information in terms of facial expressions when learning to reproduce sounds, much like a hard-of-hearing student is taught to speak. Other programs break down each task into small units. It may be that the load on the neurological system is reduced in this way, which may, in turn, make it easier for a weak localized area to perform at optimal level. These methods are exceptionally time consuming, and integrating such specialized learning into the total reading act still may be difficult. Most instructors at some point have observed children who had been drilled on phonics because of a disability in this area until they are actually somewhat skilled in reproducing the sounds of the letters or in breaking words down into their component phonetic parts. But, when these students are asked to apply phonic knowledge to the reading of connected discourse, they are unable to perform. Although the phonetic difficulty has been remediated, they still have reading problems, because of their inability to integrate this knowledge with the rest of the reading process. Because of these concerns, it is believed that caution must be used when using any remedial technique, in that this technique should probably be used only in conjunction with instruction founded on strength-based models and only after some reading fluency has been observed.

Aptitude–Treatment Interactions

Regarding aptitude–treatment interactions, Cronbach and Snow (1977) discussed at some length the rather disappointing results of investigations aimed at finding the right instructional strategies for the right populations. They concluded, however, that the search should not be abandoned, that the idea of programs fitting the needs of certain subgroups but not others was a sound one. They stated that the disappointing research may be because researchers have been looking at the wrong variables. It would be interesting to look at aptitude described previously in terms of the treatments described here subsequently. The following attempt to match instructional strategies with inferred neurological organization is, at this time, of a theoretical nature. It has not yet been proven that this system will work any better than putting all dyslexic children into one program and teaching them as if they had the same problem. It is hoped by offering this approach that research will be done that will either validate or invalidate its efficacy.

At this point, there needs to be a model for determining which educational strategy would be best for certain types of disorders. This model is based on the dyslexic subtypes previously mentioned and some reading strategies that are currently being used in classrooms around the country.

PROPOSED MODEL FOR TEACHING

The steps in the model area are as follows:

1. Determine a profile of strengths and weaknesses in the subject matter of concern. If known subtypes are available, try to classify the child into one subtype, noting peculiarities that do not fit.
2. Infer neurological processing that may be required for the normal performance of the task, using what research has shown about basic neurological organization (i.e., the functional system of reading previously mentioned).
3. Determine at what point the subject's processing breaks down in terms of this system. Determine the way the system appears to function for the child (i.e., as in Figure 2).
4. Find instructional strategies that match the student's specific learning style.

These steps, while simply put, may be difficult to follow without a great deal of knowledge at one's disposal concerning both cerebral organization and instructional strategies. Obviously, more-specific information about the functional system of reading would be more helpful in finding or designing adequate programs. However, we must use what knowledge we have at hand to begin testing our ideas. If what we derive from our investigation works, then we are validating the usefulness of the theory.

Instructional Strategies—Dyslexic Subtypes

Table 1 is a listing of a number of techniques commonly used to teach word recognition and comprehension of text (C. Hynd & G. Hynd, 1984). To the right of this list are the neurolinguistic subtypes described previously. The purpose of this table is to demonstrate which subtypes would profit from each instructional technique based upon a compensatory model. As can be seen, neurolinguistic subtypes lend themselves to instruction in comprehension.

Many of these techniques will seem familiar to reading or learning-disabilities instructors. However, because some of these may not be, further explanation is necessary.

Word-Recognition Approaches

Crossmodal

Regarding word recognition instruction, there are several methods that are said to be crossmodal—that is, requiring the use of several sensory modalities. The rationale for this type of approach is that weak modalities will be strengthened by being paired with strong modalities (i.e., a visual-processing deficit would be strengthened by adding a kinesthetic component to the word-recognition task. The child not only sees the word, but traces it. Recent research has provided evidence that seeing, tracing, spelling, then saying the word is most effective for a group of undifferentiated dyslexic children. (Hulme & Bradley, 1984).

The explanation the author gives for this finding is that phonological encoding is bypassed using this method. It can be fairly safely assumed that most of these children had difficulty with grapheme–phoneme correspondence, because surface dyslexia is considered to be rather rare in children, compared to auditory–linguistic types of dyslexia (phonological or deep dyslexia) (Pirozzolo, 1979). It also makes sense from a neurological perspective. Children with phonological or deep dyslexia have functional systems that appear to bypass the angular gyrus (the area of phoneme–grapheme correspondence), so this aspect of word recognition would be the weak link in the chain.

It can be seen that crossmodal systems as a whole could be adapted to any of the subtypes listed, based on variations that are used. The *VAKT* (visual, auditory, kinesthetic, and tactile) approach (Fernald, 1943) involves each of these modalities. The child looks at the word, says the word, and traces it on a rough surface (tactile and kinesthetic). This method would be best for dyslexics whose rapid whole-word recognition systems were intact.

TABLE 1

Remediation based on strength/compensatory model

Treatment method	Surface dyslexia	Deep dyslexia	Phono-logical dyslexia	Direct dyslexia	Dysnomia/dysphasia[d]
Word recognition					
Crossmodal[a]	Yes	Yes	Yes	Yes	Yes
VAKT					
Aaron's seven-step method					
Cunningham's method					
Visual–Imageable	No	Yes	Yes	Yes [b]	Yes
Whole-word					
Fading					
Sight-vocabulary (Edmark)					
Syllabary					
Rebus readers					
Phonetic	Yes	No	No	Yes[b]	No
Distar					
Orton-Gillingham					
Hegge-Kirk & Kirk					
Letter strings or linguistic					
Linguistic-spelling patterns	Yes	No	Yes	Yes	NA
Morphemic Analysis	No	Yes	Yes	Yes	NA
Context Clues	No	Yes	Yes	No	NA
Compare–contrast	Yes	No	No	Yes	NA
Comprehension					
Visual	No	Yes	Yes	No	Yes
Structured overviews					
Herringbone					
Schema-Based	Yes	Yes	Yes	No	No
Language experience					
List-group-label					
Possible sentences					
Anticipation–reaction					
Directed reading–thinking activity (DRTA)					
Visual/Language Based					
Auditory Discrimination in Depth (A.D.D.)	Yes[b]	Yes[c]	Yes	Yes[b]	Yes[c]
Fitzgerald keys	No	Yes	Yes[b]	No	Yes
McGinnis	Yes	No	No	Yes[b]	Yes[c]

TABLE 1 (*Continued*)

Treatment method	Surface dyslexia	Deep dyslexia	Phono-logical dyslexia	Direct dyslexia	Dysnomia/dysphasia[d]
Compensatory					
Glossing	Yes	Yes	Yes	Yes	NA
Slicing	Yes	Yes	Yes	Yes	NA
Guided listening	Yes	No	Yes	Yes	NA
Guide-o-rama	Yes	Yes	Yes	Yes	NA

[a] Depending on modifications, can be adapted to most subtypes.
[b] not necessary
[c] used with difficulty
[d] Abbreviation NA = Not Applicable

Aaron's (n.d.) seven-step method of word recognition involves the following: (1) The word is said by the examiner and put into a meaningful context (language development). (2) The child is asked to say the word (visual/auditory memory). (3) He is shown (visuospatial analysis) several versions of the word, which have letters missing, wrong, or reversed, and is asked to supply what is in error and say the word correctly. Then several versions of the word are orally spelled with errors (auditory analysis) and read with missing letters or syllables and the child is asked to supply what is missing. (4) The child says the word when it is flashed (speeded recall). (5) The child traces (kinesthetic–tactile) the word and writes it from memory. (6) He demonstrates knowledge of word meaning by reading the word in context (in a language experience story, a basal reader, or a rebus). (7) Finally, he demonstrates comprehension of the word in written context. This method, as one can see, uses most available modalities and requires the reader to use visuospatial information as well as phonetic information to demonstrate knowledge of the word. It can, however, be adapted to either a surface dyslexic or a phonological dyslexic. The surface dyslexic might not be required to complete all of Step 3, or Step 3 could be made more kinesthetically oriented. The phonological dyslexic might bypass the last part of Step 3. It is unlikely that the hyperlexic would need word-recognition instruction this tedious, but he could perform well on all steps except the last, where the hyperlexic would be required to put the word in context, and hence demonstrate understanding of the meaning of the word. This step could be made more concrete by using a picture or a diagram in step one. The reliance on word meaning, particularly if the word were more concrete, would be helpful to the deep dyslexic, as would tying the other steps to the kinesthetic modality.

P. M. Cunningham's (1980) method for word recognition is an adaptation of Aaron's seven-step method. The word is introduced in the context of a story, and the child holds up a word card with the target word on it every time he or she hears it in the story. Next, the child cuts the word up into individual letters and is required to spell the word using the scrambled letters. He writes the word from memory, puts it in written sentences, and, finally, uses it in a story. Again, this method would probably work best for students with phonological dyslexia because of its reliance on letter strings and the visual analysis of words. The deep dyslexic would need a graphic image of the word meaning such as a picture or a demonstration of the use of the word, so that he or she can access the word in question.

Visual–Imageable Approaches

Visual-imageable approaches to word recognition may rely more on the right hemisphere processing of words than do phonological approaches. *Whole-word* techniques, such as Look–Say, which are context based, and *fading* (where a word is presented with a picture and the picture is gradually removed) should work especially well with phonological and deep dyslexics. Concrete nouns will be the easiest for the deep dyslexic to master. If verbs, abstract nouns, prepositions, et cetera can be illustrated in some sort of graphic way, however, the student should be at a better advantage to learn these words.

Dinnan and Lodge (1976) content that many heretofore unteachable students can be taught to read if we abolish the notion of the function word. They believe that students should be taught that all words have meaning, and that the meaning can be demonstrated by pairing the word with its opposite and by later putting the word in its proper space along a spectrum or words. Dinnan and Lodge believe that words can be classified into having to do with matter, time, space, or amount. As an illustration, they say that *is* is a time word whose opposite is *was*. It would be placed in a continuum (e.g., was . . . is . . . will). Actually, this system has a great deal of merit for the phonological or deep dyslexic, because of its emphasis on meaning and categorization of words, which are areas of strength for these subtypes.

Sight–Vocabulary programs (i.e., Edmark Reading Program, Edmark Associates) are available that are as close to a pure visuospatial whole-word approach as one could possibly get. The method might be as follows: A word (e.g., *boy*) is presented and pronounced by the teacher and the student as the student points to the word. The direction of the teacher is to say, "Find 'boy.' Say 'boy.' " Then the word is paired with a very dissimilar word (e.g., "boy—forest") and the teacher says again, "Find 'boy.' Say 'boy.' " The number of words that are presented with the target word is increased and the visual differences are decreased until the child can pick out the word from five closely similar words. At this point, the child is required to demonstrate understanding of the meaning of the word. The child matches the word to a picture, reads it in a sentence, and reads a story that uses the word. The Edmark approach would be useful to the phonological or deep dyslexic. The hyperlexic would not need the intensive word recognition, but could profit from the approach to comprehension.

A *syllabary* (Gleitman & Rozin, 1973) is a pictorial representation of the syllables in a word. In a syllabary, the word *before* might be presented as 'b' 4. The rationale for this type of approach is that the reader could decode words by proceeding from known word parts to unknown word parts. This approach removes the phoneme–grapheme correspondence component to word identification. P. M. Cunningham (1975–1976) has demonstrated successfully that the use of the syllabary can be a means to improve word recognition skills, and Gleitman and Rozin (1973) recommend that the syllabary could be used as a word-recognition technique when students have an inability to master phonics.

To teach using this approach, the teacher might begin by depicting simple one-syllable words and word parts such as the aforementioned. When the student knows parts such as *pen, sill,* and *wind,* the parts could be combined to make words like *pencil, silly, windy, windowsill.* The store of words can gradually be increased in size, and the ability to use the words should become easier with practice. Of course, the words should be incorporated into an appropriate context when they are mastered. The syllabary approach would be useful for students whose linguistic awareness was not impaired. There could conceivably be some phonological or deep dyslexics who would not be able to recognize word parts as separate morphemic units that are in the memory store. The imageability and concreteness of these word parts is important for the deep dyslexic.

Rebus Readers (Woodcock, 1967) use a graphic approach to teaching reading; that is, pictorial and context clues are used to aid in the recognition of words. Words are actually made into pictures, much like in the syllabary approach, which are then systematically withdrawn to effect the transition to standard orthography. This system seems almost tailor-made for the deep dyslexic, who relies on context and imageability of words.

Phonetic Approaches

Phonetic approaches, on the other hand, are necessarily going to be more effective with the surface dyslexic who has the ability to read non-words through phonetic analysis better than reading real words that are phonologically irregular. Any method that breaks words down into phonological units and builds them back up through the use of well-established phonological rules (synthetic phonics) would be good for this group of disabled readers. Also, the hyperlexic would be able to profit from this approach, but because the hyperlexic's word-recognition skills are so developed, it is not likely that he or she would need such intensive instruction as the surface dyslexic.

Distar (Science Research Associates) is a widely used, extremely structured program that uses a letter-by-letter synthetic blending approach. The *Orton-Gillingham* method (Gillingham, 1970) is a multisensory approach that uses phonics as its base rather than the whole word, as does Fernald. The students are taught (1) the names and sounds of the letters; (2) to blend the letters into words; (3) to make sentences and stories using the words; and (4) to read other material. To teach letter names and sounds, teachers use flash cards and have students trace, then copy from memory each word. When they have learned the names and sounds of 10 letters, they blend these letters into words and keep them as they progress, learning more sounds and blending more words—learning one or two new sounds per day. When students can read and write phonetically regular three- and four-letter words, they begin reading simple, highly structured stories. They must read these stories silently first and are required to read without mistakes. After a major portion of the phonics program has ended, the student is allowed to pursue independent reading.

The *Hegge, Kirk, and Kirk (1970)* method is also a multisensory approach that relies on synthetic phonics as its base, emphasizing a sound blending and kinesthetic experience. The method proceeds as follows: After the student is instructed in blending, he reads orally long lists of words or word families containing the vowel sound under study. These drills contain all the reported common vowel sounds, consonant sounds, combination sounds, and advanced sounds. There are also supplementary exercises that deal with exceptions to the drills.

Example:

cat	mat	sat	rat	fat
can	man	pan	tan	fan
cap	tap	rap	sap	lap
tab	cab	gab	jab	nab

There are other synthetic phonics approaches that are not listed here. However, to be synthetic, they must all have the essential element of blending sounds into words. Only students who will be able to perform this task efficiently should use this technique. What this approach does is offer students a way to call words, regardless of their meanings. It is assumed that meaning will be attached to these words after the words are decoded. However, a word of caution must be stated. Surface dyslexics are generally poor comprehenders, as are hyperlexics. So, while a synthetic phonics approach may get these students calling words in a fairly short period of time, they will not be attending to the meaning of what they are reading. It is, therefore, imperative that these students be given comprehension instruction suitable to their disability from the moment in which reading instruction begins. Otherwise, *purposeful reading*—reading to get information or to be entertained—will be obscured, and reading will become nothing more than a word-calling exercise. (Comprehension instruction for the surface dyslexic is discussed later in some length.)

Letter Strings or Linguistic Approaches

Approaches using letter strings or patterns are used with the rationale that they provide help with pronunciation of words while making minimal use of phonics. Linguistic approaches were common in the 1960s, with the *Merrill-Lynch Linguistic Readers* being fairly popular in regular reading instruction. It is the linguistic approach that is used in text like "Dan sat in the tan van," and it is this approach that is at the base of many of the programmed reading materials also common in the late 1960s and early 1970s. The assumption is that there are word families, such as "at" that can be blended with beginning sound such as /b/, /c/, /f/, and /m/, to form words such as *bat, cat, fat,* and *mat*. Instruction is centered on discovering and using word patterns and then building on these known patterns with minimal variation. Although there are different ways word families can be used, the most common is the use of a medial-position word family, where building takes place on the first, then the last part of the word (Tierney, Readence, & Dishner, 1980).

Example: an   tan   ban   fan   tank   fang   bang

Certain prior concepts must be mastered for the word-family approach to work. Students must (1) have a small bank of known words, (2) be sensitive to rhymning words, and (3) know consonant sounds. They need the small bank of words to provide the known—so that they can generalize to the unknown. That is, if they know *bell,* they can also read *well, tell, fell,* et cetera. Secondly, they have to be able to see that the spelling patterns that are the same (e.g., *ell*) have the same sound. Finally, they have to be able to replace one consonant sound with another. Hence, they must know the sounds the consonants make. Following this model, surface dyslexics, hyperlexics, and some phonological dyslexics might profit from using this approach, but the deep dyslexic might not.

Structural or *morphemic analysis* deals with the breaking down of words into meaning units—prefixes, suffixes, and roots. There is some controversy in the literature about the phonological dyslexic's ability to use knowledge of suffixes and prefixes in word-recognition strategies. It appears that some may be able to and some may not. Many phonological and deep dyslexics are able to pick out meaningful parts of words. Therefore, the problem of using prefixes and suffixes might be that they have not been learned as units with meaning. If this is the case, it stands to reason that, if they are taught as meaningful units, this approach should be viable for use with these dyslexic subtypes. The strategy is especially helpful for longer words. When the student comes to a word he or she doesn't know, the student will break the word into its meaningful subunits, and then build the word back up again. For instance, the word *telephone* is broken into *tele,* meaning some kind of communication across distances, and *phone,* which has to do with sound. So a telephone is a device with which you can communicate over distances that involves sound.

Teaching the use of *context clues* to word recognition can be done by the fill-in-the-blank method. The student can be provided with sentences with one word or more missing. He would then be asked to guess what the word might be, based on the other words in the sentence. There could be more than one correct choice, or only one. Students could be provided with clues such as a first letter to the word, or be asked to pick the correct word from a list of distractors, depending on their skill levels. The emphasis is on word meanings.

There is another word-recognition strategy similar to the syllabary that needs to be mentioned. The *compare–contrast* strategy involves having the student learn a list of five key words such as *at, her, an,* and *went.* By using these words and consonant substitution, the student can read words such as *manner* (an-her) *serpent* (her-went), et cetera. When they have this strategy mastered, they can learn more key words in groups of five. The problem with this method is that it requires consonant substitution and is not meaning based. Deep dyslexics and some phonological dyslexics might not be able to use this technique, although surface dyslexics could. As said before, however, the surface dyslexic student should be taught comprehension using other methods (Tierney et al., 1980).

Comprehension Instruction

Visual Approaches

Regarding comprehension instruction, some approaches rely on a visual representation of abtract ideas, in the form of a graph, a chart, a diagram, et cetera. The rationale is that the visual representation will strengthen meaning by involving more spatial processing of the information. Hence, these approaches would be most beneficial to the phonological and deep dyslexic, who seem to be able to rely on right-hemisphere processing strategies.

Structured Overviews (Readence, Bean, & Baldwin, 1981; Earle & Baron, 1973), or graphic organizers, are comprehension devices that rely on visual organization of information found in text. They can be used in the teaching of technical vocabulary and in illustrating the relationships among concepts, and can be used both pre and postreading. The relationships can be of several types:

1. *Cause–effect:* The interrelationship of two or more events, objects, or ideas.

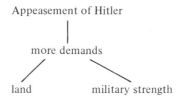

Tree 10.1

2. *Comparison–Contrast:* Similarities and differences among two or more events, objects, or ideas.

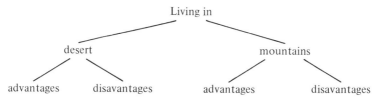

Tree 10.2

3. *Time Order:* Chronological ordering of two or more events, objects, or ideas.

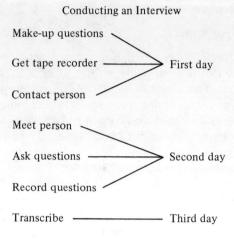

Conducting an Interview

Tree 10.3

4. *Simple listing:* Two or more objects, events, or ideas listed sequentially, according to the author's criteria.

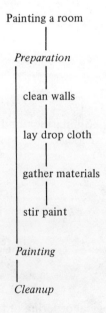

Tree 10.4

5. *Problem solution:* The interaction of two or more factors—one indicating a problem and the other a solution.

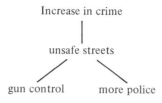

Tree 10.5

The teacher can begin using graphic organizers in a very structured way with students, in that the teacher could provide the topic, type of organization, and part of the organizer filled in. The student would be required to fill in the rest. As the student becomes more proficient, he can fill in more and come up with his own organization patterns, possibly using a combination of the preceding patterns.

With the *Herringbone* technique (Herber, 1970), the student fills in a graphic representation of text by answering "who, what, when, why, where, and how" questions.

Students who have difficulty with the sound of language but can visualize relationships and meaning (such as the deep dyslexics) might profit from using these techniques. Younger children could be encouraged to pay attention to illustrations, make their own series of illustrations, and put them in some kind of sequence to tell a story or depict relationships. They might also be asked to demonstrate comprehension by picking the correct picture or performing appropriately to a written command.

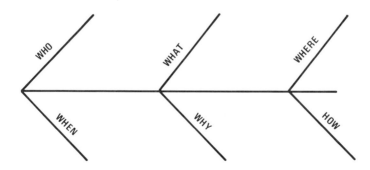

Figure 3. Example of a herringbone.

The surface dyslexic would seem to do better relying on regular comprehension instruction such as having the teacher verbally ask questions about the text.

Schema-Based Comprehension Strategies

Schema-based comprehension strategies rely on invoking the reader's background of information. The idea is that new information will be tied to what is known and hence meaningful. In the *language-experience approach* (Allen, 1976), the student has an experience (orchestrated, at times, by the teacher), talks about the experience while the teacher writes down what he says, and reads what has been dictated—his own words.

List–group–label (Taba, 1967) is an approach in which the student is asked to generate as many words as he can think of regarding a particular topic, place the words into meaningful categories, and apply an appropriate label. For instance, the concept of "snow" could evoke words such as *sled, skis, jackets, mittens, shovel, ice scraper, boots,* et cetera. When they are organized, they might look like this:

clothing to wear	leisure equipment	equipment to work with
jackets	sled	shovel
mittens	skis	ice scraper
boots		

Possible sentences (Readence et al., 1981) is a strategy in which, after vocabulary relating to topic is presented by the teacher, the student comes up with sentences that might possibly be used in the text. The student then reads to confirm or reassess his guesses while reading.

Anticipation–reaction (Readence et al., 1981) is a prereading–postreading strategy that gets the student thinking about the text, in that the teacher lists some controversial statements having to do with the subject and has the student tell whether he agrees or disagrees with these statements. After the selection is read, the student goes back to these statements and sees whether he has changed his opinion because of what was read.

Example:	Anticipation	Reaction	
	——	——	Reading is a multistage process.

The directed reading–thinking activity (Stauffer, 1969) was developed as an alternative to the *directed reading lesson,* the type of reading lesson suggested in most basal readers. In this technique, the reader makes predictions about what will be in the text, much as was done in *possible sentences,* then confirms or changes those predictions while reading through the text. There are two parts to the lesson: a process cycle and a product. In the *process cycle,* purposes for reading are set, the rate is adjusted, the material is read to verify purposes, and understanding is evaluated. Students are encouraged to use context and picture clues to aid in word identification. The *product* stage involves the extension and refinement of students' ideas and thinking.

Request (Manzo, 1969) is a technique that involves the teacher and the student taking turns asking each other questions before the prediction period. The teacher chooses appropriate material, then finds points where predictions could be made. The method is explained, reciprocal questioning takes place, predictions are elicited, and silent reading of the rest of the passage takes place to see if the predictions were right.

All of these comprehension techniques require enough prior knowledge so that the reader can make judgments and predictions. They all also rely on reading to confirm the predictions. The teacher using these methods should be sure to introduce difficult vocabulary in context and build background as necessary. Contextual readers (phonological and deep dyslexics) can profit from these techniques because, having an idea of what to expect from the material allows them to be able to use contextual clues to the fullest. Surface dyslexics can profit from these techniques because they tie previously learned words to personal experiences. A strategy like *list–group–label* or some of the others would be nonbeneficial to someone with not just reading difficulties but also difficulties with spoken language, such as a dysnomic aphasic. Persons with aphasic speech might have great difficulty generating words or ideas.

Visual–Language-Based Methods

Visual–language-based methods have been devised for use with deaf or hearing impaired students or aphasics. These techniques rely on the use of strong visual clues to written language, and may be helpful for use with deep dyslexics or students with severe phonologic and language difficulties.

Auditory Discrimination in Depth (A.D.D.) is a program that teaches letter sounds, blending, and words, through the use of a letter tray and tile letters, with one sound per letter. The difference with this approach is that the child learns to produce the sound of each letter by watching the face, mouth, and throat of the person who tells him the sound, and then practices making this sound while looking in the mirror. In other words, it is essentially a lip-reading technique for teaching phonics. One should be cautioned that it would probably take a great deal of time for the deep dyslexic to master phonics using this technique. However, he could be taught reading using another strategy, and use A.D.D. as a remedial tool.

The *Fitzgerald Keys* (Fitzgerald, 1966) are generally used with deaf or hard-of-hearing students. They are a visual representation of words in correct sentence position. This is not a reading method, but a language method. Fitzgerald maintained that deaf children need visual guides to follow when structuring sentences. The keys consist of headings that comprise various sentence patterns (i.e., who, what, whose, how many, what kind of, color, whom, what). As words are introduced, they are immediately classified under the proper headings. Actually, a child can master the use of the key without knowing how to speak. The headings themselves are taught using real objects, pictures, then just words. This is an interesting approach because the deep dyslexic often will say a word in the same category as the target word when making an oral reading error (e.g., lion—tiger).

McGinnis (1963) worked with language-delayed aphasics. Her approach to language is called "the association" method. It is also not a reading method, but the written form of words is taught through a phonetic approach. Precise articulation is emphasized, along with an association with the letter symbol. Expression is used for the starting point in building language, and sensorimotor association is used.

Compensatory Methods

Glossing (Otto, White, Richgels, Hansen, & Morrison, 1981) involves having the instructor use margins to emphasize key ideas, explain concepts in an easier fashion, define troublesome words, et cetera. Depending on the level and type of gloss, this technique could be profitable for all subtypes. (Deep and phonological dyslexics could be provided with more visual aids, such as charts, diagrams, pictures, illustrations, while surface and hyperlexic dyslexics could be provided with gloss which emphasizes tying concepts to personal experiences). *Slicing* simply involves breaking the task up into smaller units.

Guided Listening, an adaptation of Guided Reading (Manzo, 1975), is a technique where the teacher actually reads the text to the student. The student listens and tries to remember everything. The teacher jots down these student memories after the text is read. They then go over the selection again and amend or confirm what was remembered. Next, the organize the memories in a meaningful way. Thought-provoking questions are asked, and students are asked to demonstrate their knowledge through a test. (From the organized list, the teacher could go a step further and ask the student to dictate a synoposis of the selection. This dictated version of the text could then be read by the student.) The deep dyslexic might not profit from this approach because of the lack of right-hemisphere processing unless the concepts were very concrete. This technique would be most helpful to the surface dyslexic and hyperlexic and could be used with the phonological dyslexic, also. *Guide-O-Rama* (O. Cunningham & Shablak, 1975) is simply a guide to go along with the text, which emphasizes key ideas. As with the other techniques, this technique could be made applicable to any subtype, depending on the way in which the key ideas were presented.

SUMMARY

In summary, it is plain that each instructional activity must be thought of in terms of the skill requirements so that a match can be made between the requirements of the technique and the strengths of the person who is to be taught. In many cases, standard techniques fit a number of different learning styles with some slight modification. Knowing the students' strengths and weaknesses, based on a neurolinguistic model, can make the matching process easier. Too, with enough students exhibiting the same patterns or subtypes of reading behaviors, instructors could be helpful in validating or revising theory. If they were able to successfully use knowledge of neurological organization to provide the match with materials with these subtypes of students, they would demonstrate the validity of this neurolinguistic system. If not, they could experiment to find what worked, and possibly provide meaningful theoretical revisions. The neuropsychologist who works with school-aged populations is in the position of initiating recommendations based on neurological knowledge. They are, therefore, the key to this validation process. Through their work with instructors, they can be an invaluable aid in providing proper matches between learning style and techniques used.

REFERENCES

Aaron, R. (n.d.). *Seven critical steps in teaching sight words*. Baldwin, NY: Barnell Loft.

Allen, R. V. (1976). *Language experiences in communication*. Boston: Houghton Mifflin.

Annett, M. (1973). Laterality of childhood hemiplegia and the growth of speech and intelligence. *Cortex, 9*, 4–35.

Bakker, D. J. (1973). Hemispheric specialization and stages in the learning to read process. *Bulletin of the Orton Society, 23*, 15–27.

Bastian, H. C. (1898). *Aphasia and other speech defects*. London: H. K. Lewis.

Berlin, C. I., Hughes, J. R., Lowe-Bell, S. S., & Berlin, H. L. (1973). Dichotic right ear advantage in children. *Cortex, 9*, 394–402.

Boder, E. & Jerrico, S. (1982). *The Boder Test of Reading–Spelling Patterns*. New York: Grune & Stratton.

Coltheart, M. (1980). Deep dyslexia: A right hemisphere hypothesis. In M. Coltheart, K. Patterson, & J. C. Marshall (Eds.), *Deep dyslexia*. London: Routledge & Kegan Paul.

Cronbach, L. J., & Snow, R. E. (1977). *Aptitudes and instructional methods: A handbook for research on interactions.* New York: Irvington.

Cunningham, O., & Shablak, S. (1975). Selective reading guide-o-rama: The content teacher's best friend. *Journal of Reading, 18,* 380–382.

Cunningham, P. M. (1975–1976). Investigating a synthesized theory of mediated word identification. *Reading Research Quarterly, 11,* 127–143.

Cunningham, P. M. (1980). Teaching 'were,' 'with,' 'what,' and other four-letter words. *Reading Teacher,* pp. 160–163.

Decker, S. N., & Defries, J. C. (1981). Cognitive ability profiles in families of reading-disabled children. *Developmental Medicine and Child Neurology, 23,* 217–227.

Dennis, M. (1977). Cerebral dominance in three forms of early brain disorders. In M. E. Blaw, I. Rapin, & M. Kinsbourne, (Eds.), *Topics in child neurology* (pp. 189–212). New York: Spectrum.

Dinnan, J. A., & Lodge, R. (1976). *Communication: A meta theory of language.* Athens, GA: Jaddy Enterprises.

Duffy, F. H., Denckla, M. B., Bartels, P. H., & Sandini, G. (1980). Dyslexia: Regional differences in brain electrical activity by topographic mapping. *Annals of Neurology, 7,* 412–420.

Earle, R. A., & Baron, R. F. (1973). An approach for teaching vocabulary in content subjects. In H. L. Herber & R. F. Barron (Eds.), *Research in reading in the content areas: Second year report.* Syracuse, NY: Syracuse University, Reading & Language Arts Center.

Fernald, G. M. (1943). *Remedial techniques in basic school subjects.* New York: McGraw-Hill.

Fitzgerald, E. (1966). *Straight language for the deaf.* Washington, DC: Volta Bureau.

Funnell, E. (1983). Phonological processes in reading: New evidence from acquired dyslexia. *British Journal of Psychology, 2,* 159–180.

Furniss, D. W., & Graves, N. F. (1980). Effects of stressing oral reading accuracy on comprehension. *Reading Psychology, 2,* 8–14.

Galaburda, A. M., & Kemper, T. L. (1979). Cytoarchitectonic abnormalities in developmental dyslexia: A case study. *Annals of Neurology, 6,* 94–100.

Galaburda, A. M., Sherman, G. F., & Geschwind, N. (in press). Developmental dyslexia: Third consecutive case with cortical anomalies. *Science.*

Gilbert, J. H., & Climan, I. (1974). Dichotic studies in two and three year olds: A preliminary report. *Speech Communication Seminar* (Vol. 2). Stockholm: Almqvist & Wiksell.

Gillingham, A. (1970). *Remedial training for children with specific disability in reading, spelling, and penmanship* (7th ed.). Cambridge, MA: Educators Publishing Service.

Gleitman, L., & Rozin, P. (1973). Teaching reading by use of a syllabary. *Reading Research Quarterly, 8,* 447–483.

Goodman, K. S. (1968). *The psycholinguistic nature of the reading process.* Detroit, MI: Wayne State University Press.

Graesser, A. C. (1981). *Prose comprehension beyond the word.* New York: Springer-Verlag.

Harris, A., & Sipay, E. R. (1975). *How to increase reading ability.* New York: Longmans, Green.

Hécaen, H. (1976). Acquired aphasia in children and the ontogenesis of hemispherical functional specialization. *Brain and Language, 3,* 114–134.

Hegge, T. G., Kirk, S. A., & Kirk, W. D. (1970). *Remedial reading drills.* Ann Arbor, MI: George Wahr.

Herber, H. L. (1970). *Teaching reading in the content areas* (2nd ed.). Englewood Cliffs, NJ: Prentice-Hall.

Hinshelwood, J. (1900). Congenital word blindness. *Lancet, i,* 1506–1508.

Hinshelwood, J. (1902). Congenital word blindness, with reports of two cases. *Opthalmic Review, 21,* 91–99.

Hinshelwood, J. (1909). Four cases of congenital word blindness occurring in the same family. *British Medical Journal, ii,* 1229–1232.

Holmes, J. M. (1973). *Dyslexia: A neurolinguistic study of traumatic and developmental disorders of reading.* Unpublished doctoral dissertation, University of Edinburgh, Edinburgh.

Hulme, C., & Bradley, L. (1984). An experimental study of multi-sensory teaching with normal and retarded readers. In R. M. Malatesha & H. A. Whitaker (Eds.), *Dyslexia: A global issue* (pp. 431–444). The Hague: Nijhoff.

Hynd, G., & Hynd, C. (1984). Dyslexia: Neuroanatomical/neurolinguistic perspectives. *Reading Research Quarterly, 4,* 482–498.

Hynd, C., & Hynd, G. (1984). Recent neuropsychological research: Do practical implications exist? *Journal of Educational Neuropsychology, 5,* 1–7.

Hynd, G., & Obrzut, J. (1977). The effects of grade level and sex on the magnitude of the dichotic ear advantage. *Neuropsychologia, 15,* 289–692.

Jastak, J. F., & Jastak, S. R. (1978). *Wide Range Achievement Test.* Wilmington, DE: Jasktak & Associates.

Kertesz, A. (1979). *Aphasia and associated disorders.* New York: Grune & Stratton.

Kertesz, A. (Ed.). (1983). *Localization in neuropsychology.* New York: Academic Press.

Kinsbourne, M., & Hiscock, M. (1977). Does cerebral dominance develop? In S. J. Segalowitz & F. A. Gruber (Eds.), *Language development and neurological theory.* New York: Academic Press.

Kinsbourne, M., & Hiscock, M. (1978). Cerebral lateralization and cognitive development. In M. Grady & E. Luecke (Eds.), *Education and the brain.* Chicago: University of Chicago Press.

Lashley, K. S. (1938). Factors limiting recovery after CNS lesions. *Journal of Nervous and Mental Diseases, 88,* 733–755.

Lenneberg, E. H. (1967). *Biological foundations of language.* New York: Wiley.

Levine, D. M., Hier, D. B., & Calvanio, R. (1981). Acquired learning disability for reading after left temporal lobe damage in childhood. *Neurology, 31,* 257–264.

Lyon, R., & Watson, B. (1981). Empirically derived subgroups of learning disabled readers: Diagnostic characteristics. *Journal of Learning Disabilities, 14,* 256–261.

Manzo, A. V. (1969). The request procedure. *Journal of Reading, 13,* 123–126.

Manzo, A. V. (1975). The guided reading procedure. *Journal of Reading, 18,* 287–291.

Marshall, J. C. (1984). Toward a rational taxonomy of the developmental dyslexias. In R. N. Maletesha & H. A. Whitaker (Eds.), *Dyslexia: A global issue.* (pp. 45–58). The Hague: Nijhoff.

Marshall, J. C., & Newcombe, F. (1973). Patterns of paralexia: A psycholinguistic approach. *Journal of Psycholinguistic Research, 2,* 175–199.

Marshall, J. C., & Newcombe, F. (1980). The conceptual status of deep dyslexia: A historical perspective. In M. Coltheart, K. Patterson, & J. C. Marshall (Eds.), *Deep dyslexia* (pp. 1–21). Boston: Routledge & Kegan Paul.

McClure, P., & Hynd, G. (1983). Is hyperlexia a severe reading disorder or a symptom of psychiatric disturbance? *Clinical Neuropsychology, 5,* 145–149.

McGinnis, M. (1963). *Aphasic children: Identification and education by the association method*. Washington, DC: Volta Bureau.

Molfese, D. R., Freeman, R. B., Jr., & Palermo, D. (1975). The ontogeny of brain lateralization for speech and non-speech stimuli. *Brain and Language, 2*, 356–368.

Morgan, W. P. (1896). A case of congenital word blindness. *British Medical Journal, ii*, 1378.

Orton, S. (1937). *Reading, writing, and speech problems in children*. New York: Norton.

Otto, W., White, S. R., Richgels, D., Hansen, R., & Morrison, B. S. (1981). *A technique for improving the understanding of expository text* (Theoretical Paper No. 98). Madison: University of Wisconsin, Wisconsin Center for Education Research.

Pearson, P. D., & Spiro, R. J. (1982). Toward a theory of reading comprehension instruction. In K. G. Buttes & G. P. Wallach (Eds.), *Language disorders and learning disabilities* (pp. 71–88). Rockville, Md: Aspen Systems.

Petrauskas, R. J., & Rourke, B. (1979). Identification of subtypes of retarded readers: A neuropsychological multivariate approach. *Journal of Clinical Neuropsychology, 1*, 17–37.

Pirozzolo, F. J. (1979). *The neuropsychology of developmental reading disorders*. New York: Praeger.

Porter, R. J., & Berlin, C. I. (1975). On interpreting developmental changes in the dichotic right ear advantage. *Brain and Language, 2*, 186–200.

Rapin, I. (1982). Developmental language disorders and brain dysfunction as precursors of reading disability. In G. B. Wise, M. E. Blaw, & P. G. Procopis (Eds.), *Topics in child neurology* (Vol. 2). New York: Spectrum.

Readence, J. B., Bean, T. W., & Baldwin, R. S. (1981). *Content area reading: An integrated approach*. Dubuque, IA: Kendall/Hunt.

Saffran, V. M., Bogyo, L. C., Schwartz, M. F., & Martin, O. S. M. (1980). Does deep dyslexia reflect right hemisphere reading? In M. Coltheart, K. Patterson, & J. C. Marshall (Eds.), *Deep dyslexia*. Boston: Routledge & Kegan Paul.

Satz, P., Bakker, D. J., Teunissen, J., Goebel, R., & Van der light, H. (1975). Developmental parameters of the ear asymmetry: A multivariate approach. *Brain and Language, 2*, 171–185.

Schulman-Galambos, C. (1977). Dichotic listening performance in elementary and college students. *Neuropsychologia, 15*, 577–584.

Sevush, S. (1983, February). The neurolinguistics of reading: Anatomic and neurologic correlates. Paper presented at the Annual Conference of the International Neuropsychological Society, Mexico City.

Silberberg, N., & Silberberg, M. (1967). Hyperlexia: Special word recognition skills in young children. *Exceptional Children, 34*, 41–42.

Sladen, B. K. (1970). Inheritance of dyslexia. *Bulletin of the Orton Society, 20*, 30–40.

Spache, G. D. (1973). *Investigating the issues of reading disabilities*. Boston: Allyn & Bacon.

Stauffer, R. G. (1969). *Teaching reading as a thinking process*. New York: Harper & Row.

St. James-Roberts, I. A. (1981). A reinterpretation of hemispherectomy findings without functional plasticity of the brain: I. Intellectual function. *Brain and Language, 13*, 31–53.

Taba, H. (1967). *Teacher's handbook for elementary social studies*. Reading, MA: Addison-Wesley.

Temple, C. M., & Marshall, J. C. (in press). A case study of developmental phonological dyslexia. *British Journal of Psychology*.

Tierney, R. J., Readence, J. E., & Dishner, E. K. (1980). *Reading strategies and practices: A guide for improving instruction*. Boston: Allyn & Bacon.

Wilson, B. D., & Wilson, J. J. (1980). Language disordered children: A neuropsychologic view. In B. Feingold & C. Bank (Eds.), *Developmental disabilities of early childhood*. Springfield, IL: Charles C. Thomas.

Woodcock, R. W. (1967). *Peabody rebus reading program*. Circle Press, MN: American Guidance Service.

Chapter 11

Behavioral Neuropsychology with Children

ARTHUR MACNEILL HORTON, JR.*

*Veterans Administration Medical Center
Baltimore, Maryland 21212
and
The Johns Hopkins University
Baltimore, Maryland 21218*

ANTONIO E. PUENTE

*Department of Psychology
University of North Carolina at Wilmington
Wilmington, North Carolina 28403*

INTRODUCTION

As noted by Gaddes (1981), the realization that there is an overlap between neurology and learning is not new. He asserts that the famous English neurologist Hughlings Jackson suggested that there should be a recognition of both mind and body as early as 1872. Indeed, Gaddes (1981) attributes the current concepts of learning disabilities to research by neurologists in the nineteenth century who began the exploration of the complex relationship between language and neuroanatomy.

---

* Dr. Horton's contribution has been submitted in an independent capacity and is neither endorsed nor supported by the Veterans Administration.

CHILD NEUROPSYCHOLOGY, VOL. 2

More recently, there has been an explosion of interest in brain–behavior relationships. In addition to the striking illustrations of the cross-cultural validity of neuropsychological data (Luria, 1966; Reitan & Davison, 1974) the applications of neuropsychological knowledge in the schools (Hynd & Obrzut, 1981) have contributed to this trend. Clearly, there is the potential for the study of brain–behavior relationships to be of great relevance to the practice of psychology with school-aged children.

Given this background, it would appear that the integration of neuropsychology to learning would be most appropriate. It is of interest that some efforts along these lines have already been accomplished. A specialty that integrates the principles of behavior therapy with neuropsychology has developed. It has been referred to as *behavioral neuropsychology*. It is expected that this area of clinical and research interest will prove of value to psychologists and educators involved in behaviorally oriented intervention with school-aged children who have learning problems related to neuropsychological functioning.

The intent of this chapter is to review this new area of development and to examine supporting clinical and research evidence. In order to realize this objective, it would seem appropriate to clarify what is intended by an integration of behavior therapy and neuropsychology. At present, the new field has been termed *behavioral neuropsychology* by Horton (1979). Administratively, a specific interest group under this name was founded in 1978 at the Association for Advancement of Behavior Therapy (AABT) meeting in Chicago, Illinois and has continued to be active in AABT since that time. A tentative definition has been proposed. It follows:

> Behavioral Neuropsychology may be defined as the application of behavior therapy techniques to problems of organically impaired individuals while using a neuropsychological assessment and intervention perspective. This treatment methodology suggests that inclusion of data from neuropsychological assessment strategies would be helpful in the formulation of hypotheses regarding antecedent conditions (external or internal) for observed phenomena of psychopathology. That is, a neuropsychological perspective will significantly enhance the ability of the behavior therapists to make accurate discriminations as to the etiology of patients' behaviors. Moreover, the formulation of a cogent plan of therapeutic intervention and its skillful implementation could, in certain cases, be facilitated by an analysis of behavior deficits of higher cortical functioning. (Horton, 1979, p. 20).

This definition may be somewhat arbitrary. Moreover, the preceding definition makes a number of assumptions regarding neuropsychology and behavior therapy that are controversial (Hynd, 1981; Sandoval & Haapanen, 1981).

The remainder of this chapter is devoted to the specific application of behavioral neuropsychology with children. These aspects are organized into four sections. The first is concerned with theoretical issues and attempts to make a distinction between traditional and contemporary behaviorism. The second section focuses on treatment planning and includes the Lewinsohn model for intervention with the brain-injured. Basic behavioral neuropsychology guidelines (Horton & Wedding, 1984) that deal with topographical organization of human neuroanatomy and a brief discussion of basic child neuropsychology profiles, based on the work of Hartlage (1975), are presented. The third section selectively reviews the existing empirical research on the application of behavioral methods with two populations (i.e., learning disabled and brain damaged). The fourth and final section serves as a summary statement but also includes some speculations about the future directions that behavioral neuropsychology with children may take.

THEORETICAL ISSUES

Behavioral Issues

As previously mentioned, two major conceptual concerns relative to the blending of behavior therapy and neuropsychology are discussed. The first theoretical issues to be considered are reconciliation of neuropsychology and its subject matter of inferred variables with traditional behaviorism and its concept of the "black box." The second theoretical issue that is discussed is how contemporary concepts of behavioral assessment and treatment can be integrated into behavioral neuropsychology. These comments are relatively concise; however, more elaborate discussions can be found elsewhere (Horton, 1979, 1981).

The traditional behavioral model is sometimes characterized as viewing the human mind as a "black box." There is a time-honored theoretical view within traditional, including radical, behaviorism that the sum total of human behaviors can be adequately explained in terms of observed stimulus–response paradigms (Watson, 1913). This perspective asserts that the behavior of human organisms can be accounted for without reliance on unobserved or covert factors (Skinner, 1938). This is of course a radical behaviorist position, which has been extensively described previously (Marr, 1984; Mozer, 1979).

Simply put, a traditional behaviorist would argue that variables that are not observable as stimulus–response actions are not useful to explain behavior. It is important to remember that *inferred variables*, that is, variables that may not be observed (i.e., "black box"), are disregarded as valueless by many traditional behavior therapists. There are some behavior therapists, however, who would postulate that there are legitimate inferred variables in the functional analysis of human behavior (Mahoney, 1974).

At this point, it is important to reconsider that inferred variables come in two varieties: intervening variables and hypothetical constructs (Craighead, Kazdin, & Mahoney, 1976). Moreover, the differences between these two types of inferred variables are straightforward. Somewhat oversimplified, *intervening variables* are conceptual abstractions because they exist only in theory. A thought, of course, would be an example of an intervening variable. At present, it is impossible to directly observe thoughts; nevertheless, they are used to explain human behavior (e.g., "I won't think about that today, for tomorrow is another day."). Hypothetical constructs are quite different. Again grossly over simplified, *hypothetical constructs* have a physical substitute or a process substitute, which, while unobservable, from time to time can be verified if particular efforts are taken. As observed by Horton (1981).

> Hypothetical constructs in neuropsychology tend to have physiological referents and can, if so desired, be verified. If a child evidences certain characteristics, it might be postulated that there is damage to the right parietal lobe. In this case, our hypothetical construct is based on our knowledge of the brain–behavior relationship and can be verified through neurosurgery" (p. 368).

The main point of the preceding statement is that neuropsychological data may be considered as hypothetical constructs. Because neuropsychological data are hypothetical constructs, they are in a different class of events than the intervening variables. Therefore, it can be argued that there are theoretical grounds for the inclusion of neuropsychological data in an enlarged behavioral paradigm (Horton, 1979). While the ultimate test is of course empirical, still it should be clear that neuropsychological factors cannot be dismissed on the grounds that they are unscientific or inaccessible to measurement.

At this point, the second conceptual concern is considered. In a few words, the concern is, "How do contemporary views of behavioral assessment and treatment blend with behavioral neuropsychology?" From the outset, it should be recalled that contemporary behavior therapy has been marked by debate over the role of cognitive factors (Wolpe, 1973; Beck & Mahoney, 1979). While this is not the place to review this debate, it should be remembered that there is at least some willingness to use inferred variables as legitimate concepts in the functional analysis of human behavior (Mahoney, 1974). Moreover, contemporary behavior therapy is characterized by evolving clinical acumen. Part of that increased sophistication is seen in improved behavioral assessment techniques. Some would say, for instance, that behavior therapy is, to a large measure, defined by the techniques used. Hayes and Zettle (1980) have observed that some would classify techniques like self-monitoring as behavioral, while holding that a MMPI was non behavioral. It might be argued, however, that such a distinction is artificial and arbitrary, not to mention nonempirical.

In a seminal paper, Hayes and Zettle (1980) outlined a more progressive conceptual paradigm. The basis of their argument rests on the distinction between *conceptual* ("how to talk about doing X") and *technical* ("how to do X") dimensions of behavioral assessment and treatment. As these authors stress, the most rational guideline is to use the conceptual rather than the technical dimension when making clinical decisions about behavioral assessment and treatment. That is to say, if a technique or procedure can be talked about in terms of behavioral principles and is empirically testable, then it could be classified as behavioral. In the viewpoint of this perspective, who originated the technique or the topographical details of the procedure is not the criterion for judgment. Rather, relying on the conceptual dimensions of behavioral assessment and treatment, the crucial point is to view the antecedents and consequences of a behavior in order to deduce the intended purpose of the action. Listing the physical details is an assessment only to the degree that it enables one to understand the intended purpose of the behavior of interest.

The instances where the aforementioned conceptual perspective of behavioral assessment and treatment are applied, some implications of behavioral neuropsychology are evident. Using a conceptual criterion allows neuropsychological assessment devices such as the Halstead–Reitan Neuropsychological Test Battery, the Luria–Nebraska Neuropsychological Battery, and the Kaufman Assessment Battery for children to be considered as behavioral assessment instruments and therefore suitable to include in a database to plan and evaluate behavioral treatment. Failure to imply such a perspective would constitute the problem of limiting the efficacy of behavior therapy: That is to say, only techniques (such as self-maintaining sheets or fear surveys) that were originated by self-identified behavior therapists would qualify as behavioral. If one's goal is a clinically relevant science (Hayes & Zettle, 1980), then the advantages of the conceptual criterion of behavioral assessment and treatment appear to far outweigh any possible disadvantages. As observed by Horton (1981):

> Whether or not such a blend of neuropsychology and behaviorism proves a potent addition to the current professional arsenal of concepts and techniques of school or other applied psychologists, remains an empirical question, which in the best tradition of behaviorism should be objectively tested. (p. 369)

In such a manner, the neuropsychological perspective would be, if provided the necessary basis of empirical evidence, integrated into an enlarged and clinically sophisticated contemporary behavioral paradigm.

Neuropsychological Issues

In planning behavioral interventions for neuropsychologically impaired children, several additional issues should be considered. The development of appropriate treatment strategies depends on an appreciation of both the developing brain and the typical effects of neural dysfunction on children's behavior.

An area that is often overlooked but provides considerable information on these issues is the animal literature on developmental neuropsychology. According to Miller (1984), there are several conclusions that may be drawn after reviewing these findings. These include the following:

1. Regardless of intervention, a specific recovery pattern is to be expected.
2. Developmentally immature subjects show both behavioral and neural resiliency (plasticity?).
3. Overlearned skills tend to be less disrupted.
4. Intervention, especially when initiated close to the time of injury, will probably influence its outcome.

Thus, there is strong support, according to Miller (1984), for indicating that some recovery will occur regardless of posttrauma experience or intervention. Nevertheless, both pre- and postmorbid variables have a significant impact on the outcome of the perceived behavioral deficit. Presumably, the implication for treatment planning includes careful behavioral analysis of premorbid skills with immediate intervention to be initiated after the behaviorally disrupting event.

Another factor that should be considered in the development of behavioral interventions with children includes an understanding of predisposing factors as well as the common sequalae of brain injury. According to Klonoff, Crockett, and Clark (1984) epidemiological and natural-history data gathered at the University of British Columbia provides some answers to these issues. Their findings include the following:

1. Boys have a higher predisposition than girls to central nervous system injury.
2. There is a poor relationship between medical history and predisposition to head injury, although a significant relationship between environmental factors and brain injury does exist.
3. The sequelae of brain injury in younger children includes emotional

and personality changes, while the sequelae for older children includes headaches and dizziness, as well as learning and memory difficulties.

While the gender findings may not have an important bearing on treatment programming, the relationship between environment and head injury has strong implications for planning. Specifically, treatment planning should take into consideration environmental factors such as actual physical environment as well as family structure in order to minimize future occurrences of neural impairment, as well as to maximize the generalizability of the office- or institution-based treatment program. Finally, an understanding of expected sequalae is an important addition (often the primary or only source of information) to appropriate and comprehensive neuropsychological assessment.

The development of most treatment programs hinges on the acceptance that neuropsychological injury produces neuropsychological impairment and that the role of the neuropsychologist is to provide either restitution of desired behavior (Luria, 1966) or amelioration (Golden, 1981) of undesirable behavior. Underlying this assumption are the beliefs that neural trauma results in behavioral deficits and that a lesion in a specific location results in behavior directly reflective of the impaired structure. This simplistic approach, as seductive as it may appear, is inappropriate and results in an incomplete understanding of neural and behavioral reorganization or reintegration.

Whether complete (restitution) or partial (amelioration) recovery is the goal, the intent of treatment is to work directly on deficits. Reynolds (1981), among others, has proposed that a more robust approach would be to focus on the assets of the child, rather than on the deficits. Strategies capitalizing on the child's best-developed processing approaches will yield more effective results than focusing on the amelioration, for example, of the deficits produced by the neural impairment. Another issue relative to this approach is the assumption discussed earlier that accepts the belief that specific lesions produce specific behavioral deficits. The complexity of the brain as well as the lack of understanding of most specific structures of the brain (often due to limited technological sophistication) makes this belief invalid. A more appropriate approach would be to consider that a specific lesion should be interpreted behaviorally as what can the rest of the brain do in the absence of that specific structure. Considering both of the preceding arguments, then the approach that appears best suited for the treatment of the developing brain would be to focus not on the deficits (alone) but on the assets as a way to maximize treatment efficacy and to more accurately understand the rehabilitative process.

TREATMENT STRATEGIES

Lewinsohn's Model

With his associates at the University of Oregon Neuropsychology Clinic, Lewinsohn had done important clinical and research work (Lewinsohn, Dancer, & Kikel, 1977; Glasgow, Zeiss, Barrera, & Lewinsohn, 1977) on the remediation of memory deficits in brain-damaged individuals. In the course of this work, Lewinsohn and his colleagues have developed a useful paradigm for clinical work with brain-damaged individuals, which could be well applied to work with children. Essentially, it involves four steps, as follows:

1. General assessment of neuropsychological functioning
2. Specific assessment of neuropsychological functioning
3. Laboratory evaluation of intervention techniques
4. In-vivo application of intervention techniques (after Glasgow et al., 1977).

Basically, the first step requires the use of standard neuropsychological assessment devices. For example, in the case of Ms. J., Glasgow et al. (1977) administered the Wechsler Adult Intelligence Scale (WAIS) and the Halstead–Reitan Neuropsychological Test Battery (HRNB) after an intake interview. Interestingly, this woman, who had received a concussion in an automobile accident $3\frac{1}{2}$ years earlier and complained of school-related memory problems, earned a WAIS full-scale IQ of 114 and a Halstead Impairment Index of .25. The purpose of the first step, as seen in this case, is to obtain normative psychometrics and a global view of the client's–patient's neuropsychological functioning. Clearly, a hypothesis-testing approach is avoided at this stage, although, presumably, hypotheses about the client's brain functioning are derived after completion of this general assessment.

The second step is to examine in detail the specific parameters of the problem. In the case of Ms. J., selections from a reading-skills training program of the aforementioned presentations and narrative were used to elucidate the actual dimensions of her semantic memory functions. To a degree, this step is very similar to a behavioral assessment of neuropsychological-impaired child. Whether the approach is psychometric (as with the HRNB) or open-ended (e.g., Luria), the goal is to focus on the deficits (and assets) in order to better understand the goals of the treatment plan.

In the third step, specific intervention techniques are introduced in the context of a controlled (or laboratory) setting. In the case of Ms. J., oral rehearsal and a study organization strategy were selected. After the demonstration of intervention effectiveness, then generalization efforts can be initiated. Clearly, intervention strategies (whether focusing on deficits or assets) are developed from the data gathered during the first two steps of the intervention.

In the fourth and last step, application of the successful laboratory intervention to the real-world problem is accomplished. In the case of Ms. J., this involved her applying the PQRST technique to her academic performance problems. Evaluation of the in vivo application was assessed by self-monitoring of negative and self-critical thoughts that were directly stimulated by her memory performance and also by her self-rating of recall of newspaper articles, immediately, 24 hours, and 7 days after reading. A final measure of outcome was Ms. J remaining in school and enrolling for an increased number of credit hours.

Thus, it can be seen that Lewinsohn's paradigm provides a general framework for conceptualizing the longitudinal aspect of clinical behavioral therapy with the brain injured. The general framework and specific evaluation, as well as specific intevention and generalization, provides a robust model for the behavioral intervention of children with brain injury. It should be kept in mind that while the WAIS and HRNB were used in this illustration, there is no reason that this should always be the case. Rather, general assessment should be taken to imply that use of any quantitive (as well as qualitative) neuropsychological measuring devices is acceptable. Indeed, it is possible to contemplate the use of neuropsychological devices in this context with no conceptual difficulties. In order to elucidate the exact parameters of the adaptive behavior deficits secondary to brain injury, it might be expected that considerable manipulation of stimulus–response dimensions will be necessary.

In order to illustrate some of the issues presented, it would be desirable to discuss some of the conceptual issues involved in the Lewinsohn model, particularly Steps 2 and 3. To a degree, these conceptual issues are overlapping with some recent thinking in behavioral assessment. The particular framework is drawn from the work of Goldfried and Davidson (1976). Essentially, when considering variables associated with maladaptive behavior, Goldfried and Davidson (1976) discuss four types. These are as follows: (1) stimulus antecedents, (2) organismic variables, (3) response variables, and (4) consequent variables.

Stimulus antecedents are considered as demands, often environmental. These demands and their perception determine the strategy and success of the coping process (Lazarus & Folkman, 1984).

On one hand, this category refers to the various neuropsychological abilities that need to be assessed. However, to just think of neuropsychological abilitites in the classic sense of memory, abstraction, and concept formation would fail to do this category justice. Also, as outlined by Goldfried and Davidson (1976), a therapist must consider expectations, attributions, and self-reinforcement standards to maximize treatment efficiency.

In this category, the focus is on the residual response abilities. To cite an oversimplified example, if a brain-damaged individual is unable to comprehend verbal stimuli, it is futile to expect him or her to answer the telephone. Goldfried and Davidson (1976) make the point that assessment of response variables should include situation-specific samples of the behavior under study, as well as data concerning its duration, frequency, intensity, and magnitude.

It is the sine qua non of behavior therapy that consequences influence behavior (Skinner, 1981). Basically, the reinforcing or punishing consequences of actions play a role in determining whether or not the particular action will increase in frequency. Various parameters such as immediacy, type, content, and ratio of reinforcement to response are of critical importance for behavior initiation, increase, maintenance, and generalization. In this context, it might be well to consider the classical distinction between ability and performance. Just because a brain-damaged individual fails to perform an action does not mean that he or she is incapable of performing the action. It could be that the person simply does not want to perform the action because he or she is receiving more reinforcement for doing some other sort of action, as in secondary gains, for example.

At this point, consideration is devoted to treatment planning. It would be fair to observe that at this point in the development of behavioral neuropsychology treatment, planning for children is most appropriately labeled an art rather than a science, in large part due to the lack of data-based information. Also, it should be noted that this presentation focuses on general considerations in treatment planning. More detailed discussion of specific training strategies of neuropsychological deficits are available in other sources (Golden, 1981; Luria, 1963; Miller, 1984). The general considerations discussed include (1) self-efficacy, (2) personality × treatment interaction, (3) resources, and (4) intrusiveness to setting.

Bandura (1969) has advanced that an individual's perceived effectiveness is an explanatory mechanism for therapeutic behavioral change. Put another way, all behavior-change methods that are successful work by creating and strengthening a person's conviction of personal effectiveness. This individual belief in self-effectiveness determines activities children engage in, as well as the amount of and persistence of effort in the presence of aversive experiences. Essentially, four sources of data shape self-mastery beliefs. These are successful personal behavioral performance, observed successful performance of others, states of physiological arousal, and verbal persuasion. Previous research by Bandura (1969) and his associates has demonstrated that successful personal behavioral performance appears to be the most influential variable for radical modification of self-efficacy beliefs. Implications for treatment planning are straightforward.

Essentially, whenever possible, successful in vivo performance should be the focus of therapy with the brain-damaged child. Of course, with the brain-injured and inattentive child, often providing prompt and salient feedback is a difficult proposition. Wherever possible, assistance devices or techniques to provide self-effectiveness feedback should be used. To a large degree, motivation for change is a function of both the reward or reinforcement to accomplishing an action or task and also the probability by which the child assesses his or her likelihood of accomplishing the action or task successfully (i.e., motivation = reinforcement × subjectively assessed probability of success). Thus, it can be seen that influence of personal beliefs is a crucial process in treatment and must not be neglected.

With respect to personality × treatment interaction, this refers to patient–client characteristics that potentiate certain therapeutic methods. For example, Goldfried and Davidson (1976) note difficulties with patients who are "brighter and more psychologically sophisticated" in reporting actual behavioral samples. In addition, these authors mention the great importance of knowing client's–patient's personal standards for self-reinforcement. In many cases, a major criteria for treatment planning is the ability to make quick progress. Early success has a major effect on building sustained motivation through the self-efficacy mechanism alluded to earlier.

With respect to resources, this refers to environmental characteristics of the treatment setting (medical center and/or community and/or home) as well as either personal qualities or skills of the therapist(s). For example, the availability of family to serve as mentors and therapists is quite important. Also, knowing the limits of the child's situation both at home and at school prevents the construction of an unrealistic treatment plan.

With respect to intrusiveness to setting, this refers to economic, cultural, and social barriers to treatment. For example, aversive therapy procedures are often quite effective but are often seen as intrusive, in that they violate certain commonly held expectations regarding preferred methods of treatment by the parents and lay public. Conversely, the use of self-monitoring procedures, because they are relatively innocuous might be seen as minimally intrusive. To a large extent, the point is that, at least on a surface level, psychological interventions must deal with the issue of parental and lay expectations.

In summary, careful behavioral analysis and subsequent behavioral treatment intervention for neuropsychologically impaired adults using the Lewinsohn models appears readily transferable to children. Notwithstanding the limitations of complex interaction, such as plasticity (Bigler & Naugle, 1985), this approach provides a basic yet robust framework from which to launch a successful behavioral neuropsychological program for children.

Behavioral Neuropsychology Guidelines

The generation of suggestions for the behavior therapy of children with learning disabilities or brain damage is a difficult task. While in no way meaning to provide a complete answer, some guidance might be gained from consideration of basic neuroanatomical parameters. Meier (1974) described the neurocortex as exemplifying three primary dimensions. These are (1) left to right, (2) front to back, and (3) top to bottom. More specifically, the left-to-right dimension has been termed *laterality,* the front to back dimension has been described as *caudality* while the top-to-bottom dimension has been termed *dorsality* (Horton & Wedding, 1984). These terms are used in a unique manner in the context of this discussion. Moreover, the terms were chosen for ease of behavioral expression rather than an attempt to precisely identify microneuroanatomy. Also, the following suggestions make the assumption of fairly circumscribed and localized mental impairment. In addition, it might state that some of these guidelines are postulated on the basis of clinical findings. As emphasized in a later section of this chapter, additional research is needed.

Laterality

As noted by Horton and Wedding (1984):

On a clinical level, hemispheric specialization can provide a model for treatment planning. The two cerebral hemispheres process information in different ways. Assuming right handedness, the left hemisphere is logical and language oriented while the right hemisphere is intuitive and concerned with spatial aspects of stimuli. (p. 216)

Given these two modes of hemispheric mental asymmetrical functioning (see also Glass, in press), there are implications for the selection of therapy–remediation tasks and the therapeutic management of learning-disabled and structurally brain-damaged children. Hartlage (1975) and others (Boder, 1973; Mattis, French, & Rapin, 1975; Pirozzolo, 1979, 1981) have eloquently argued that there are subtypes of reading disability and that a neuropsychological assessment is crucial for the adequate differential diagnosis and resulting recommendations for appropriate educational intervention. While it is clear that there is evidence supporting the existence of multiple different subtypes of reading disability (Pirozzolo, 1979), there is some consensus (Boder, 1973; Horton & Wedding, 1984) that the two most common subtypes present with auditory–linguistic and visuospatial elements (Pirozzolo, 1981). In order to illustrate these subtypes and to also provide an example of the power of a conceptualization of lateralization with respect to possible emotional correlates, suggested educational intervention and prognosis examples of three basic neuropsychological profiles for children drawn from the work of Hartlage (1975) are presented in Table 1.

It should be noted that Hartlage identifies type I children as typifying left-hemisphere dysfunction, type II children are exhibiting right hemisphere dysfunction, and type III children are characterized as having generalized cerebral dysfunction syndrome. While this categorization, like many attempts to relate research to clinical practice, represents an oversimplification of the actual clinical situation, it does provide an initial attempt at rational intervention procedures.

Caudality

As observed by Horton and Wedding (1984)

Caudality refers to localization within the anterior–posterior dimension. There is some agreement that the frontal lobes involve the planning, execution, and verification of behavior while the posterior sections are involved with the reception, integration, and analysis of sensory information. (p. 219) (emphasis added).

As earlier noted by Luria (1966), whether or not the prefrontal regions of the cerebral cortex have sustained substantial impairment is of great clinical importance. Others have, of course, eloquently described the behavioral effects of frontal lobe lesions and the resulting affective and psychosocial consequences (Struss & Benson, 1984). There is clear consensus that compromised frontal-lobe functioning can reduce the degree of novel problem solving a patient may be able to perform. Consequently, individuals with frontal-lobe impairment often show deficits in self-management skills. Luria (1966), for example, has observed that when a brain-injured soldier of World War II had suffered impairment that included the frontal lobes, the prognosis for returning to independent function was dismal. Horton and Wedding (1984) have suggested that a brain-damaged patient with intact frontal lobes will often demonstrate more successful behavior adjustment than a patient with frontal-lobe impairment even, in cases where the non-frontal-lobe-impaired patient may show a higher degree of overall brain damage on objective indices of neuropsychological functioning.

TABLE 1

Basic neuropsychological profiles for children[a]

	Type I child	Type II child	Type III child
Neuropsychological profile	Comparatively lower WISC-R verbal than performance IQ score, with consistently lowered language ability (i.e., depressed, ITPA and PPVT scores) relative to perceptual–motor skills (i.e., Bender–Gestalt or VMI)	Comparatively lower WISC-R performance than verbal IQ and consistently lowered perceptual–motor ability relative to language skills	No consistent pattern of WISC-R; strength and weakness or clear superiority of either language or perceptual–motor abilities and skills
Neurological syndrome	Left hemisphere dysfunction	Right hemisphere dysfunction	Generalized cerebral dysfunction
Emotional correlates	Reserved, tentative, and uncertain of self-efficacy	Impulsive and uncritical of personal performance	Restless, irritable, and hyperactive
Educational intervention	Whole work or look–say reading programs and perceptually oriented instructional modes	Linguistic and aural instruction modes	Extreme structure and special placement
Prognosis	Persistent problem during academic career (after third grade) but relatively good adjustment in nonacademic pursuits	Difficulty in early school grades (K–2) but tend to do better in later elementary grades (3–6) with generally successful academic career	Little ultimate academic success

[a] From *Clinical and Behavioral Neuropsychology: An Introduction* by Arthur MacNeill Horton, Jr. and Danny Wedding. Copyright © 1984, Praeger Publishers. Reprinted by permission of Praeger Publishers.

In terms of therapeutic applications with children, the role of cognitive behavioral treatment strategies appear to have significant potential. For example, Meichenbaum (1977) has developed the use of self-instructional therapy to develop self-contracts with children who exhibited difficulties with impulse control. Adaptation of self-instructional therapy and developmentally appropriate verification, such as the turtle technique (Schneider & Robin, 1976), are worthy of detailed study in this population.

Dorsality

Dorsality refers to the top-to-bottom dimension of the neuroaxis. There is theoretical work (MacLean, 1973) to suggest that there are interactions among evolutionally distinct layers of neuronal tissue. The clinical implication is that the depth of brain impairment could have great relevance. It should be freely admitted that at present, the knowledge of brain–behavior relations, relative to dorsality, is not adequate to generate many meaningful treatment suggestions for impairment to developing brains.

CONCLUSIONS

As earlier outlined, recent decades have seen exceptional growth in the neurosciences. New diagnostic technology and dramatic conceptual insights have set the stage for even more impressive progress in the coming years. This chapter has been focused on the prospects of a particular subfield of the neurosciences—behavioral neuropsychology. Specifically, we were interested in the application of this subfield to the cognitive, affective, and behavioral problems of children who are suspected of being organically impaired.

In an attempt to provide a summary of the chapters, the following comments are proposed. First, there is ample evidence that behavioral methods are effective with brain-injured and learning-disabled children. Second, there is a wealth of data supporting the diagnostic and prognostic value of neuropsychological assessment techniques with brain-injured and learning-disabled children despite the fact that it has not been elucidated. These studies form a mature body of research literature and are well accepted by experts in child development and pediatric neurology. Third, treatment validity is an area that will require much additional research. There is minimal data supporting the use of neuropsychological assessment instruments to select behavioral treatment methods. With few exceptions, the mass of data is at a case study level. Clearly, the great need is for the conceptualization and execution of well-controlled and methodologically sophisticated research.

It would appear straightforward that the ultimate worth-assessment of behavioral neuropsychology with children will rest on its ability to make significant contributions to the amelioration of cognitive, affective, and behavioral problems of children who are suspected or confirmed to have organic brain impairment. Of crucial importance will be the issue of appropriate interface with traditional systems of socialization and educational attainment. The expectation and hope is that this chapter will have been of some value in the challenge to alleviate emotional distress and to promote academic accomplishments with children who have suffered or who are presumed to have problems in learning that are neuropsychologically based.

> . . . it is clear that much additional work will need to be done in order to effectively integrate neuropsychology and behavior therapy with school-aged children. At the same time, there is some cause for cautious optimism. Initial efforts on both conceptual and research fronts have demonstrated significant promise. Whether or not this promise will be fulfilled is a question only the future may answer. (Horton, 1981, p. 371).

REFERENCES

Bandura, A. (1969). *Principles of behavior modification.* New York: Holt, Rinehart & Winston.

Beck, A., & Mahoney, M. J. (1979). Schools of thought. *American Psychologist, 34,* 93–98.

Bigler, E. D., & Naugle, R. I. (1985). Case studies in cerebral plasticity. *International Journal of Clinical Neuropsychology, 7,* 12–23.

Boder, E. (1973). Developmental dyslexia: A diagnostic approach based on three atypical reading–spelling patterns. *Developmental Medicine and Child Neurology, 15,* 663–687.

Craighead, W. E., Kazdin, A. E., & Mahoney, M. J. (1976). *Behavior modification: Principles, issues and applications.* Boston: Houghton Mifflin.

Gaddes, W. H. (1981). Neuropsychology, fact or mythology, educational help or hindrance? *School Psychology Review, 10*(31), 322–330.

Glasgow, R. E., Zeiss, R. A., Barrera, M., Jr., & Lewinsohn, P. M. (1977). Case studies on remediating brain damage deficits in brain damaged individuals. *Journal of Clinical Psychology, 33,* 1049–1054.

Glass, A. (Ed.). (in press). *Individual differences in hemispheric asymmetry.* New York: Plenum.

Golden, C. J. (1981). *Diagnosis and rehabilitation in clinical neuropsychology.* Springfield, IL: Charles C. Thomas.

Goldfried, M. R., & Davidson, G. C. (1976). *Clinical behavior therapy.* New York: Holt, Rinehart & Winston.

Hartlage, L. C. (1975). Neuropsychological approaches to predicting outcome of remedial educational strategies for learning disabled children. *Pediatric Psychology, 3,* 23–28.

Hayes, S. C., & Zettle, R. D. (1980). On being "behavioral": The technical and conceptual dimensions of behavioral assessment and therapy. *the Behavior Therapist, 3*(3), 4–6.

Horton, A. M., Jr. (1979). Behavioral neuropsychology: Rationale and research. *Clinical Neuropsychology, 1,* 20–23.

Horton, A. M., Jr. (1981). Behavioral neuropsychology in the schools. *School Psychology Review, 10*(3), 367–372.

Horton, A. M., Jr., & Sautter, W. (in press). Behavioral neuropsychology. In D. Wedding, A. M. Horton, Jr., & J. S. Webster (Eds.), *Handbook of clinical and behavioral neuropsychology.* New York: Springer.

Horton, A. M., Jr., & Wedding, D. (1984). *Clinical and behavioral neuropsychology.* New York: Praeger.

Hynd, G. W. (1981). Rebuttal to the critical commentary on neuropsychology in the schools. *School Psychology Review, 10*(3), 389–393.

Hynd, G. W., & Obrzut, J. E. (Eds.). (1981). *Neuropsychological assessment and the school-aged child: Issues and procedures.* New York: Grune & Stratton.

Klonoff, H., Crockett, D. P., & Clark, C. (1984). Head injury in children: A model for predicting course of recovery and progress. In R. E. Tarter & G. Goldstein, (Eds.), *Advances in clinical neuropsychology.* (Vol. 2). (pp. 139–157) New York: Plenum.

Lazarus, R. S., & Folkman, S. (1984). *Stress, appraisal, and coping.* New York: Springer.

Lewinsohn, P. M., Dancer, B. G., & Kikel, S. (1977). Visual imagery as a mnemonic aid for brain-damaged persons. *Journal of Consulting and Clinical Psychology, 45,* 717–723.

Luria, A. R. (1963). *Restoration of function after brain injury.* New York: Macmillan.

Luria, A. R. (1966). *Higher cortical function is man* (B. Haigh, Trans.). New York: Basic Books.

MacLean, P. D. (1973). *On the evolution of three mentalities.* Toronto: University of Toronto Press.

Mahoney, M. J. (1974). *Cognition and behavior therapy.* Cambridge, MA: Ballinger.

Marr, M. J. (1984). Conceptual approaches and issues. *Journal of the Experimental Analysis of Behavior,42,* 353–362.

Mattis, S., French, J. H., & Rapin, T. (1975). Dyslexia in children and adults: Three independent neuropsychological syndromes. *Developmental Medicine and Child Neurology, 17,* 150–163.

Meichenbaum, D. H. (1977). *Cognitive behavior modification.* New York: Plenum.

Meier, M. J. (1974). Some challenges for clinical neuropsychology. In R. M. Reitan & L. A. Davison (Eds.), *Clinical neuropsychology: Current status and application.* (pp. 289–323) New York: Wiley.

Miller, E. (1984). *Recovery and management of neuropsychological impairment.* New York: Wiley.

Mozer, M. H. (1979). Confessions of an ex-behaviorist. *the Behavior Therapist, 3*(3), 3.

Pirozzolo, F. J. (1979). *The neuropsychology of developmental reading disorders.* New York: Praeger.

Pirozzolo, F. J. (1981). Language and brain: Neuropsychological aspects of developmental reading disability. *School Psychology Review, 10*(3), 350–355.

Reitan, R. M., & Davison, L. A. (Eds.). (1974). *Clinical neuropsychology: Current status and applications,* Washington, DC: Hemisphere.

Reynolds, C. R. (1981). Neuropsychological assessment and the habilitation of learning. Considerations in the search for aptitude × treatment ineraction. *School Psychology Review, 10,* 343–349.

Sandoval, J., & Haapanen, R. M. (1981). A critical commentary on neuropsychology in the schools: Are we ready? *School Psychology Review, 10*(3), 381–388.

Schneider, M., & Robin, H. (1976). The turtle technique: A method for self-control of

impulsive behavior. In J. D. Krumbolts & C. E. Thorenson (Eds.), *Counseling methods.* (pp. 157–163). New York: Holt, Rinehart & Winston.

Skinner, B. F. (1938). *The behavior of organisms.* New York: Appleton-Century-Crofts.

Skinner, B. F. (1981). How to discover what you have to say—A talk to students. *Behavior Analyst, 4,* 1–7.

Struss, D. T., & Benson, D. F. (1984). Neuropsychological studies of the frontal lobes. *Psychological Bulletin, 95,* 28–33.

Watson, J. B. (1913). Psychology from the standpoint of a behaviorist. *Psychology Review, 20,* 158–177.

Wolpe, J. A. (1973). *The practice of behavior therapy.* New York: Pergamon Press.

Index

317